Regulating How We Die

*The Ethical, Medical, and Legal Issues
Surrounding Physician-Assisted Suicide*

Edited by Linda L. Emanuel

Harvard University Press
Cambridge, Massachusetts
London, England
1998

Printed in the United States of America

Library of Congress Cataloging-in-Publication Data

Regulating how we die : the ethical, medical, and legal issues
  surrounding physician-assisted suicide / edited by Linda L. Emanuel.
    p.   cm.
  Includes bibliographical references and index.
  ISBN 0-674-66653-4 (cloth)
  ISBN 0-674-66654-2 (pbk.)
  1. Assisted suicide—Moral and ethical aspects.
  2. Assisted suicide—Law and legislation—United States.
  3. Euthanasia—Moral and ethical aspects. I. Emanuel, Linda L.
  R726.R445 1998
  174'.24—dc21   97-38892

Contents

CONTRIBUTORS

Marcia Angell, M.D.
Executive Editor
New England Journal of Medicine

George J. Annas, J.D., M.P.H.
Professor and Chair,
Health Law Department
Boston University School of Public Health

Margaret P. Battin, Ph.D.
Professor of Philosophy
University of Utah

James F. Childress, Ph.D.
Kyle Professor of Religious Studies
and Medical Education, University of Virginia

Ezekiel J. Emanuel, M.D., Ph.D.
Chief, Department of
Clinical Bioethics,
Warren G. Magnuson Clinical Center,
National Institutes of Health

Linda L. Emanuel, M.D., Ph.D.
Vice President for Ethics Standards
American Medical Association

Erich H. Loewy, M.D.
Professor of Bioethics
University of California, Davis

Edmund D. Pellegrino, M.D.
Director, Center for Clinical Bioethics
Georgetown University

Paul J. van der Maas, M.D., Ph.D.
Professor of Public Health
Erasmus University, Rotterdam

Susan M. Wolf, J.D.
Professor of Law and Medicine
University of Minnesota Law School

PREFACE

Physician-assisted suicide and euthanasia may appear to be hot new topics. But the questions have been debated since before Hippocrates. Some of the arguments change, but mostly they do not. And yet the questions are urgent, and answers must be rendered anew for society's current context.

This volume aims to clarify and balance the arguments concerning physician-assisted suicide and euthanasia and to direct attention to the root issues that motivate calls for their use in our own time. In Parts One and Two the cases for and against physician-assisted death are debated. Angell powerfully describes the deep desire to help those who suffer physically and request assistance in dying. Battin argues that physicians have a moral duty, if not a legal obligation, to assist in securing the death of patients—sometimes even if it is against the physician's own principles. Loewy notes the difficulty of denying assistance to those who, by reason of disability, cannot but would have committed suicide. On the other hand, Pellegrino argues that ideal palliative care can manage almost all suffering adequately, and that physician-assisted suicide does not serve the individual patient or the larger society well. Wolf points out that physician-assisted suicide and euthanasia are all too likely to be born of an ambivalent or nonauthentic request, especially in cases involving children. Both Wolf and Childress note that many bioethicists and theologians believe euthanasia to be a generally misguided interpretation of mercy.

Part Three attempts to put these points and counterpoints into empirical, historical, and legal perspective. Van der Maas directs our attention to the question, What empirical evidence currently exists, or would be helpful in the future, to support or undermine the arguments pro and con? He draws extensively on studies of the Dutch and U.S. experience with physician-assisted suicide and euthanasia, as well as on findings in the behavioral and social sciences, epidemiology, and ethnology. Ezekiel Emanuel asks, Why have physician-assisted suicide and euthanasia become such prominent issues in our time? In the course of answering this question, he provides a history of these practices through the ages. On the legal question of whether patients have a constitutional right to assistance with suicide, George Annas provides a historical account of various state rulings and, most recently, a ruling by the United States Supreme Court.

In my concluding chapter, to help weigh the opposing positions, I juxtapose the main arguments in the debate in a series of point-counterpoint analyses. To assist the reader for whom these questions have personal relevance, I examine a series of practical points for an interested person to consider, whether the decision to be made pertains to an individual or to public policy, and whether the person making the decision is the one who is dying, a family member, the physician, or a public servant. I also articulate a personal position on policy that developed during the process of reviewing the arguments in this volume and watching the evolving public, professional, and legal debate. It is a position I have taken with present-day society—and with patients from this society—in mind.

The topic of this book is somber and speaks a great deal of the circumstances surrounding death. The contributors and I hope that this book will help to guide those who must make very difficult decisions, whether at the level of public policy, in their personal practice, or among their own family members. We hope that it will benefit those whose suffering needs better understanding and redress. If the book succeeds in this way, it will be an honor to all who contributed.

This book is respectfully dedicated to my colleagues in the health professions who have committed themselves to providing patients with comfort in the face of dying—and to all who, grappling with the fact of mortality, have sought to make something of this essential condition of life.

PART ONE

Considerations in Favor

1

Helping Desperately Ill People to Die

MARCIA ANGELL

I first thought about euthanasia when I was an intern in 1967. I realized then for the first time that medicine did not have all the answers, that there was suffering for which there was no relief.

Two patients brought this fact home to me. One was Mr. C., a blue-collar worker in his 50s, whose terminal lung cancer had spread to his spine. He lay on his back waiting to die, paralyzed from the waist down, in constant pain, and desperately short of breath. When I suggested increasing his morphine, with the intention of hastening his death as well as relieving his pain, I was overruled by the resident, on the grounds that this would depress the patient's respiration. (Fortunately, the resident was in turn overruled by the attending doctor.) But even with more morphine, the patient was still unable to move, short of breath, and miserable.

The second patient, also a man in his 50s, was a physicist on the faculty at Harvard University. He had multiple myeloma, in those days an untreatable form of cancer. The disease had spread throughout his skeleton, causing excruciating pain. In addition, the man was profoundly weak and tired. Both the professor and his wife repeatedly asked me whether there was anything I could do to hasten his death. I said that I could increase his dose of morphine until it depressed his respiration. Doing so might cause him to get pneumonia, which I would then not treat. This was the only option, and it was not clear whether it would work. In both these cases, the intention was to bring about death as well as to relieve pain. But these patients' suffering was hardly limited to pain. In both cases there was also immobilization, shortness of breath, weakness, and a sense of utter despair and pointlessness.

In those days, physicians and their instructors paid little formal attention to the dying process. I do not remember a single mention of it in the medical school curriculum. It was as though dying were a medical failure and thus too shameful to be discussed. We were to succeed, not fail. When we came up against the reality of dying patients and their suffering, as I did in my internship, we were largely on our own. If patients asked for help in dying, they might or might not receive it. Whether they did depended more on us—our compassion, courage, and ingenuity—than it did on the patient's condition. In most cases, a patient's death was hastened without an explicit request by the patient or the family, although often there was an implicit understanding. For example, patients would say that they would rather be dead than continue pointless suffering, and families would ask the doctor whether "something" could be done. A doctor at that point might stop antibiotics or transfusions or whatever life-sustaining treatment was being given, often adding large doses of morphine as well.

Many doctors thought it was wrong to stop life-saving treatment, however, even if the patient requested it. They believed that their job was to extend life whenever possible. In those days, little distinction was made among the various methods of shortening life. All were forbidden. Most doctors also had an exaggerated fear of the addictive properties and side-effects of morphine. Furthermore, medical practice was highly paternalistic. Doctors rarely spoke with patients about decisions at the end of life; they simply made them. Seeking explicit agreement to hasten death would have been seen as unkind, as well as incriminating and unnecessary. In any case, the matter was far removed from public discussion, much less a subject of political controversy. What happened in any given case was at the doctor's discretion. It was all very private, and no policies or procedures governed the situation.

Enormous changes have occurred since then. For one thing, the consumer movement, fostered by the legal doctrine of informed consent, has greatly limited the ability of doctors to act alone. So, too, has the development of a team approach to hospital care. Increasingly, decisions must be discussed not only with patients but among all members of the health care team. More important, the issue became a public matter in 1975, when Joseph Quinlan went to court to ask for the authority to discontinue all "extraordinary procedures" keeping his daughter, Karen Ann, alive.[1] Suddenly the "right to die" was not just a private matter but a legal, ethical, and social issue.

Other legal cases followed the Quinlan case. As these poignant stories were publicized, large numbers of healthy people for the first time began to think about whether extending life might produce more suffering than benefit. They became aware that modern medicine was a two-edged sword, capable of dramatically rescuing some people from death, while damning others to prolonged suffering. Beginning in 1976, the state legislatures, one by one, enacted Natural Death Acts, which gave doctors immunity from prosecution if, under certain circumstances, they complied with a patient's living will and withheld or withdrew life-sustaining treatment. President Reagan established a Commission for the Study of Ethical Problems in Medicine, which in 1983 issued its report, *Deciding to Forego Life-Sustaining Treatment*.[2] In it, the Commission laid out principled procedures for approaching the problem of suffering at the end of life. These supported the concept of withholding life-sustaining treatment under defined circumstances. Physician-assisted dying had become a public issue, and doctors could no longer act alone on a case-by-case basis.

With increasing attention to the manner of dying came explicit distinctions that had not always been recognized. Withholding life-sustaining treatment, such as an artificial respirator, dialysis, or antibiotics, was held to be morally different from assisting in suicide by writing a prescription for large amounts of barbiturates, for example. And both of these acts were different from euthanasia, that is, actively causing death by giving a lethal injection. It became generally accepted that withholding life-sustaining treatment was permissible, but euthanasia was not. Assisting suicide—making it possible for a patient to take his own life—remains more contentious. It is thought by some to be appropriate under certain circumstances, but many believe it is always wrong.

The ambiguous position of assisted suicide is mirrored in the law. Suicide is not illegal, but in most, though not all states, assisting in suicide is.

The purpose of all three acts—withholding life-sustaining treatment, assisting suicide, and euthanasia—is the same: to hasten death. They are often thought of as constituting a continuum from passive to active. To withhold life-sustaining treatment simply means to refrain from initiating a treatment or to withdraw a treatment that has already been initiated. Thus, not placing a patient on an artificial respirator would be passive, even though it resulted in death, as would removing a respirator from a patient already using it. Writing a prescription for an overdose is seen as more active. Even though it is up to the patient to actually take the overdose, the doctor has actively supplied the means. Euthanasia is the most active, in that death is caused by an explicit act.

Paradoxically, however, from the patient's perspective, euthanasia is probably the most humane of the three events, since it is fast and painless. Withholding life-sustaining treatment may be much less humane, in that it extends the dying process and accentuates symptoms (such as suffocation or fever) until death occurs. Despite the differing moral status of the three methods of shortening life, it is often difficult to appreciate the differences in practical terms. For example, withdrawing a respirator requires removing the machine and a period of agonal struggle for breath as the patient dies. This is not a "passive" scene—it is stressful for the patient, for attending physicians and nurses, and for family members at the bedside. Furthermore, if it occurred against the wishes of the patient, it would constitute murder. By contrast, injecting an overdose of morphine into an intravenous line produces a quiet, peaceful death, even though doing so constitutes "active" euthanasia.

There is another confusing element. Both withdrawing treatment and euthanasia do not require the participation of the patient. Either could be done without the patient's cooperation. In contrast, assisted suicide—the morally "intermediate" act—*does* require the patient's participation. To die, the patient must swallow the pills—a voluntary act of a necessarily aware patient. Thus, the traditional moral distinctions are entirely based on what the doctor does, not on the consequences of the doctor's action for the patient. The question asked is the nature of the doctor's act: Is it passive or active or intermediate? The moral judgment is divorced from the patient's perspective. We do not usually ask how the patient is affected. Because the patient seems left out of the moral equation, the distinctions seem to me somewhat artificial and ultimately unpersuasive.

Until a decade or so ago, none of the methods of hastening death was generally accepted. Now, withholding life-sustaining treatment is not only accepted but commonplace. The controversy is about more active means of hastening death. But in discussions of the risks and benefits of permitting physician-assisted suicide and euthanasia—sometimes lumped together under the rubric physician-assisted dying or aid-in-dying or assisted death—the evolution of our attitude toward withholding life-sustaining treatment can be illuminating.

Stopping Life Supports

Since the Quinlan case was settled in 1976, a large body of case law and of legal and ethical opinion gradually grew around the issue of withholding life-sustaining treatment.[3] Three cases in particular are of interest because they well illustrate some of the important principles that have emerged since the Quinlan case, principles that have been buttressed again and again in other cases. In discussing them, I do not mean to imply that the courts should be the final arbiters of medical ethics. Far from it. I believe that there is entirely too much court-watching and too much confusion between what is legal and what is right. But these three cases are now a part of a medical and ethical consensus as well as a legal one. For this reason, they serve as a useful framework for discussing the issue of withholding life-sustaining treatment. They also illustrate the fact that the most important question is usually not what the decision should be but who should make it.

The first case, *Lane v. Candura*, was decided by the Massachusetts Court of Appeals in 1978.[4] Mrs. Candura was a 77-year-old woman whose leg was gangrenous. She was told that she would die unless the leg was amputated. She nevertheless refused the amputation. Her daughter, Mrs. Lane, took her mother to court to compel her to undergo the amputation. The court ruled in favor of the mother. She was found to be competent to make her own decision and was not required to have medical treatment against her will, even though the treatment was thought to be life-saving.

This case illustrates three important principles. First, a competent patient may, with few exceptions, refuse any medical treatment—even if it is life-sustaining—for any reason whatsoever. Competence in this context is defined as understanding the nature of the decision and its likely consequences. It does not mean making a decision that most of us would find sensible. Second, the case illustrates the primacy of self-determination (often termed patient autonomy) as the standard to be applied to such decisions. Is this what the patient truly wanted? No other standard takes precedence over it—not even consideration of the patient's best interests. Autonomy in this context is grounded in the constitutional right of privacy and the common law right of self-determination. It is also inherent in the doctrine of informed consent: if a patient must consent to a medical procedure, then the right to refuse is implied. In 1990 the U.S. Supreme Court, in the *Cruzan* case, affirmed the right to refuse treatment, basing it on the liberty clause of the Fourteenth Amendment.[5] Third, *Lane v. Candura* illustrates the proper role of the family in such a decision. A family member, no matter how loving the intent, should not be permitted to usurp a competent patient's rights.

The second court case involved a patient who, unlike Mrs. Candura, was clearly not competent. This case, *Brophy v. New England Sinai Hospital,* was decided by the Massachusetts Supreme Judicial Court in 1986.[6] It involved a 49-year-old firefighter and emergency medical technician, Paul Brophy, who after a ruptured aneurysm in his brain was in a coma from which he would never recover—a condition termed a "permanent vegetative state." Brophy's life was maintained by a feeding tube in his stomach. In the course of Brophy's work, he had seen several people in similar states, and he had repeatedly told his family and friends that he would not want to live that way. When it became clear that Brophy would never regain consciousness, his wife asked to have the feeding tube removed to comply with his earlier expressed views. The hospital refused, on the grounds that removing the tube would lead to Brophy's death and therefore would not be in his best interests. The Massachusetts Supreme Court ruled in favor of Mrs. Brophy, Brophy was transferred to another facility, the feeding tube was removed, and Brophy died. The feeding tube was considered simply another form of medical treatment, a view upheld by the U.S. Supreme Court. Earlier opinion held that artificial feeding was different from other life-sustaining treatment, in that it had important symbolic value. Although this distinction is no longer generally accepted, there are still those who believe that stopping artificial feeding is tantamount to euthanasia.

The Brophy case illustrates two principles. First, it shows the use of what is known as "substituted judgment" as the standard to be applied to decisions when self-determination is not possible. Substituted judgment refers to a decision made by someone else—usually a family member or close friend—on the basis of the patient's preferences or values as expressed before he or she became incompetent. In this case, Brophy had once been competent and made his wishes known clearly. Mrs. Brophy then acted as his substitute. It helped that his 90-year-old mother and five grown children agreed with the decision. Second, the Brophy case illustrates the appropriate role of the family in such decisions. When the patient cannot speak for himself, the family can exercise substituted judgment. In such cases, the range of permissible decisions is wide, depending on how explicit the patient's advance directives were, but the range is not quite as wide as when an individual decides for himself. For example, it is unlikely that a family would be allowed to refuse glucose to treat insulin shock in a diabetic.

The third case is the most celebrated—the case of Karen Ann Quinlan, decided by the New Jersey Supreme Court in 1976. This was the first of the widely publicized right-to-die cases. Quinlan was a 21-year-old woman in a permanent vegetative state reportedly as a result of an accidental overdose of tranquilizers and alcohol. She was thought to require a respirator, and when it became clear that she would never recover, her father asked to have the respirator removed. The hospital went to court, not because the doctors disagreed with Mr. Quinlan but because they were uncertain about their legal liability and wanted the court to give them immunity. The court upheld Mr. Quinlan, and the respirator was removed. As it turned out, Karen Ann was not respirator-dependent, and she lived another ten years because her parents were not willing to stop artificial feeding.

Unlike the Brophy case, the Quinlan case was not decided on the basis of the substituted judgment standard. Instead, the New Jersey Supreme Court invoked what is now known as the "best interests" standard. According to this standard, when a patient is no longer competent and has never expressed views on the subject—or when the patient is a child or is a mentally retarded adult—medical treatment must be in accord with the patient's best interests. Best interests are defined as being consistent with what most reasonable people would choose in a similar situation. In the Quinlan case the court also made it clear that such decisions did not, in its view, belong in the courts at all. It held that Quinlan's parents could have made the decision at the bedside, provided a hospital-appointed committee agreed that Karen Ann's condition was irreversible.

The treatment options permitted under the best-interests standard are much more limited than those permitted under the other two standards—self-determination and substituted judgment. The best-interests standard by definition does not allow for eccentricities or idiosyncrasies. Instead, it appeals to a majority view. If, for example, Mrs. Candura had not been competent and therefore had been treated according to the best-interests standard, she would probably have had her leg amputated, since this is what most reasonable people would want in her situation. But despite the narrowness of the best-interests standard, it usually does allow for some latitude. And within this more limited range of options, most common law holds that the decision rests with the family, as it did in the Quinlan case. Quinlan's father could have decided either way—to remove the respirator or not—since most people would presumably have found either decision reasonable.

What can we learn from the above cases? First, that competent patients may refuse any treatment whatsoever. Second, advance directives or living wills—expressed either orally or, more compellingly, in writing—carry great weight. Nevertheless, there are still some uncertainties, mostly having to do with who should be the decision-maker for incompetent patients who did not leave advance directives.

We also see that there is a hierarchy of decision-makers: first, the patient or a designated proxy; second, the family with the advice of the doctor; and finally—to resolve disputes—the courts. Most hospitals have created what are known as ethics committees to consider such cases. Although they can be valuable in resolving disputes so that they do not have to go to court, it is important to recognize that they are not themselves decision-making bodies. Patients do not cede their civil rights to institutional committees just because they are sick and in the hospital. The cases that come before the courts usually do so because a subordinate decision-maker sought inappropriately to be the primary decision-maker. This is what happened when Mrs. Lane tried to usurp her mother's prerogative, and when New England Sinai tried to usurp the Brophy family's prerogative.

We can also think of a hierarchy of ethical standards to apply in making these kinds of decisions: first, self-determination; second, substituted judgment; and third, the best-interests standard. Here again, problems have arisen when a subordinate standard was used inappropriately—as when Mrs. Lane invoked the best-interests standard for her mother, rather than deferring to Mrs. Candura's right to self-determination.

The courts are best reserved for settling disputes—not for granting immunity or providing advice and certainly not for making decisions. What sorts of disputes might usefully reach the courts? First, there is sometimes an issue of who should be the guardian for an incompetent patient, especially when the patient does not have close family members. The court is the proper place for this decision to be made. Second, a serious disagreement about a medical decision may have to be adjudicated in the court. The disagreement may be among family members, or it may arise from a caregiver's belief that the family's decision is outside the permissible range or based on improper motives. If these sorts of disputes cannot be resolved within the institution, perhaps with the help of the ethics committee, then any of the interested parties may appeal to the courts.

The importance of these three cases in considering assisted

suicide and euthanasia is that they consistently affirm the right of individuals to have maximal control over their own life and death. And they also indicate that the traditional commitment to life at all costs was explicitly breached in the 1970s. Most of the disputes over withholding treatment that have reached the courts have concerned incompetent patients—such as Brophy and Quinlan—for whom a proxy decision-maker was necessary. In such cases, once the decision is made, its implementation is usually not difficult. Patients in a permanent vegetative state require artificial feeding. Stopping it—as in the case of Brophy—causes death without suffering, since such patients cannot feel anything.

But what of the people who are conscious and competent and who want desperately to die because they face prolonged suffering and increasing helplessness? Such patients far outnumber ones like Brophy or Quinlan who are incompetent. Indeed, the American Hospital Association estimates that 70 percent of the 1,300,000 hospital deaths each year occur after a decision is made to withhold life-sustaining treatment. Most of those patients are competent at the time the decision is made, although sometimes it is implemented later, after the patient is no longer competent. That's nearly a million deaths each year, compared with about 10,000 people who at any given time are in a permanent vegetative state.[7] These numbers give a clear indication of the dimensions of the problem.

In these cases we know who the decision-maker should be and we know what the decision is. As demonstrated in the *Candura* case, a competent patient is the decision-maker. But how can the decision to hasten death be implemented? Obviously, it is now accepted that we may refuse life-sustaining treatment, and many of us do. But is that enough to solve the problem of prolonged dying? For many of us, the answer is no.

Major problems arise when we rely on our right to refuse life-sustaining treatment to ease the dying process. For one thing, doing so assumes that there will be some life-sustaining treatment to be withheld. That is not always the case. For example, a person might be suffering from advanced cancer but have no immediately life-threatening condition, such as pneumonia, for which a treatment, such as penicillin, could be withheld. Such a patient is thus dependent for a merciful death on the happenstance of developing such a complication. In a 1996 decision declaring unconstitutional New York's law against physician-assisted suicide, the Second Circuit Court of Appeals based its argument on this fact.[8] The court held that the New York law violated the constitutional right of equal protection under the law, since it denied help in dying to those without life-sustaining treatment, while permitting it for those who were receiving such treatment.

Even when there *is* life-sustaining treatment to be withheld, doing so can entail a period of agony for someone who is conscious. Removing a respirator produces suffocation; terminating dialysis produces the symptoms of uremia; refusing feedings produces the symptoms of dehydration or starvation. What is passive for the doctor may not be so passive for the patient. For many years, of course, we have relied on caregivers to ease the last hours or days of suffering by giving large doses of morphine or barbiturates, but this is often done parsimoniously and erratically, by the grace of the doctors and nurses.

Relying on our right to refuse treatment also does not speak to the needs of people who would like the option of choosing death not just near the end of a terminal illness but at the beginning, before they have undergone a long deterioration and become helpless. This was true of Janet Adkins, the first person Dr. Jack Kevorkian helped to commit suicide. She had early Alzheimer's disease and wanted to act while she was still able to.

Because of these problems, which are appreciated by most people intuitively if not explicitly, our attention has turned increasingly toward physician-assisted suicide or euthanasia as a means to hasten death. After all, the thinking goes, if the intent in withholding life-sustaining treatment is to cause a merciful death, why not accomplish the purpose faster and more humanely and at the time of our choosing, without relying on chance?

Death Goes Public

The issue was brought powerfully to public attention by the actions of three people. In 1988 an anonymous young resident confessed in the *Journal of the American Medical Association* to an episode of euthanasia.[9] He claimed to have administered a lethal injection to a young woman suffering from terminal cancer of the ovary. He had been called to see her for the first time while he was on night duty at a hospital. There was no discussion with the patient or her companion. He simply killed her.

Then in 1991 Dr. Timothy Quill, an internist in Rochester, New York, described in the *New England Journal of Medicine* the assisted suicide of his patient, Diane.[10] Diane was suffering from acute leukemia and asked Quill to provide enough sleeping pills to end her life when she found it intolerable. Quill, who had been Diane's doctor for eight years, was unable to dissuade her, and so he complied with her request. Four months later, Diane killed herself.

In the meantime, Dr. Jack Kevorkian, the retired Michigan pathologist, had launched his incredible career helping people to commit suicide. People came to him for the purpose, from all over the country. He did not know them before they came to him requesting his help in committing suicide.

Most doctors and ethicists seemed to approve of Dr. Quill's act, while disapproving of the anonymous resident and of Dr. Kevorkian. Indeed, a grand jury in New York, where, at that time, assisting suicide was illegal, refused to indict Quill. But in Michigan, where it was not illegal, a law was crafted specifically to stop Kevorkian. The anonymous resident's act was nearly universally condemned. Yet, what are the essential differences? Quill and Kevorkian both assisted suicides. To be sure, Quill was Diane's longstanding doctor and is blessed with a more circumspect manner, but are these circumstances enough to render the same act acceptable in one case and unacceptable in the other? As for the resident, he performed euthanasia, not assisted suicide. Although the patient's death may have been welcome, it is in my view clearly immoral to have acted unilaterally. If she had requested euthanasia, the question would be much more difficult.

Regardless of how we see these acts, assisted suicide and euthanasia—once taboo subjects—are now openly aired and debated in medical journals as well as in the popular media. A great deal of attention in these debates is given to the experience in the Netherlands. There, euthanasia has been openly practiced for two decades. Although still technically illegal, the practice is protected by case law. It is subject to stringent guidelines put forth in 1984 by the Dutch Medical Association.[11] These guidelines stipulate that euthanasia must be performed only for competent patients who are suffering intolerably with no possibility of relief, and who consistently and repeatedly request euthanasia over a reasonable time. The patient need not be terminally ill, but there must be a medical illness. Euthanasia is not permitted for depression, which is treatable, nor as a response to unhappiness—although a violation of this prohibition was featured on a Dutch television documentary on the subject. The intent is that euthanasia not be an option for patients with reversible illnesses or intractable suffering. The usual method of euthanasia in the Netherlands is to induce sleep with a barbiturate, then to administer a lethal injection.

The consequences of the Dutch acceptance of physician-assisted dying are controversial. Indeed, not much was known about them until a government-appointed group—the Remmelink Commission—studied the matter in 1991.[12] It found that 35 percent of deaths in the Netherlands involved either withholding life-sustaining treatment or giving enough morphine to shorten life. (Recall that in the United States the comparable figure is 70 percent of hospital deaths.) But 1.8 percent of all deaths were the result of euthanasia, and 0.3 percent the result of assisted suicide. Of particular note was the fact that in an additional 0.8 percent of deaths, euthanasia was performed after the patient was no longer competent, in violation of the guidelines. In addition, there have been reports of euthanasia being performed on children, also a violation of the guidelines. The report of the Remmelink Commission was variously reassuring and alarming, depending, it seemed, on the prior position of those reacting. Some felt it was as good a record as could be expected; others saw the Netherlands well on its way down a slippery slope.

In the United States, assisted suicide is illegal in most states and euthanasia is illegal in all of them, but since 1988 we have seen a series of efforts to change that. The voters in three states—California, Washington, and Oregon—have been asked to approve measures that would permit physician-assisted dying under certain circumstances.[13] California, which twice voted on the issue, and Washington both rejected the initiatives. But the margins were not great. In 1994 Oregon passed its initiative by a narrow margin, becoming the first place in the world to legalize physician-assisted dying. After the failure of court challenges to reverse the Oregon law, the state legislature mandated a new referendum to consider the matter. In 1977 the voters once again approved physician-assisted suicide, this time by a wide margin.[14]

The defeat of the California and Washington initiatives and the initially narrow margin in Oregon are puzzling in view of public opinion polls showing that at least 60 percent of the public support some form of physician-assisted dying.[15] Many observers believe that the reason for the discrepancy is concern over inadequate safeguards in the provisions, but this is speculation. One might equally speculate that the lengthy safeguards that were present in the referenda were worrying to the voters. Any proposal so couched in conditions and qualifications implies grave risks. Voters may have been frightened at the last minute.

The Oregon bill was sharply limited to physician-assisted suicide. Euthanasia was not a part of it. It was thought that this would make the measure more palatable to the voters. Many thought that the Washington and first California initiatives were defeated because of the failure to distinguish between these forms of physician-assisted dying. That, too, is speculation. We simply do not know whether the failure to distinguish between suicide and euthanasia was a problem for the voters. At least one poll indicated that, although many doctors and ethicists make much of the distinctions between methods of hastening death, the public does not.[16]

In 1996 two federal appeals courts took the matter out of the hands of the state legislatures in their jurisdictions. The U.S. Court of Appeals for the Ninth Circuit declared unconstitutional Washington's law against physician-assisted suicide. A month later, the Court of Appeals for the Second Circuit declared unconstitutional a similar law in New York. Both were reversed by the U.S. Supreme Court. The Ninth Circuit Court had invoked the due process clause of the Fourteenth Amendment; the Second Circuit based its decision on the equal protection clause. But both courts, like the people in the public opinion poll, found no moral distinction between assisted suicide and withholding life-sustaining treatment.[17] Many believe that, quite apart from the merits of the arguments, the courts were arrogating to themselves decisions that properly belonged to the legislatures. Others believe that since decisions at the end of life are essentially private decisions involving individual rights, the courts are the proper forum.[18]

The most frequent argument against permitting assisted suicide is that it would inevitably lead to a gradual erosion of our respect for life. According to this view, there is no landmark on this slippery moral slope to tell us we've gone too far and no purchase to stop the slide. I find this argument unpersuasive in the abstract. Life is full of slippery slopes, and one of our more interesting duties is negotiating them. If we stayed off them altogether, we could accomplish very little.

But the argument is much more persuasive in the particular case of the United States at the end of this century. Unlike the situation in other Western democracies, caring for a family member with a long illness in the United States can be financially devastating. And we do little as a society to help with the other difficulties of caring for the chronically ill. Given the heavy burdens, then, mightn't there be pressures on sick people with expensive illnesses to ask to die? And wouldn't this pressure be greatest among the very old, the poor, and the handicapped—who may be too weak to resist the pressure? And in this social context, with all its economic harshness, mightn't voluntary euthanasia, requested by the patient, be extended to involuntary euthanasia of incompetent patients, first for their own sakes, then for the sake of their families, then for the budget of the health care system? These are the practical slippery-slope concerns that I have. They do not apply with nearly the same force to a country such as the Netherlands, where there is a universal and comprehensive health care system and where a lingering illness does not bankrupt the family.

The Case for Physician-Assisted Suicide

Despite these concerns, it seems to me that the problem of aiding people who face prolonged dying is so great that we cannot ignore it. Any of us may be in the situation some day, and it behooves all of us to develop our thinking on the matter. We cannot avoid the slippery slope; in fact, with the growing acceptance since *Quinlan* of the right to withhold life-sustaining treatment, we are already on it, like it or not. The issue now is simply where and how to find a purchase. The 1996 decision of the Ninth Circuit Court of Appeals declaring unconstitutional Washington's law against physician-assisted suicide emphasized this point.

I believe there are two alternative ways we might deal with the problem, while preventing a headlong slide downhill. The first is to permit physician-assisted suicide under certain circumstances, but not euthanasia. By definition, suicide requires the patient to act; euthanasia does not. By limiting assisted dying to suicide, patients retain ultimate control and they can change their minds at any time, as was emphasized by the Second Circuit Court of Appeals. To be sure, an occasional, ambivalent patient may succumb to outside pressures, but no system of safeguards for any workable endeavor is absolutely foolproof. The crucial point is that, unlike either euthanasia or withholding life-sustaining treatment, suicide requires a deliberate action by the patient.

An alternative way to negotiate the slippery slope would be to draw the line strictly between voluntary and involuntary euthanasia. Euthanasia would be permitted, but only for competent patients who request it, as in the Netherlands. Unlike assisted suicide, it would not exclude patients who, because of their illness, cannot swallow pills. It would, however, exclude patients who are not competent, such as Brophy and Quinlan, and it would also exclude children, as well as adults with advanced Alzheimer's disease. But perhaps these limitations are the price of preventing abuse. Indeed, euthanasia so restricted might be a second stage in legalizing physician-assisted dying, to be considered only after we as a society, perhaps in only a few states, have had some experience with legally sanctioned physician-assisted suicide.

Whatever our approach, the problem of dying in agony will not go away. In my view, it is time to incorporate physician-assisted suicide into our medical armamentarium, to be used infrequently under certain well-defined circumstances. It should be available for those, like Janet Adkins, facing slow disintegration, and for those overwhelmed by the infirmities of old age, as well as for those in the throes of advanced disease. As in the Dutch guide-lines, it should not be used as an answer to depression or other treatable illness. Modern medicine now performs great miracles, but it also produces great anguish, not all of which can be relieved even by the most assiduous attempts to treat pain.

Polls of doctors indicate that a majority of them, like the public at large, believe assisted suicide or euthanasia is sometimes appro-priate. But among these doctors, about half believe that the act should be performed by someone else, not a doctor. They believe that a doctor's function must be to extend life, never to shorten it. To them, an absolute proscription against physician-assisted dy-ing prevents confusion on the part of doctors and distrust on the part of patients. Doctors need never wonder whether they should be extending life or cutting it short, and patients need never wonder what their doctor is up to. I find this position peculiarly divorced from the real business of medicine—to provide care in whatever way best serves the patient's interests. If acceding to a patient's request to hasten death seems appropriate to the doctor, how can he or she justify withdrawing from the patient's care at that point? The greatest harm we can do is to abandon a desperate patient.

Most of the arguments against physician-assisted suicide place the doctor at the center of the issue. Is the doctor's act one of omission or commission? Is it consistent with the doctor's role? If this is the focus, it is reasonable to argue that withholding life-sus-taining treatment is permissible but not assisted suicide or eutha-nasia. If we shift the focus from the doctor to the patient, however, the calculus changes. Suppose instead of asking about the doc-tor's act, we ask whether the *patient's* act is one of omission or commission—that is, is the patient required to perform the final action or can it be done by someone else, perhaps without the patient's full knowledge or consent? If we wish to maximize self-determination for the patient, assisted suicide is more reasonable than either euthanasia or merely withholding treatment.

A second question would be whether the patient's death will be as quick and painless as possible or whether there will still be a period of suffering. If degree of suffering is the standard, then euthanasia is probably the best form of assisted dying. The point is that by placing the patient, not the doctor, in the center of the picture, we may come to very different conclusions about the moral status of the ways doctors might help suffering patients to die.

Permitting physician-assisted suicide might have positive effects in addition to minimizing suffering. Some patients facing an irreversible progressive disease take their own lives while they are still in reasonably good health, because they fear that if they wait, they will find themselves unable to do so—either because they are too impaired to act or because they are confined to a hospital. Knowing that assisted death would be available when they needed it would undoubtedly lead many incurably ill people to postpone ending their lives. They would thus live longer and, even more important, they would live in more peace.

This effect was clear in Quill's account of his patient, Diane. Once she had the prescription for a lethal dose of sleeping pills, her anxiety subsided and she was able to enjoy wholeheartedly her remaining months with her family. The same phenomenon was described in a 1995 article in *The New Yorker* by Andrew Solomon.[19] Solomon recounted the story of his mother's death from ovarian cancer. Only after she stockpiled enough sleeping pills to kill herself was she able to achieve some measure of happiness in the time remaining to her.

The problems of prolonged dying are not new, but they have become more urgent in recent years because we now have the technology to extend life long after some people would wish to be dead. There is little precedent for the kinds of decisions we need to make. Merely having the right to refuse life-sustaining treatment does not solve the problem of prolonged dying for all patients. We need to do more for them. To be sure, we must choose our way carefully, mindful of the possibilities of abuse. But paralysis is not an answer, and moralism is no substitute for compassion.

2

Is a Physician Ever Obligated to Help a Patient Die?

MARGARET P. BATTIN

Physician-assisted suicide will probably soon become legal on a state-by-state basis, culturally tolerated, and openly practiced. But while this change will resolve some moral issues, it will raise others. One particular question which, I suspect, covertly fuels many physicians' anxieties about legalization of physician-assisted suicide is this: Is a physician ever *obligated* to help a patient die? If physician-assisted suicide were to become legal or legally tolerated, would the patient have a right to assistance, a right held against the physician for performance of this duty?

It may seem obvious that physicians can never be obligated to do something they regard as morally wrong—especially not something that may seem to them to be as profoundly morally wrong as contributing to the self-killing of their patient. Whatever the law says, for some physicians, conscience still may not permit it. All proposals for the legalization of physician-assisted suicide that have been proposed to date take this stance: that the physician may elect to help, but is not obligated to do so. In voter initiatives in Washington, California, and Oregon, in state legislative initiatives, in model statutes such as that of the Boston Working Group,[1] and so on, all proposals have opt-out provisions, or "conscience clauses," that permit the physician to refuse to participate in a suicide. Oregon's Measure 16, which passed at the polls in November 1994 and withstood a repeal measure in 1997, is representative. It says: "No health care provider shall be under any duty, whether by contract, by statute or by any other legal requirement to participate in the provision to a qualified patient of medication to end his or her life in a humane and dignified manner."[2]

But the basis of opt-out clauses—the ubiquitous assumption that a physician's scruples provide adequate justification, legally and morally, for excusing him or her from assisting in suicide—is rarely challenged. Furthermore, there is little challenge to the informal understanding that if the practice of assisting suicides were to remain extralegal but still become widely accepted, physicians could nevertheless choose to opt out, based on their conscience or any other personal consideration. It is just this assumption that I wish to examine here. It is my view that even the physician with the most profound moral scruples against physician-assisted suicide can, in certain circumstances, incur an obligation to provide this assistance. But when this turns out to be the case, it is almost always the product of that physician's own doing, and thus could have been avoided.

I hasten to add that I support the legal recognition of opt-out provisions in legislation concerning physician-assisted suicide. But that does not mean that a physician has no *moral* obligation to help, even if there is no legal one. Opt-out clauses, whether explicitly stated in legal documents or informally embedded in culturally understood social expectations, cannot always provide moral protection, even if they do shield a physician from legal action or social blame.

This paper has two principal parts: a long background section that examines the argument over physician-assisted suicide and shows how a positive right to assistance is generated from two basic moral principles, and a more sharply focused applications section that examines how a patient's right to assistance in suicide can impose an obligation on the physician to assist, even if the physician has scruples against doing so.

To address the question of physician obligation, we must first review the principal arguments for and against physician-assisted suicide in terminal illness, since these arguments establish whether the dying patient has rights to assistance in suicide.

These rights would at a minimum include the "negative" right not to be interfered with or prevented from committing suicide if the means are available from a willing physician, and they might also include the "positive" right to require a physician to provide such help if requested.[3] If there are such rights, do they impose obligations upon physicians, even when as physicians they do not want to participate and even when the law provides opt-out clauses protecting them from any legal obligation to do so?

The Case for Physician-Assisted Suicide

The moral argument in favor of permitting physician assistance in suicide is grounded in the conjunction of two principles: self-determination (or, as bioethicists put it, autonomy) and mercy (or the avoidance of suffering). The moral right of self-determination is the right to live one's life as one sees fit, subject only to the constraint that this not involve harm to others. Because living one's life as one chooses must also include living the very end of one's life as one chooses, the matter of how to die is as fully protected by the principle of self-determination as any other part of one's life. Choosing how to die is part of choosing how to live.

The second component of the moral argument in favor of physician assistance in suicide is grounded in the joint obligations to avoid doing harm and to do good (the principles of nonmaleficence and beneficence, as bioethicists often put them). In medical-ethics discussions, some writers call this the principle of patient interests or patient welfare, but in the specific context of end-of-life questions, I like to call this the principle of mercy—the principle that one ought both to refrain from causing pain or suffering and act to relieve it.[4] The principle of mercy, or avoidance of suffering, underwrites the right of a dying person to an easy death, to whatever extent possible, and clearly supports physician-assisted suicide in many cases. Suicide assisted by a humane physician spares the patient the pain and suffering that may be part of the dying process, and grants the patient a "mercifully" easy death.

The principle of mercy is relevant in two general classes of cases, one comparatively unproblematic, the other far more disputed. In the first case, the dying patient is currently enduring

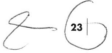

pain or other intolerable physical symptoms (such as continuous breathlessness, nausea, vomiting) or is suffering from emotional and psychological anguish. In the second case, the patient with a terminal illness anticipates and seeks to avoid pain and suffering, knowing that they are highly likely to occur in the future course of the disease. Narrow constructions of the principle of mercy are typically interpreted to support just the patient's right to avoid current pain and suffering; the requirement that the patient be undergoing "intolerable suffering" is often read in this way. Broader constructions support preemptive strategies intended to avoid anticipated pain and suffering before they begin.

Of course, with modern pain-management techniques—especially those pioneered by the hospice movement for treating pain before it develops, on a regular schedule, rather than as needed after the patient already experiences it—most pain in terminal illness can be avoided. Other symptoms caused either by the disease itself or by the treatments employed to arrest it (including diarrhea, itching, restlessness, confusion, hallucinations, and many others) can also be controlled at least to some extent with adequate management. And suffering—that constellation of emotional and psychological factors often described as anguish, despair, hopelessness, fear, and dread—can be greatly relieved by sensitive counseling and plain old-fashioning caring.

But not all pain, symptoms, and suffering are amenable to treatment or actually receive treatment. The 1995 SUPPORT study, for example, showed that about half of patients dying in five major teaching hospitals experienced moderate to severe pain at least 50 percent of the time during their last two or three days of life.[5] Many other studies both in the United States and worldwide document inadequate treatment of pain from cancer and other causes. Sometimes this failure is due to fears of creating addiction to narcotics, sometimes to ignorance of contemporary escalating or "ladder" methods of pain management, and sometimes to lack of adequate drugs, facilities, personnel, and other resources. Whether or not nearly all pain *could* be controlled, the reality is that much pain in dying patients is not effectively treated.

It is always possible to relieve pain, other symptoms, and suffering by producing partial or complete unconsciousness through sedation. But some patients do not want this sort of relief, even if it could be effectively managed over time. They regard as repugnant programs that stress the heavy use of analgesics, especially opiates, because this treatment does not accord with their conceptions of death with dignity, or with the sort of easy passage they wish for themselves and for the family members who will be close observers of it. They do not want a medicalized, drugged dying process; they do not want "terminal sedation." They want a death they can meet consciously, in the company of their family, at a time and place and in a manner of their own choosing.

It is these two basic moral principles, self-determination and mercy, in which the right to suicide in terminal illness is grounded. Like rights of self-determination generally, the right to suicide in terminal illness is initially the negative right (sometimes called a liberty right) not to be interfered with; patients retain the right to control what is done to them in the sense of preventing what they do not want. That is what liberty, in the negative-right sense of the term, is. In the circumstances of terminal illness, however, self-determination may become a positive right as well—a right to require someone to help, a right to request or demand what one actively wants. This transformation can occur because endstage terminally ill patients, dying of degenerative processes in a long, debilitating illness, may not be able to exercise their right to influence the circumstances of their death without assistance from another person. They are often institutionalized in a hospital or other facility or bedridden at home, with constant surveillance ("care"), perhaps in pain or with other disturbing symptoms. And while some terminally ill patients do find alternative means of committing suicide—shooting themselves or jumping from buildings—for most of them this is completely unrealistic or utterly repugnant. The right to control one's own dying as far as possible in order to avoid suffering or pain is the right to seek an *easy* death. It is not merely the "right to die"; it is the right to try to die without suffering and with what is often called dignity, in a way, perhaps, that underscores the importance of the very end of life. But this is a right nullified without the assistance of someone who can provide both technical and emotional support.

The most plausible party for providing such assistance is the physician. It is the physician who has access to drugs, who has specialized knowledge of appropriate dosages, and who knows how to prevent side effects such as nausea and vomiting.[6] Equally important, the physician can be a source of emotional support for both patient and family. Seen in this light, the right to assistance in suicide is plausibly construed as the dying patient's right to help from his or her own physician, at least where there is a personal physician who knows the patient well, who has been directly, extensively, and intimately connected with and responsible for that person's care, who may know the family, and who understands, better than any other physician or other party able to provide assistance in suicide, that person's hopes, fears, and wishes about how to die.

The realistic physician also knows how the sort of death the patient seeks is likely to contrast with the expected course of events if assistance is not provided. Not only is the right to suicide in order to achieve an easier, more acceptable death not much of a right if one cannot exercise it by oneself, but it is only fully supported where such help is provided by the most effective person in this role, the patient's own physician, or, if there is no such arrangement, the physician currently responsible for providing the patient's terminal care.

It is important to recognize that in serving as the basis for the rights of dying patients, self-determination and mercy do not function as independent principles, each sufficient in itself. A mere request for physician-assisted suicide by a perfectly healthy person does not justify a physician's assistance. Similarly, the mere fact of pain or suffering in a terminal patient does not license a physician to end that person's life, if the person does not seek physician-assisted suicide.[7] Fears that legalization would license assisted suicide for a healthy person without pain or suffering, or involuntary or nonvoluntary mercy-killing, are often expressed by those who oppose it, but this is to misunderstand what the bases of a patient's right would be under any of the current proposals. *Both* principles, self-determination and mercy, must be applicable for the patient to have any substantial claim on the physician's help.

In practice, these two principles do not always function in independent ways. The principle of self-determination may play a large role in what constitutes acceptable and unacceptable forms of pain relief to the patient. The principle of mercy likewise plays a role in what the patient conceives of as an easy death, taking into consideration both his or her own comfort and the comfort of family members or others who will be observers of the death or directly affected by it.

A person's background views about the significance of the final parts of one's life—the last months, weeks, days, hours—may also influence how patients exercise their rights. In a contemporary secular view, perhaps borrowed from medieval theology but often (though not always) cleansed of its religious underpinnings, these last moments are given special weight in a way that makes the physician's role particularly important. In medieval Christian theology, the final moments of life were the last chance for repentance, perhaps made in the religious ritual of extreme unction but in any case held within the conscience of the dying person. Repentance and complete acceptance of God in the last moments of life were held to be crucial, in that they might pave the way for salvation. A lot rode on these last moments.

The modern secularized version of this scene recognizes, at a minimum, that the very last part of one's life can be of paramount emotional, reflective, and social significance; it can be viewed as the conclusion, the resolution, the culmination of a life now completely lived. That is the reason some people choose to end their lives directly, so that they can finish their lives as themselves, able to think, communicate, and (for some) to pray, rather than be overtaken by pain or sedated into oblivion.

Thus we begin to see the basic structure of the argument about physician-assisted suicide. The side favoring physician-assisted suicide argues from the conjunction of the moral principles of self-determination and mercy to establish the right to direct assistance in dying—a right which in turn generates obligations on the part of the physician. At a minimum, the physician is obligated to refrain from attempting to prevent the suicide, whether by threat, force, or involuntary hospitalization. And insofar as the patient's right becomes a positive claim to assistance, the physician, as the party most knowledgeable in medical matters, must provide help in doing what the patient seeks. And because the patient's trust and comfort with a familiar caregiver is also crucial in seeking an easy death, the obligation to assist is particularly strong for the patient's own physician.

To be sure, relabeling might take some of the sting out of this obligation. Were the physician's role redescribed as "attending" in a "patient-directed" or "self-enacted" death, rather than "assisting" a "suicide," it might not seem so controversial or so difficult for physicians with scruples against "suicide" to comply with.[8] That is why the practice is often called "aid-in-dying" or other less freighted names, and why legislative measures, including Oregon's Measure 16, can insist that what is authorized "shall not constitute a suicide."

But relabeling is not the point. The point is that if the patient has a right to physician-assisted suicide, aid-in-dying, or whatever the act is called, the two underlying moral principles clearly show that at least in some circumstances, the patient's personal physician has a corresponding obligation to provide the assistance the patient seeks—despite whatever opt-out legal clauses or social expectations may be available.

The Case against Physician-Assisted Suicide

If the patient has the right to seek an easy, merciful death, including death by means of physician-assisted suicide, the corresponding obligation on the part of the physician to provide assistance can be overridden only by other relevant considerations of equal or greater weight. The two basic arguments most frequently used to oppose physician-assisted suicide are the slippery-slope argument, which points to the likelihood of abuse, and the principled argument, which points to the intrinsic wrongness of killing.

The slippery-slope argument, backbone of the literature opposed to physician-assisted suicide, claims that legal and societal recognition of physician-assisted suicide will lead by gradual degrees to outright abuse: from a few sympathetic cases of suffering, we will move to the coercion of dying patients by malevolent family members who harbor long resentments or fragile ones who cannot bear the stress, to the callousness of cost-cutting insurers and health-maintenance organizations, and the greed, arrogance, or impatience of physicians who for a variety of reasons do not take adequate care of their dying patients. Finally we will reach the point where patients with disabilities or chronic illnesses or other conditions requiring extraordinary care are forced into "choosing" suicide when that would otherwise not have been their choice.

Focusing on physicians, the slippery-slope argument points to inadequate training in terminal care, fatalism about patients who are dying, overwork and severe time pressures in clinical settings, endemic racism, prejudice against the elderly, the disabled, those who have mental illnesses, and those who do not speak English, frustration with patients who are not improving, and many other factors which, it claims, will lead physicians to nudge, push, or force their patients in this direction. In its extreme forms, the slippery-slope argument predicts that we will end with medical holocaust: widespread involuntary killing, disguised only by the fact that its victims are not herded into concentration camps but remain dispersed in various hospitals, nursing homes, long-term care facilities, and bedrooms of their own homes. Patients will be killed against their will, it is argued, once we open these floodgates.

Slippery-slope claims have been the focus of most objection to legalization of physician-assisted suicide. But claims of this type are notoriously difficult to defend, since they require both adequate evidence of causal factors that will lead to the feared future circumstance and reasons for thinking there are no adequate ways to prevent the predicted slide. But while cost pressures within a currently chaotic medical care system may provide reason for expecting manipulative pressures on terminally ill patients to choose suicide (in addition to or in spite of equally manipulative pressures to extend treatment), there are many resources for erecting barriers to abuse—waiting times, documentation of requests, prohibition of fees, mandatory counseling, and the analysis of records after the fact to identify deviant patterns of physician practice.[9] Certainly, we must be continuously alert to the risks of abuse. But this risk, like most risks in slippery-slope arguments, is not predictable with sufficient probability to warrant the undercutting of terminally ill patients' basic rights to a physician's assistance—especially their own physician's assistance—in suicide if they choose.

The second moral claim of the opposition to physician-assisted suicide, that killing is intrinsically wrong, is often presented with religious defenses. This argument is not so much concerned with future abuse but with the very fact of killing that physician-assisted suicide involves right now. Killing, it is argued, has been repudiated by religious codes from ancient times to the present; killing violates the sanctity of life; killing destroys the Creator's work. That killing is wrong, it is asserted, is a basic moral principle, regardless of whether it is set in a religious context or not and regardless of whether one kills another or kills oneself. While the argument concerning the wrongness of killing is more often used against active euthanasia, it is also employed against physician-assisted suicide.

Most religious and ethical systems recognize some forms of killing as justified: killing in war, killing in self-defense, killing in capital punishment, and so on. In discussions of physician-assisted suicide and euthanasia, the claim that killing is intrinsically wrong is often transmuted into the claim that *doctors* should not kill. Though it might be permissible for soldiers in combat, jailers acting at the orders of the justice system, and innocent persons defending themselves from aggressors to kill in specific circumstances, it is never permissible for doctors, acting *as doctors*, to kill. It is simply outside the physician's role, a basic violation of it, in fact. Healing, the doctor's professional task, precludes killing.

But does the physician's role really preclude direct involvement in a patient's death? Clearly the physician's role centers on healing, but when healing is no longer possible and the patient is dying (after all, everyone must die eventually), what is the physician's role in this circumstance? Historical precedent will not resolve the issue: while physicians in some time periods have at least officially rejected assistance in a patient's suicide, physicians have at other times accepted it. For instance, the mainstream Greek physicians of ancient times regarded it as part of their role to provide patients whom they could not treat with a lethal drug, either at the patient's or the family's request; hemlock was developed for this purpose.[10] At the same time, the Hippocratic school of medicine held that the physician ought not to do this; this view is the one incorporated in the Hippocratic Oath. Indeed, there has been dispute about this issue throughout Western medical history.

But the issue here is not just whether doctors throughout the ages do or do not agree about their roles in caring for a dying patient and whether that may include direct killing. Such a determination would hardly answer an issue about *rights*. It is possible that physicians throughout the ages have rejected any involvement in ending life; it is also possible—and there is much evidence to suggest this—that they have been quietly willing to do so in sympathetic circumstances. One thinks, for instance, of Freud's physician, who promised and delivered a lethal drug at Freud's request after Freud had endured many years of oral cancer. But that possibility is changing as physician roles vis-à-vis the dying become a matter of broad public concern.

In the late twentieth century in the developed world, most people face death from diseases with characteristically prolonged downhill courses (cancer, cardiovascular conditions, organ failure at various sites, neurological diseases, and so on), and these often involve extended pain, limitation of function, and suffering. Physician-aided death has always been an issue, but not a frequent one, since previously there were not many cases in which dying took this extended, more difficult form; now, at the end of this century, it is becoming an issue of massive scope.

It is also important to observe cultural differences in notions about the proper duties of physicians. Doctors in the Netherlands, where physician-assisted suicide and euthanasia are broadly accepted and legally tolerated, take direct aid-in-dying to be among the duties of the conscientious doctor. While many physicians report that performing euthanasia is personally difficult, they say they believe it to be part of the physician's role, and expect one another not to desert their patients at the end. As the Remmelink Commission, which examined the practice of euthanasia and physician-assisted suicide in that country, reported, under certain circumstances, "a large majority of physicians in the Netherlands see euthanasia as an accepted element of medical practice."[11]

Nor is the religious conception of "innocence" of much help in explicating the principle of the wrongness of killing. Especially within Catholic teaching, this principle holds that it is wrong to kill the innocent, not that it is wrong to kill altogether. But not only is it difficult to separate the innocent from the guilty in any nontheological sense that could be used in public policy (aside from singling out convicts, enemy soldiers, and assailants of nonaggressive people), it would also mean, applied in the context of assisted suicide in terminal illness, that it was just the guilty, not the innocent, who could hope to have their pleas for assistance in suicide answered. But this, of course, seems backwards: if anyone is to be forced to suffer when they choose not to do so, it should not be the innocent but the guilty.

Are these arguments—the slippery-slope argument concerning abuse and the argument from the wrongness of killing—sufficient to undercut the patient's rights of self-determination and mercy that jointly support a moral right to physician assistance in suicide? It is crucial that the arguments favoring physician-assisted suicide and the arguments opposing it are of different structures. The arguments in favor of assisted suicide appeal to the conjunction of two fundamental moral principles: self-determination and mercy. These two basic moral principles are acknowledged by all parties, including physicians, patients, and observers (both opponents and proponents of physician-assisted suicide), as just that: basic moral principles. Even physicians who oppose physician-assisted suicide accept the principle of self-determination—it is, after all, what underlies the opt-out conscience-clause provisions in legislation concerning physician-assisted suicide.

The same principle is also recognized by the patient seeking help as the basis of his or her own right of self-determination. Physicians and patients alike also recognize obligations of mercy: relieving pain and suffering is a central part of the physician's task, as well as what the patient seeks from the physician.

Furthermore, opponents of physician-assisted suicide also appeal to both these principles: autonomy or self-determination is the basis of the right not to be killed against one's will (feared as the consequence of the slide down the slippery slope) and mercy is the basis of the patient's right to avoid the fear and emotional pain that the prospect of being killed against one's will would involve. All sides, then, recognize these two fundamental moral principles, though they may differ about their relevance in the issue of physician-assisted suicide.

The arguments *against* physician-assisted suicide, however, have a different structure; they are not based on fundamental moral principles. The principle "do not kill" cannot be directly defended without qualification, it is widely assumed, since it would also prohibit killing in war, self-defense, and capital punishment. Even the more limited principle of not killing the innocent, though defensible elsewhere, backfires in terminal-illness contexts. The more focused application "doctors should not kill" is not usually treated as an argument in principle, since it would run afoul of historical and contemporary cross-cultural variation, but as a form of slippery-slope argument. Why shouldn't doctors kill? The answers characteristically point to the bad consequences that would ensue if doctors were to kill or assist in the suicide of even those patients who asked for this help. Patients, it is said, would no longer be able to trust their doctors. Doctors would overstep the bounds of legally permitted assistance in suicide, moving on to killing that is in no way sanctioned by law. Perhaps the law, too, might expand its scope, permitting doctors to kill patients, especially patients with disabilities, where there were no acceptable moral grounds for doing so. Furthermore, the integrity of the medical profession would be threatened.

But when the question is pursued in this way, a principle-based argument is thus transmuted into a consequentialist one that points to the harms killing might cause. Unless it is held that *all* killing causes harm sufficient so that it cannot be permitted (a view almost never consistently advanced by opponents in the current public discussions of physician-assisted suicide), it is difficult to show why, if their dying patients earnestly request it in preference to irremediable suffering, physicians in particular should not kill, without appealing to a consequentialist argument. But this is not an argument in principle; it is an argument about possible future practice.

Given this difference in the structure of the arguments for and against physician-assisted suicide, we may conclude that the burden of proof runs in favor of recognizing dying patients' rights to physician-assisted suicide if they are suffering intolerably or if they anticipate intolerable suffering. Only principle-based claims of equal or greater weight, or predictive proof that widespread bad consequences and medical holocaust would really ensue, can override this right. Moreover, claims about possible harms cannot be merely conjectural, speculative guesses about what could happen but must provide clear, incontrovertible evidence of genuine threats that can be avoided in no other way. Slippery-slope arguments against rights succeed only if they can provide good evidence that the projected future harm is really great and truly inevitable.

Claims about abuse in Holland are often used to try to make this point, but many of those given broadest circulation in the United States involve substantial distortion of the facts. Despite claims about the notorious "1,000 cases" in which suffering patients were euthanized without a current explicit request, there is no evidence of abuse that would be sufficient to prove that allowing physician-assisted suicide and euthanasia leads to medical holocaust.[12] Indeed, many observers think protections for patients in the Netherlands are improving as legal regulation and social recognition of a formerly underground practice increases. There is no sound evidence of a pattern of generalized abuse.

The overall structure of the argument invites (though does not require) proponents of the physician-assisted suicide to show that widespread, serious abuse will not result, and this, I think, they are able to do. Certainly the possibility of abuse should always be taken seriously, by proponents and opponents alike, regardless of the structure of the argument. Even with the weight of principle on their side, proponents have been working to show that it is possible to devise adequate barriers against abuse. No compelling case has been made by opponents that legalizing or otherwise accepting physician-assisted suicide will cause overridingly great harms, sufficient to override the patient's basic rights of autonomy and mercy in the first place, and much of their argument has involved the kind of diffuse threat often employed in slippery slope argumentation but without real corroboration. But if the opposition cannot reasonably establish that substantial harms would ensue, it has not produced a case strong enough for overriding a right.

The error many interpreters of the physician-assisted suicide debate have made, sizing up the arguments concerning self-determination and mercy on one side and the arguments concerning the wrongness of killing and the possibility of abuse on the other, is to treat these as equal, not just in content but in structure. But they are not equal in structure; the self-determination and mercy side is logically stronger, being grounded in basic moral principles, while the argument from the wrongness of killing (which is focused in practice, as we have seen, on the wrongness of *doctors'* killing and is argued primarily on slippery-slope grounds, or grounds of projected consequences) and the slippery-slope argument itself function as challenges to it. This structure of rights grounded in basic moral principles and correlative obligations (articulated by proponents) and reasons for overridings (articulated by opponents) captures all the elements of both sides of the argument.

The Physician's Obligation

This elaborate analysis, based on the structure of the arguments for and against physician-assisted suicide, may seem entirely irrelevant to the practicing physician. What bothers the physician is the claim that patients have a *right*—a right "against" the physician—for performance of an "obligation" to help patients kill themselves. Actual clinical situations in the real world are often not simple, and the relevance of ideals such as self-determination and mercy are far from clear. Even among physicians who recognize a moral obligation to assist dying patients with suicide, putting that policy into practice in actual situations is often problematic.

For example, a patient may seek help in suicide because of anticipated pain and suffering that lies in the future but has not yet occurred. Honoring this request is likely to be a problem where statutes define eligibility for physician-assisted suicide in terms of time to projected death. Oregon's Measure 16 and most other U.S. proposals make eligibility for assistance a function of expected outcome (death within six months), but they do not specify what degree of medical deterioration must already have occurred. What if the physician cannot be certain that death will occur in six months? Or what about a suffering patient who articulated a wish for suicide in the past but has since become incompetent? This is the problem with more than half of the notorious 1,000 Dutch cases, where wishes for euthanasia had been expressed but there was no current explicit request. What should physicians do about conscious, competent patients who earnestly wish assistance in suicide and are enduring irremediable pain or suffering but cannot administer the means of death to themselves—for instance, patients who are unable to take oral drugs, or who are too disabled to use other means of administration such as self-injections or suppositories? Here, if the physician feels a moral obligation to provide assistance, it must be by physician-administered euthanasia, not physician-assisted suicide.

Of particular relevance is the situation some Dutch physicians report in assisting patients with suicide. Though the suicide may begin with the patient's self-administration of a lethal oral solution, suppository, or pills, if the effect is not complete or if vomiting occurs (as sometimes happens with oral drugs not preceded by an antiemetic), or if the effect cannot be complete because the volume required for one-time administration would be too large (as with patients who have difficulty swallowing), the physician must be prepared to perform euthanasia at the end.

Other situations also make things far less clear, as is the case with patients who are chronically but not terminally ill, or who suffer from paralysis, or who have some but not overwhelming pain, or whose suffering is exclusively anticipatory, at some distant and undetermined point in the future, and so on. Each of these mixed, difficult cases presents a different challenge.

The obligations of physicians in these situations are best expressed in terms of a double axis of continuums: the stronger the patient's current wish for a physician-assisted death (this is the self-determination axis) and the greater the patient's experience of unrelievable pain and suffering in the process of dying (this is the mercy axis), the stronger the dual basis of the patient's right, and hence the stronger the physician's correlative obligation to provide the patient with assistance in dying. At the other end of this double axis of continuums, where the patient does not want to commit suicide and is not suffering from a terminal illness, the physician has an obligation *not* to assist the patient's death. Intermediate points yield a range of somewhat weaker to somewhat stronger claims on the physician. In many of these, a physician may choose to respond to a patient's request for assistance but is not morally required to do so. Only toward that end of the continuum, where earnest request and a real need for mercy coincide, where the patient seeks an easier death but cannot accomplish this with ease or dignity acting alone, does the possibility of obligation to the dying patient arise. Thus, obligation to assist a patient in suicide may be a comparatively rare thing, but it nevertheless can arise. It is this obligation which, I think, physicians' scruples are too easily assumed to defeat.

What about the physician who objects? Even where physician-assisted suicide has been fully legalized and no legal penalty or other harm to the physician, family members, or others is anticipated, and where there are no issues about borderline cases like those above, a physician may still have scruples against participating in this practice. The opt-out clauses that are part of all current public initiatives and legislative proposals permit the physician to decline to participate. But in order to evaluate the moral weight of these opt-outs and determine whether they outweigh a patient's rights, we must know something about the reasons for them.

Consider the sorts of explanations various physicians might provide for declining to meet a patient's request for assistance in suicide. Some explanations involve doubts about the psychological and medical appropriateness of ending life in the specific case, such as "The patient is ambivalent" or "The patient's pain could still be alleviated." These reasons, in effect, challenge the criteria of eligibility by asserting that self-determination and mercy do not in this case fully apply. Other reasons could involve points of self-interest or self-protection, such as "It's too time-consuming," "I'll lose respect around the hospital," or "I don't want to dirty my hands." Reasons of self-interest may include both reasons of trivial concern, like "It takes too much paperwork," and concerns about more substantial personal risks, as in "I don't want to subject myself or my family to social ostracism or legal risk."

But some of the reasons a physician might offer, if being truthful, for not wishing to participate are rooted in more basic moral scruples: the beliefs that it is contrary to the physician's religion, that it is sinful, that it is a violation of the law, and that it is profoundly morally wrong. These are not trivial or merely self-interested excuses but serious, earnest reservations. It is important not to minimize the force of some physicians' objections or the range of behaviors such objections might proscribe. Kevin Wildes, a Jesuit, points out that because suicide is held in the Roman Catholic tradition to be inherently evil, so is assisting in a suicide.[13] But Wildes also argues that for a physician to refer a patient to another, more compliant physician would likewise be complicity in evil, and hence evil itself. A conscientious believer not only would make use of an opt-out clause but would refuse to have anything to do with the suicide at all, not even providing advice, confirming a terminal diagnosis, or transferring a patient's records to another physician (as most opt-out clauses, including that of Measure 16, would require), for this too would be tantamount to complicity in evil itself.

It may seem self-evident that scruples of this intensity should be honored without reservation, perhaps especially where they have a religious basis. Clearly, it would do substantial psychological, emotional, and spiritual harm to physicians to force them to violate their own consciences, and under most circumstances this would be unnecessary: after all, patients may be easily able to find other physicians willing and prepared to provide the aid they seek. In such cases, the patient's rights of self-determination and mercy would still be satisfied, though by some other physician, and real harm to the physician with scruples would be avoided.

While genuine scruples on the part of the physician should be honored whenever possible, there are circumstances where the patient's right overrides these scruples. The patient may have a particularly strong relationship with the original physician, and may find it impossible to achieve such a relationship with another. Or there may be no other physician available with equal technical skill in terminal care or similar specialization in the patient's particular disease. Or there may be no other physician available at all. Or there may be no other physician available who is willing to assist in a suicide, a circumstance particularly likely in a practice area or facility where physicians tend to share the same values and views. If all physicians were to decline to participate, this would render the patient's right to assistance nil.

While in many situations it will be comparatively easy for a patient to find a physician willing to assist in suicide, especially if full legalization has occurred, there still may be circumstances in which a particular physician is the only one who could reasonably be called upon to provide assistance. Because in these circumstances the patient cannot find an alternative, the case for expecting this physician to cooperate, despite his or her scruples, is far stronger.

This may seem to be a rare circumstance, but it is closely related to another, far more common situation in which the physician does not tell the patient about his scruples until quite late in the downhill course of the disease. By this time the patient is often seriously incapacitated and in substantial need of ongoing medical care. As the patient deteriorates, it becomes increasingly difficult for the patient to transfer to the care of another physician—with whom, in any case, there would be no longstanding relationship or pattern of mutual understanding. By not informing the patient of his or her scruples in a timely way, the physician has in effect made himself or herself the only one available to this patient.

Nor can it be supposed that it is the patient's responsibility rather than the physician's to bring the matter up early on (though the prudent patient will certainly do so). The patient cannot be expected to understand the probable course of the disease, the likelihood of pain or other symptoms that are inherently untreatable, possible limitations of the physician's capacity to relieve pain and suffering (whether because of a lack of skill, a lack of information, or institutional priorities), or other factors in the medical course that lies ahead. The effect of delay is compounded if the physician—perhaps seeking to avoid "dirty hands" or any complicity in "evil"—refuses to consult, refer, confirm a diagnosis, transfer records, or cooperate in any way.

In short, because it has become too late for the patient to switch to another doctor to receive that aid to which the patient has a right, it has likewise become too late for the doctor to announce any principled reservations he or she may have. Although the individual physician with serious reservations may not have an obligation to assist in the suicide of a patient where it is easy for the patient to transfer, in this case it is the physician's own behavior that has led to a situation in which that physician has become the patient's only choice.

Furthermore, the patient may have come to rely on expectations that the physician will help. Consciously or unconsciously, physicians often foster a patient's trust in their capacity to negotiate a peaceful, dignified death. Especially if physician-assisted suicide is legal, patients may come to expect that their physician will provide assistance in suicide if asked to do so. Furthermore, the physician may even believe there is some medical reason to encourage this expectation, since evidence suggests that when patients believe they can count on the physician to provide aid-in-dying on request at a later date, this expectation allows them to extend their lives longer.[14] The patient who believes that help will be available whenever it is finally needed will often hang on until the very last minute.

Of course, the obligation may be different when the patient's terminal condition is of sudden onset or could not be foreseen: for instance, in unexpected, massive stroke, in accidental trauma, and in various other conditions. But the majority of cases are not like this. In the contemporary world, at least in developed countries, most dying involves a downhill, deteriorative trajectory, the general outlines of which the experienced physician can readily foresee. This includes virtually all cases of cancer, much cardiovascular disease, most neurological conditions, most organ disease or failure, virtually all AIDS, and so on. It may be particularly true when the patient is hospitalized or institutionalized in a nursing home or other health care facility (as is the case for the vast majority of deaths occurring in the United States) or otherwise under close surveillance. The physician *can* foresee what is coming and how the patient is likely to die; by remaining in a position of care for the patient, the physician incurs a growing obligation, as the patient's capacity for self-determination diminishes and the need for mercy grows, to assist in easing the patient's death in the way that the patient desires.

To put this in another way, the physician's obligation to help arises primarily within a relationship that develops during the course of providing care for a dying patient. As time goes on and the patient's condition declines, the patient's rights grow stronger both on grounds of self-determination and of mercy, and thus the physician's obligation grows correspondingly more difficult to evade.

Nor is it adequate to argue that the patient's death can always be softened by either of the two principal means of negotiating death that are already legal and already widely employed: first, the withholding or withdrawing of treatment without which the patient will die, such as respiratory support or artificial nutrition or hydration, and second, the over-ample use of pain-relieving drugs, especially morphine, which, although ostensibly used with the intention of relieving pain, also decrease respiration and thus hasten death. These two strategies, now ubiquitous in U.S. medical practice, are not adequate means of satisfying the physician's obligation to the dying patient who seeks assistance in suicide, since the physician's obligation is rooted not just in the principle of mercy, which these means of negotiating death might provide, but also in the principle of autonomy or self-determination. Of course, if these strategies are satisfactory to the patient, then the physician's obligation to assist the patient in dying can be met in this way. But to repeat, some patients find these strategies distasteful or repugnant and, as an expression of their basic right of self-determination, seek means of dying they perceive as more dignified and more humane, more in keeping with their own basic values. They reject a form of dying they perceive as drawn-out, overmedicalized, drugged, undignified, and cruel, and they are not willing to settle for this, even to salve the physician's conscience—especially if they believe the physician's conscience or religious commitment is being used to trump their own rights.

Many physicians try to avoid such situations with promises like "I won't let you suffer," seeking to reduce the patient's fears and to give the patient the courage to continue. But the physician's obligation is *strengthened,* not relieved, by such tactics. If the physician proves unable to treat the patient's pain or suffering adequately, this simple, consoling phrase actually reinforces the obligation the physician now incurs. It is mercy that is promised in that little phrase, and it is the need for mercy that is part of the basis of the patient's right to assistance in dying.

"I won't let you suffer" may covertly promise something else as well—a period of dying that is not only pain-free but lived in a conscious, alert, still-autonomous way. This promise is certainly not explicit; but to at least some patients, "not suffering" does not suggest the absence of conscious experience, as in terminal sedation, but rather the enjoyment of conscious experience in which suffering does not occur. To some, at least, "I won't let you suffer" will seem to mean "I'll see that you can remain alert, still capable of emotion, communication, and other things that may be important to you, like final goodbyes or prayer, in a way that is not distorted by suffering."

The development of increasingly stronger rights on the part of the patient as the patient's condition declines and correspondingly stronger obligations on the part of the physician caring for the patient during that decline is exacerbated by medicine's tendency to delay decision-making as long as possible, waiting until a crisis or change of status to raise most questions about withholding or withdrawing treatment, using opiates for pain management, or addressing other elements of terminal care.[15] This may reinforce patients' tendencies to evade and delay discussion of issues they find it painful to think about, especially if denial is part of their defense against bad news. But it is not only hesitation, fear of raising painful issues, or perhaps even cowardice on the part of both the patient and the physician that favors postponing discussion of these issues. Longstanding institutional practice contributes as well. Despite legal requirements like that imposed by the Patient Self-Determination Act, which requires hospitals and other institutions to ask patients if they have advance directives, and despite other recent changes, the institutional ethos of medicine tends to put decision-making about end-of-life situations off as long as possible, until virtually the last minute at which an effective decision can be made. Not only do these patterns of delayed decision-making tend to displace responsibility away from the patient onto the physician, family members, and others, as the patient becomes increasingly incapacitated and less and less capable of genuine participation in them, but these patterns also tend to put physicians into an increasing moral bind and make them still more vulnerable targets for moral blame—though blame of a different sort, and even harder to see for a physician who objects in principle.

If decision-making is postponed long enough, the patient who would perhaps have requested the physician's assistance in suicide may become incompetent, delirious, or comatose. As these final stages of deterioration occur, self-determination and mercy—the principles that formed the basis of the patient's original right to aid—cease to be relevant in any direct way. The incompetent or delirious patient is no longer capable of current, self-directing autonomous choice and cannot effectively request assistance in suicide, and may not be able to carry it out even if assistance were provided; and if unconscious, the patient is no longer capable of experiencing suffering or feeling pain. Since neither autonomy nor mercy is relevant any longer, the patient's original right to assistance in suicide may seem to evaporate, and with it the physician's obligation to assist. Thus, it may seem, if the physician with scruples delays long enough, he or she is home free.

But I think not. There is a new basis for moral blame here, and blame of a stronger sort. The physician no longer merely fails to meet the obligation a patient's right to assistance generates, but now is blameworthy for suppression of that right as well. If the singular importance of this right is rooted in the secularized medieval view that the last moments of life can be of particular significance, it is not a trivial right that is being suppressed, and the physician's blameworthiness in doing so is greater than it would be for suppressing other rights, such as rights to information about a prognosis, or informed consent to procedures, or access to certain treatment. If the kinds of rights suppressed in caring for a patient near death are far more substantial than those that might be violated during other periods of caring for a patient who is temporarily ill but will recover, then a physician does particularly grave moral wrong in delaying, prevaricating, and eluding the patient's claim.

Conclusions

That physicians may come to have obligations to provide direct assistance in the matter of dying does not mean that they are required to honor any patient request. It is still up to the physician to assess as carefully as possible (preferably in consultation with others, especially those with expertise in diagnosing depression or other psychologically confounding states) whether the request is stable, unambivalent, uncoerced, fully informed, and reflects the patient's most basic values—in short, whether it is a rational request, rationally made. It is also up to the physician (again, preferably in consultation with others, especially experts in the treatment of pain) to ascertain that there are no alternative ways acceptable to the patient of relieving the current pain and suffering or that which is about to occur.

But where the patient's request really does originate in autonomy and in the claim to mercy, it does mean that the physician is obligated not to entrap the patient into compliance with the physician's values rather than the patient's own values, which is what happens when choices are ignored or decision-making is delayed. This will be the particular temptation (though it would not be phrased in this way) of those physicians who have the strongest reservations and scruples against killing or assistance in suicide. After all, these are the physicians who are most likely to want to avoid the issue, to delay any discussion of dying, to promise not to let the patient suffer at the end so as to avoid having the patient raise the question of suicide assistance in the first place, and to delay assistance until the patient's own deterioration renders the issue moot. Perhaps these physicians will signal, albeit unconsciously, that physician-assisted suicide is not a topic open to discussion. But in doing so, especially if physician-assisted suicide is legal or broadly accepted in the culture, they become the physicians most likely to have generated for themselves a strong moral obligation, one they will most bitterly resent. Paradoxically, it is physicians with the firmest moral scruples who may be the most likely to find themselves in this profoundly unwanted situation.

This conclusion is not a palatable one, especially for physicians who have the strongest moral reservations but who are not alert to the moral consequences of their own behavior. Physicians who entrap patients into compliance with their own values paradoxically also entrap themselves into having moral obligations they do not want. Even if the law protects these physicians from being forced to honor them, the moral obligations they have brought upon themselves will remain. Opt-out clauses may provide legal protection, but they do not guarantee moral protection too. Of course, a patient's right to assistance from a particular physician may be overridden where both the psychic damage to the physician's conscience would be genuinely grave and the disruption to the patient of transferring to another physician comparatively small, but it is not always the case that both these conditions are met. There may be little moral sympathy for physicians whose own behavior creates the dilemma they seek to avoid.

This conclusion applies not only to physician-assisted suicide but to any mode of life-ending assistance to which a patient has a right but to which a physician has scrupled objections, be it withholding or withdrawing of treatment, the overuse of opiates, the cessation of nutrition and hydration, the induction of terminal sedation, and so on. The irony is that in most situations it is fairly easy for physicians to protect themselves from such obligations. All it requires is announcing in advance—*well* in advance—what scruples one has and whether these would preclude one's willingness to assist, so that the patient can seek care somewhere else and not become dependent on aid from this physician. Ideally, such a discussion might occur at the beginning of a continuing relationship between a physician and patient, long before any evidence of terminal illness might arise, so that both physician and patient would be aware of differences in individual values that might some day be relevant in the matter of terminal care. After all, if the vast majority of people in the developed world die of diseases with characteristically long downhill courses, there is a substantial chance for any individual patient that the issue will eventually arise. Of course, in the comparatively transitory climate of contemporary medicine, the possibility of such conversations between patients and their personal physicians so far in advance may be wishful thinking; but there is no reason they could not occur far, far earlier than such conversations ordinarily do.

Physicians must also be careful not to lean too heavily on assertions of scruple by the institutions in which they practice. Catholic hospitals, Hospice, and the VA system, for example, have all articulated opposition to physician-assisted suicide, as have other organizations. Although institutional announcement of scruples in effect involves institutional refusal to honor patients' particularly important rights, the patient cannot assume that the physician's scruples track those of the institution or are significant to the physician to the same depth or degree. It may be easier for institutions than for physicians to announce scruples about physician-assisted suicide; for an institution, announcing scruples requires merely issuing a position statement or policy directive—and making sure the patient is informed of this. Physicians, by contrast, have to talk clearly, directly, even intimately with their patients—their *own* patients—who are dying. Prior, clear announcement of their own personal scruples will perhaps be less difficult for doctors in a future in which physician-assisted suicide is legal, but only if the current climate of medical decision-making also changes.

But physicians' own behavior is not the only culprit in engendering moral obligations they do not want. Public attitudes and practices contribute to this as well, paradoxically reinforcing obligation-producing behavior on the part of physicians. Believing that physicians' objections to assisted suicide excuses them across the board, the public has not demanded full, compelling evidence for any claim that would have the effect of overriding a patient's principle-based rights. Society leads physicians to assume that trivial, self-interested objections will trump patients' rights as easily as profoundly held scruples (though the Boston Working Group's model statute would not do so), and society does not notice the way in which the legal structures now being developed to protect genuine, profoundly held scruples invite this. Society does not require physicians with either trivially or profoundly held scruples to own up to them in advance, and to put them forward for the patient's inspection. And society lets physicians and institutions delay decision-making so long that the patient's rights, and the physician's corresponding obligations, are effectively eclipsed. We think that we have solved the moral problem in this way. We haven't. On the contrary, we have only made it worse.

3

Harming, Healing, and Euthanasia

ERICH H. LOEWY

Euthanasia is, in many ways, a distasteful topic. No one likes to envision the killing of others, the killing of patients by health care professionals, or a society which condones killing. And yet euthanasia, like illness and death of which it is a part, needs to be faced squarely. It will not do to obfuscate the issue or claim that what we are clearly doing is not being done. Furthermore, euthanasia and its practice all too easily become the property of what many of us would consider to be at best questionable practitioners and perhaps charlatans. Instead of furthering the discussion, as some have claimed that it does, such grandstanding has done much to detract from it.

In this discussion I wish to look closely at issues surrounding active voluntary euthanasia—defined here as a direct act of killing, done at the direct request of the person being killed. I will argue that the time has come for us as a society to consider legitimizing active voluntary euthanasia when it meets the following conditions: It must be deliberate; it must be under circumstances in which the death of the individual is reasonably felt to be inevitable, shortly at hand, and, above all, in which the time until death is filled with relentless suffering; and it must be by the request of, or at least with the consent of, the person who is to die.

Suicide and Letting Die

Active voluntary euthanasia so defined has many similarities to suicide. In suicide, rational persons, for whatever reason, decide to voluntarily end their life. In voluntary euthanasia, another person assists in carrying out the wish. Common to both is that the decision to end life is made by the person who ends up dead. In the first instance, the method chosen is direct: persons end their own life by their own means, or at least by their own hands. In the second instance, an agent is interposed between the person and the means. Even when others become the instrument of the person's desire, reason would still incline us to regard the patient's wish as suicidal. Agents who willingly serve as middlemen must now grapple with their own conscience: inevitably they become part of a causal chain at whose end is someone's death.

If we consider suicide to be ethically wrong under all circumstances, we could not find an ethical justification for the practice of euthanasia. Those who have traditionally opposed suicide have done so for reasons which either directly or indirectly appeal to religious values. Even when Kant attempts to argue against suicide on what to him seem to be perfectly rational grounds (that in committing suicide one would use oneself merely as a means and would fail to use oneself also as an end in itself), a religious motivation appears to peak through.[1]

Personal choice, individualism, and autonomy are much emphasized in American culture: too much so, some of us, including myself, would think. Nevertheless all of us would, I think, agree that personal choice and freedom to make one's own decisions deserve high standing in a hierarchy of social values. If, then, we consider respect for a person's autonomy to be at least a conditional ethical obligation—if we believe that in most instances persons have a right to self-determination as long as this self-determination does not in a significant way harm others—it is difficult to see how one would argue against an at least conditional right to commit suicide.

There are many occasions when suicide might be felt to be ethically problematic. Persons who have an important obligation and an obligation which they can reasonably fulfill toward others (for example, persons who are their family's main material or psychological support or who have a critical task to fulfill) could be argued to have an obligation not to destroy themselves and, in that process, seriously harm or even destroy others. But when we speak of patients in the final stages of a painful and debilitating illness, such considerations are hardly pertinent. Terminally ill patients certainly continue to have obligations, but in most instances such obligations are negative: to act ethically, they cannot deliberately harm others, lie, steal, or kill, and they are expected to minimize the burden they impose on others. The capacity to act in a more positive manner (the ability to support one's children, to teach one's students, or to treat one's patients) is, at the very least, attenuated if not indeed lost. In a country in which individual rights not only are respected but have, in many ways, become a national fetish, objections (especially legal objections) to suicide strike us as peculiarly inappropriate.

The argument that persons who commit suicide leave their families and friends with considerable mental anguish has often been made and, undoubtedly, is sometimes valid. Such a judgment would depend not only on the circumstances which surrounded the act itself but also on the way the act was carried out. In many instances when patients are terminally ill, the decision to commit suicide (or, in fact, in the Netherlands to undergo euthanasia) is made in the embrace of loved ones. When suicide becomes illegal or is viewed as somehow shameful or ethically illicit, the ability of the patient to discuss such an alternative with family, friends, or caregivers becomes severely narrowed, and the possibilities that those left behind would suffer mental anguish would be thereby enhanced. Stories (albeit not firm data) from the Netherlands would suggest that such an act done in the loving embrace of a consenting family is far easier for family members to bear than watching the agonizing death of a loved one.

Few today would argue that suicide under every and all circumstances is ethically wrong. Even if we objected to suicide on personal secular or personal religious grounds, most of us would grant such a right at least conditionally to others. And even most of those who think that suicide as well as voluntary active euthanasia are unethical find little wrong with not prolonging the life of moribund or severely suffering patients. Somehow, while we object to active interference, we hold that passively "allowing something to happen" is morally always quite different than actively bringing the same result about.

Patients who are suffering intensely and who have no further realistic hope of amelioration or cure (patients, in other words, who are confronted with a choice between living a bit longer with protracted suffering or having their suffering shortened by a self-chosen earlier death) do not as much wish to die as they wish not to continue living in the way that circumstances now inevitably force them to live. Such a difference is important, for it would counsel caregivers to do all in their power to return content to a life seen by the patient as not worth having. Caregivers, if they wish to prevent their patients' suicide or their patients' requests for assisted suicide or active euthanasia, should become skilled at "orchestrating death"—that is, in providing a multidisciplinary approach to the terminally ill which emphasizes life and the way it is lived rather than death.

There is, in truth, no such stage as "dying"; a patient is either alive or dead, and when still alive is never beyond some form of help. Orchestrating death may involve, besides care from the medical and nursing staff, help from social workers, psychologists, pain-control specialists, and clergy, and it must always enlist the help of family and loved ones. The primary caregiver acts like a conductor of a symphony orchestra—he or she does not play every instrument but sees to it that the instruments are coordinated. Orchestration may include assisting suicide or otherwise actively helping the patient to die. But just as efficient birth control sharply decreases the need for abortion, good orchestration at the end of life sharply decreases the need for assisted suicide or active euthanasia.

Few patients who die in hospitals today die when they do because there was no other choice. Almost always there is something that might have prolonged life another minute, another hour, or another few days. Somewhere along the line, tacitly or explicitly, the patient, surrogates, the physician, or the health care team have decided that "enough is enough."[2] When patients riddled with cancer and with no possibility of cure decide to forgo further life-prolonging treatment, they have decided that being dead is preferable to the other available options. On the patient's part, such a decision, when made under the same circumstances (and whether we like to admit it or not), bears a strong resemblance to a decision to commit suicide. When surrogates, physicians, or the health care team make such decisions, there is an unavoidable resemblance to assisting with dying or, to be blunt, killing.

There are at least two different ways of "allowing" someone to die. We may refrain from interfering in a train of events which, without such interference, inevitably will lead to death (such as not treating pneumonia with antimicrobials). Or we may become a bit more active and discontinue a therapy upon which that patient's life depends (such as removing the ventilator in a permanently ventilator-dependent patient). In either case we may claim that we did not cause the death; the patient's underlying disease, not the act, was the cause. But while such a statement most certainly has some truth in it (if it were not for the underlying condition, acting or failing to act would not have caused death), such a statement is morally disingenuous. We cannot evade the fact that our failure to act (refraining from using antimicrobials, for example) when we could easily have acted, or our action (removing the ventilator) when we easily could have refrained from acting, inevitably makes us a part of the causal chain leading to a person's death. Like it or not, acting by acting or acting by omitting when we know that what we do is one of the critical factors in bringing about or preventing a death inevitably makes us an integral and essential part in a causal chain. Had we not wished death to occur (or had we not at least been reconciled to the fact that, all things considered, death here was the lesser of the available evils), we would not have acted or failed to act as we did: it would have been simple to do otherwise.

The discussion about suicide and euthanasia is by no means a new one.[3] It dates back at least to the ancient Greeks and most probably goes back far longer than that. In the case of euthanasia, the discussion among physicians was centered more on whether physicians should be allowed to bring about a death than on the more general issue of whether anyone should ever be allowed to kill.

There is no doubt that many ancient philosophers—among them Plato, Socrates, and the Stoics—found euthanasia ethically acceptable; others, notably Aristotle (if one can infer this from his attitude toward suicide) and the Pythagoreans, did not. Hippocratic ethics, being significantly influenced by the Pythagoreans, opposed euthanasia; but only a minority of Greek physicians belonged to the Hippocratic school. Early Christians opposed all killing: indeed, killing in self-defense, in war, or as capital punishment was, to the early Christians, morally unacceptable.[4] Euthanasia, therefore, was opposed by the Church. In medieval times, many if not most physicians were priests, and medicine was quite thoroughly under Church control. Despite this, Sir Thomas More, a pious Catholic writing during the Renaissance, favored a society in which, among other rather progressive ideas, euthanasia would be available.[5] In modern times, the idea of euthanasia has become ever more popular thanks to two forces: increasing individualism and with it an increased emphasis on an individual's right of self-determination; and advances in medical science that have made the often almost indefinite prolongation of life into a practical reality.

During the Nazi era, euthanasia took on a new and far more menacing meaning—a meaning which unfortunately has continued to infect discussions about euthanasia. I want to clearly differentiate between what the Nazis (and some before them) termed "euthanasia" (and which, in fact, was generally simply murder) and what has been, and generally is today, understood by that term. The term euthanasia as generally used means the bringing about of another's death solely with the good of the person being killed in mind: any benefit, supposed or real, to family, state, or institution is not a consideration. What the person performing euthanasia considers to be a benefit to another may, in fact, not be a benefit. But at any rate and however wrongly conceived, it is the benefit of the person killed and no one else's benefit which motivated that person's acting. Euthanasia as used by the Nazis was a different matter: the "benefit" to the person killed was hardly the issue. What mattered was that killing such a person allegedly benefited the state or society. Documents are clear about this.[6] The euphemism "euthanasia" as used by the Nazis was a thin veneer for what all civilized beings would simply call "murder."

Still, such killing—whatever its terminology—raises the legitimate fear that what could arguably be morally allowable killing would open the door to what clearly could not be morally accepted. Such a slippery-slope argument, in some ways a distant cousin of the Nazi argument, says that once we take our finger out of the dike, a deluge of misuse is likely to follow. This argument is not without substance. Allowing killing, for any reason, is undoubtedly a dangerous move. It is, however, a move which we do not seem to hesitate to make when it comes to killing our enemies in war (whom we do not know personally and whom we often kill impersonally, as when we bomb cities), executing criminals, or killing in self-defense. In these instances we feel that we can isolate and distinguish such specific acts of killing sufficiently so that the social impact in promoting other forms of killing will be small. Such acts of killing, however, totally lack the main attribute that any form of conceivable euthanasia must have: when we kill in war, execute criminals, or kill in self-defense, killing is done not to benefit the person killed but to benefit an individual or corporate other.

I am not arguing that dead persons can be "harmed" any more than that they can be benefited. Any benefit (for example, cherishing their memory or honoring a prior expression of their will) or harm (such as trivializing their life's work or attributing their work to another) is benefit or harm in a purely symbolic sense. That does not make it unimportant, but it makes it important for reasons that are quite different from those for benefiting or harming another who can be aware of the benefit or harm done. Here I speak of "benefiting the person killed," not the dead person. As long as a person is dying, he is alive; and as long as he maintains consciousness, he can very much be the subject of any benefit or harm done. Benefiting the person killed is very much benefiting (or trying to benefit) the living even if it is benefiting him by stopping his life.

Many if not most of our activities, furthermore, can constitute slippery slopes. Having a glass of wine may lead to drunkenness, and eating a good dinner can be the first step on the road to gluttony. Slippery slopes are unavoidable. Rather than disallowing certain considerations or actions, the presence of the slippery slope merely counsels caution in making choices.[7] Discretion, which makes actions safer, if not safe, and better, if not good, proceeds in a social context in which choices must be made.[8]

Harming Patients: Euthanasia and Capital Punishment

Physicians are, above all else, traditionally enjoined to "do no harm." In general doing no harm is interpreted as, at least, causing only the minimal amount of avoidable or unintentional harm necessary to achieve a goal mutually desired by both patient and physician. Expecting physicians "not to do any harm" whatsoever would condemn the modern physician (and probably would have condemned his ancient counterpart) to virtual inaction. The injunction against significantly harming is what has caused health professionals serious and perhaps quite appropriate misgiving when limiting treatment in dying patients (and, therefore, allowing an earlier death to occur), and it has caused most physicians to look at any form of active killing (be it for "beneficent" euthanasia or in the service of the state) with horror.

A revulsion against killing is seen as a proper professionally- and socially-conditioned reflex, a reflex which largely safeguards both the individual patient and society. Yet "harming," as used in the ethics literature, is not always a very clear concept. We tend to equate killing with harming: to be killed is, we think, equivalent to being harmed; to have one's life saved is to be benefited. And in most, but not in all, circumstances this intuitive belief will be found correct. It will be found correct because being alive (the biological and objective fact) is the necessary condition for having a life (the subjective and biographical fact); and being able to experience our daily lives and pursue our plans is, under normal circumstances, something we all want to do.[9] Most persons associate the notion of harming with that of being injured or damaged. Having one's plans thwarted, if having one's plans thwarted could be avoided, or being caused unnecessary pain are things we associate with the concept of harm. And most certainly physicians ought not to unnecessarily thwart their patients' plans or seek to cause them unnecessary pain.

The notion of harming and benefiting in the medical context is, however, a far richer one than can be encompassed by merely curing illness, prolonging life, or alleviating suffering. When all is said and done, only the person acted upon can ultimately decide whether something harmed or benefited them. What is seen as a benefit by myself may very well be viewed by my patient as a harm. No matter how persuasive my plastic surgeon may be, her attempt to improve the appearance of my admittedly ugly nose is only a benefit if I find it to be such. There are circumstances when prolonging a life which is coming to its end and which the person whose life it is sees as a grave burden would be viewed by that person as being harmed. Likewise, patients too weak and physically dependent to kill themselves and who plead for the help of health care providers might look upon a refusal of help as a form of being harmed or, at the very least, of not being helped or benefited. The language of harm, then, does not get us very far.

The language of harm is reciprocal with the language of benefit. In the clinical situation the concept of harm or benefit can only be applied to the living: the dead are beyond being benefited or harmed. Some may, for reasons of personal philosophy or for reasons of particular circumstance, consider that having their life prolonged constitutes a benefit; others, for reasons of personal or particular circumstance, may consider having their life prolonged (or, contrary to their desire, not terminated) to constitute serious harm. The decision is one which can only be made within the context of personal belief and particular circumstance.

How the question of euthanasia is framed is critical to our discussion. If we frame euthanasia as killing or as murder, the answer we give is apt to be quite different than if we were to frame this question as one of preventing suffering or assisting the freedom of the will in those who lack freedom of action. The function of medicine is not only that of sustaining biological life but, and at least with equal force, that of relieving suffering. Which of these sometimes conflicting obligations takes precedence depends upon the situation and upon its possibilities.

When sustaining life can be done only briefly and then only at the expense of intense suffering, refraining from sustaining life is said to be morally permissible. On the other hand, when relieving suffering can only be done at the expense of terminating a biological existence no longer desirable to the patient, terminating this existence, while not necessarily morally worse than failing to sustain, is proscribed. Whether we fail to sustain the patient and allow him or her to die or actively and gently terminate that life, the patient is dead.[10] In the former instance, however, the dying may have been prolonged and agonizing; in the second, more rapid and gentler. That killing is, under all circumstances, more reprehensible than letting die is, at least in clinical medicine, not intuitively or reasonably obvious.

Neither is the notion of what it is to "do harm." What of physician's participation in capital punishment? Is that sort of helping to kill not very similar to active euthanasia, especially when the condemned (as sometimes happens) asks to be executed? The arguments used against physician participation in capital punishment often seem quite similar to the arguments used against euthanasia and especially against physician participation in this process. The general argument, at least superficially, is that physicians must not become killers.[11] But by itself that argument begs the question: Why should physicians as physicians not participate? After all, capital punishment in America is (unfortunately, in my view) held to be morally permissible. But in killing the criminal, physicians are not serving the criminals' "good" even if, under unusual circumstances, the criminal should consent or even ask for such a death. The options facing such a person are much too unknowable: he or she might be freed, or might learn to develop a host of other fulfilling interests which continue to bring joy to life. Some criminals, for example, have developed a life-long interest in birds (the bird-man of Alcatraz), others have become accomplished in law, and many have adapted in other ways.

Above all else, physicians must never utilize tools (actual as well as conceptual) acquired in the process of medical training for their patients' detriment but always for their patients' good.[12] The reason physicians must not use the tools of medicine to knowingly harm patients resides in the social contract in which physicians and their community are enmeshed. Medicine is a social task, and the mission of medicine is ultimately one which is developed by physicians and their communities in an ongoing and dynamic fashion. The assumption that physicians will seek to bring about their patients' good and never knowingly seek to do them harm has persisted throughout history and persists today. It underwrites the trust which patients must necessarily put in the health care professionals they consult.

Unquestionably, not executing healthy persons is a part of "not doing harm." It is clear that, since the options are unpredictable and wide, the good of criminals (even should they conceive otherwise) may not be served by execution. Patients dying a painful death are a different matter. Their options are few: they can either die in prolonged agony or, more mercifully, can choose to end their days more easily and earlier. Helping patients to die who, under such circumstances, seek to end their life is quite different than killing patients whose options are unknowable and who, for the most part, do not want to die.

The physician's personal belief about the probity of capital punishment is not the question. Using a noose, an electric current, or a gun to end another's life is not a skill acquired in the course of medical training and not, therefore, covered by the physician's social contract with society. Using a noose, an electric current, or a gun is quite a different act for a physician than injecting persons or advising others how, where, and how much to inject. Medical skills used in capital punishment are medical skills perverted to the detriment of a particular patient.

The claim that criminals in jail have no physician-patient relationship with their executing physician is flawed. The fact that no prior relationship may have existed is not the point. No prior relationship exists between the accident victim and the physician who happens by and renders aid; yet few would claim that no professional obligation grounded in the physician–patient relationship had been incurred. When physicians use either the tools of medicine or the technical or cognitive skills acquired in the process of their medical training, they are inevitably acting as physicians upon another, who then becomes the patient. The doctor's pledge is to do no harm, and harm in the case of capital punishment is easily defined and demonstrated.

The Four Questions

Thus, in considering euthanasia, four distinct questions must be kept separate: (1) Is the killing of a human being ever a defensible act? (2) If so, under what circumstances? (3) Is there some reason why health professionals acting as health professionals should not participate in the killing of a patient? (4) All things considered, is legalizing euthanasia a wise thing to do? These are rather separate questions. And yet the discussion about euthanasia has all too often attempted to discuss these issues all at once.

Is it ever morally permissible to kill another human, and if so under what circumstances? Most of us would concede that at the very least self-defense is morally permissible, provided the most minimal force to adequately safeguard oneself is employed. That does not make killing another in self-defense a "good" thing, but it makes it permissible because, all things considered, it is a lesser evil than allowing an innocent person (oneself) to be killed.

Although self-defense may be the most obvious kind of killing that we condone, it is not the only kind. When we set speed limits higher instead of lower or when we decide to mine coal or build high-rise buildings, we know that a certain number of deaths that would not otherwise have occurred are apt to occur. We go to war, and many of us count the killing of our enemies by our friends as acts of heroism; and in America we (unfortunately, in my view) execute criminals or those we believe to be criminals. Further, and perhaps most tellingly, we have structured and we continue to structure our society so that many are hungry, poor, homeless, and without medical care while some live in opulent luxury. And deaths due to hunger, poverty, homelessness, and lack of medical care could, at least in our society, be largely prevented. To say that we always hold the killing of other humans to be unallowable is simply not true.

What then are the minimal conditions which might make killing of humans, while not good, at least better than the obverse? There are social reasons: building high-rise buildings, mining coal, or driving cars at the legal limit are examples. But in these examples, those who will die have engaged in the activity causing their death with open eyes: construction workers, coal miners, and drivers all know that they run a risk, and they are free to take it or not.[13] Other social reasons are hardly voluntary: those who are poor, homeless, hungry, or without medical care only rarely knowingly chose their fate.

Communities can make a reasonable argument that condoning killing will encourage others to kill. There is a not unreasonable fear that the practice could brutalize society as well as the medical profession. Brutality and callousness in society and on our streets has increased. Often we fail to help persons in distress; persons being robbed, assaulted, or raped while others look on without interfering is not a rare event. Above all, we read of the hunger of children and the homelessness of families, and often shrug our shoulders. This callousness toward suffering is, in many ways, society's greatest ill. We seem to be concerned about the preservation of life and the danger of allowing a life of one who wants to die to come to an end while, at the same time, we seem to be callous to the suffering around us.

If precept is an important factor in molding attitudes, communities will arguably be encouraged to be more callous, rather than less, if we overvalue life and undervalue the importance of suffering. Forcing patients to die slowly and in pain rather than allowing them, at their own choosing, to end their existence with dignity and in peace reinforces callousness. Not permitting others to help incapacitated patients accomplish this makes the terminally ill the hostages of the medical profession and of society's own idiosyncratic viewpoint of personal morality. A society that condones killing in war, metes out death as punishment, and is at best indifferent toward the hungry, the homeless, and the poor cannot argue that life is an absolute good that must be preserved. Condoning killing as a last resort to bring about the death of those who, because of relentless suffering, do not benefit from life but long for death is far less apt to encourage brutal killing in society than are war, execution, and indifference to social conditions.

When we speak of euthanasia or of physician-assisted suicide under the conditions I have outlined here, we are speaking about killing or enabling the suicide of a patient whose only option is between an earlier and less painful and a later but a more painful death. There are important differences between physician-assisted suicide and euthanasia. Under ordinary circumstances, patients who are assisted in their suicide by a physician have the capacity to kill themselves: they can swallow medication or follow direction. Under the circumstances that form the grounds for this discussion, patients often no longer possess the strength to carry out their desires; they may be too weak, too debilitated, or too dependent upon others. This is often the case at the very end.

To deny such a person the right of such a choice appears difficult to defend. I would argue that the killing of people for their own benefit and at their own request when these are the only two options may not be a moral good: but given the choices, it can be argued to be a far smaller evil than the alternative. But just because euthanasia may, under these narrow circumstances, not be ethically impermissible does not mean that anyone is obligated to help patients achieve their end. Nor does it mean that there may not be something in the social concept of health professional which might make participation by a member of this group problematic.

Killing others who are terminally ill, at their own request when they are incapacitated and unable to implement their own wishes, is a form of assisted suicide in circumstances when nonassisted suicide is no longer possible. If we do not acknowledge the right, at any time, to take one's own life, then assisting in suicide is clearly wrong. If, however, we are to grant others, at least at certain times, the right to commit suicide, then it is difficult to see why those who aid such persons can, necessarily, be faulted. Personal morality (or the particular morality of our particular moral enclave) may or may not prevent some of us from participating, just as personal morality (or the morality of our moral enclave) may or may not prevent some of us from committing suicide or from assisting with abortion. But such personal morality is personal and difficult to generalize to an entire professional group.

Most physicians are willing to refrain from treating terminally ill patients merely to prolong their life, and most are even quite willing under such circumstances to withdraw life-sustaining therapy. Some have argued that passively allowing something easily preventable from happening is quite a different matter from bringing it about. Not treating terminally ill patients when treating an intercurrent condition is likely to be successful, or even withdrawing life-sustaining therapy, is apt to be termed "letting die" and is, as I have noted before, viewed as ethically quite different from "killing." Those of us who, like myself, cannot accept this distinction outside a specific context and situation feel that it is especially difficult to maintain in clinical medicine. The dividing line between allowing a death to occur when the means are easily at hand to prevent it and causing such a death by more direct means is blurred.

Is there some reason why health professionals, acting as health professionals, should not participate in the killing of a patient? Do the peculiar ethical precepts of health professionals preclude their participating in any active form of killing? Even if active euthanasia were to be considered a morally acceptable option and even if its legality for nonprofessionals were to be established, a severe moral problem for physicians remains. The issue "touches medicine at its moral center" and the feeling that "if physicians become killers or are even merely licensed to kill the profession will never again be worthy of trust and respect as healer and comforter and protector of life in all its frailty" is a powerful one.[14] Physicians and other health professionals are dedicated to life and to its preservation. Even if one were to acknowledge that the tradition to prolong life lacks ancient roots, it nevertheless has become a powerful motivating force for today's practicing physician.[15] Society in its social contract with healers assumes this dedication as the tacit underpinning of the contract.

Physicians, and other health professionals, were human beings and members of the community long before they entered their profession. They were part of the community in which the medical ethos is embedded and from which it is nourished. Health professionals were conditioned in their moral viewpoint by the particulars of their own peculiar background. They entered medicine with a certain set of background beliefs on which their experiences were engrafted. The medical ethos is not a linear tradition simply handed down from generation to generation, to be passively accepted by graduating physicians. Generations, and individuals, must reinterpret this ethos for themselves; and, inevitably, such an interpretation is molded by each generation's, and each individual's, peculiar background and experience.

The tradition of medicine has encompassed many changes. It has developed from eschewing the care of the dying to finding such caring to be a compelling obligation. Unquestioned paternalism, in which the "good" was interpreted on the healer's terms, has been largely replaced by a more collegial model in which the "good" is jointly sought and pursued. The tradition has evolved and grown. And the tradition, in many ways, is what we, as individuals and as a profession, interpret it as being.

To bring about a "good act of healing in the face of the fact of illness," which is undoubtedly what the profession is about, can be interpreted in many ways.[16] Not harming, alleviating suffering, as well curing disease and not causing death, are important and simultaneous obligations. Professionals, in establishing hierarchies of values, bring to that activity all the preconceived and communally derived beliefs and viewpoints which they brought to their understanding of the medical ethos. When obligations clash, when, for example, hopeless suffering can only be alleviated by causing the death of the patient, the individual's prior understanding becomes central to the issue. Determining which of these compelling obligations takes precedence is a personal decision and one which has to be made by each healer for and by himself or herself. Inevitably it will be made in the context of that particular person's background and beliefs. Such a decision will say more about the particular character of the actor than it will about the issue itself.[17]

Those who make the statement that physicians (and of course, by inference, other health professionals) should not (ever) kill make this statement from the comfort of their present, generally not severely suffering, condition. If health professionals should never kill (and if by inference killing by health professionals of their patients, at any rate, is then always to be judged evil), one must come to terms with the following documented story. During the round-up in the Warsaw Ghetto (from which Jews were sent to their extermination in Treblinka or Auschwitz), the Nazis came to the children's hospital to deport the patients. Dr. Adina Blady

Szwajger, a Jewish physician, poisoned the children and thus allowed their peaceful death rather than condoning their agonizing death in the gas chamber and all that would go before. She did so to save them from hopeless and pointless agony; she did this to prevent their suffering.[18]

Can we claim that what Dr. Szwajger did can be equated with "harm"? Those who knew of this adjudged her deed as heroic and were grateful. Many will say that such an extreme situation is one which can find no comparison in the civilized world. And, indeed, even the agonizing death of one riddled with metastatic cancer or slowly choking to death with no hope of relief may be far preferable: I do not know and cannot judge. I have neither died with metastatic cancer, choked to death, nor been exterminated in Treblinka. But I do know that those who have not undergone this experience are ill-equipped to pass judgment on either a course of action which prevents such suffering or on one which refuses to do so.

Occasionally the suggestion has been made that specially trained people who are not health care professionals should, if euthanasia were ever to be accepted, be the ones to perform the act. Health care professionals would then, so the argument goes, be able to escape the evident conflict which euthanasia poses for them. In my view, such a suggestion, superficially attractive though it may be, has severe practical drawbacks. When laypersons enter medical school, they are embarrassed or disgusted by many of the things they must see and do. As time goes on, they become used to such activities: examining naked persons or dealing with excreta becomes a matter of routine. Creating a professional group whose job would be to kill daily instead of rarely (even if such killing were done in the service of decreasing suffering) runs the danger of creating a group of people who are no longer bothered by causing death. That does not seem to be socially desirable.

Further, the person who undertakes to relieve suffering by killing a patient should know and understand the patient (and preferably the family and friends) well. It is not something to be done lightly, in the normal course of a day's work. Being causally involved in the death of another—whether it is an involvement by forgoing or withdrawing treatment or whether it is by a more direct act—should hurt. Such an act is never "good" in itself: at best, it is merely better than the alternative choices available.

There are also technical problems. Ending a life with as little suffering as possible may not be as easy as it sounds. It requires an understanding of and experience with pharmacology, physiology, psychology, and other disciplines which one cannot expect a lay person or a technician (who also must act under a physician's direction) to have. If technicians were to acquire this knowledge, understanding, and experience, they would be physicians!

Even if one were to find active euthanasia an ethically acceptable option under some circumstances and even if one were to affirm the probity of having at least some physicians voluntarily participate, the advisability of legalizing euthanasia would still be far from clear. On the whole the issue—not as much an ethical as a political one—can be briefly stated: Is it safer to outlaw a practice which will then continue to go on uncontrolled, or is it perhaps safer to permit it but to surround it with many controls and safeguards?

The practice of euthanasia is far wider spread than most will publicly admit to. What happens currently is that decisions are made idiosyncratically and are informed by personal standards, since there are no professional guidelines. Those who participate do so at enormous risk of criminal prosecution, though often physicians who have actively shortened patients' lives have, despite overwhelming evidence of their "guilt," been adjudged "not guilty" or given a slap on the hand. This leaves physicians without guidance, and renders patients powerless, confused, and insecure. Ultimately it leaves justice betrayed: a wink and a nod is no way to deal with critically important issues.

On the other hand, officially permitting euthanasia likewise has distinct drawbacks. The United States is not Holland, in which the practice of active euthanasia has (if we are to give credence to most, albeit by no means to all, reports) worked fairly well. Even in the Dutch setting, troubling problems remain: recently, proxy consent given for children and requests submitted by psychiatric patients have been honored. American culture tends to abuse many liberties, and to readily allow finances and personal or corporate profit to be the driver in decision-making. Legalizing active euthanasia, as well as not legalizing it, is not without risk.

On the whole, however, it would seem that legalizing, strictly controlling, and carefully supervising active euthanasia is safer than leaving it to personal caprice. Such strict control must be expressive of communal values and in a democracy will, for better or worse, be subject to political manipulation. Like any slippery-slope activity, it is possibly acceptable and guardedly safe only if we realize its dangers and are ready to proceed very cautiously.

Conclusions

When all is said and done, I think that we must face the following truths: No society can claim that it condemns or disallows all killing. In many cases, if not indeed in most, physicians (whether they like to admit it or not) are causally implicated in the death of their patients: somewhere along the line the decision that "enough is enough" is and will continue to be made. Persons who have no further options except either to die later with more protracted suffering or to die earlier but with shorter suffering may often choose to die earlier. Physicians, since they hold the power in the medical setting, will, as part of a trusting physician-patient relationship, be asked to help.

The better our care of terminal patients, the less will be the need for euthanasia. Orchestrating death by giving as much content and meaning to the last stage of living as to every other stage, rather than focusing on dying, can do much to reduce the need for euthanasia. Nevertheless, the need for active euthanasia will not vanish. Inevitably, part of good "orchestration" of a patient's last days may require euthanasia or assisted suicide. Laws that entirely forbid the practice appear merely to serve to sweep the activity under the carpet and remove it from social and public control.

As a society and as a profession, we must grapple with the issue and in a democratic way come up with decisions that we can live with, from which we can learn, and which we can adapt. It may be the case that society, while rigorously setting limits and controlling the practice of euthanasia, will choose to carefully allow it when patients who are terminally ill and who have no options other than living longer and suffering more or living shorter and suffering less repeatedly ask for this help. Health professionals who wish to participate would be controlled but not stigmatized; those whose moral scruples would not permit them to participate would be free not to do so.

Eventually, having learned from such a practice, our society may well make changes in either direction. We may find that euthanasia has served us well and that, perhaps, requests by advance directive or by appropriate surrogates could be tolerated. Or experience may teach us that the practice has not served us well and that it should be eliminated. Thoughtful analysis and dialogue, rather than strident appeals to mercy on the one hand and to tradition or religion on the other hand, are the only means to ensure that the concerns of patients, their physicians, and the larger society of which both are a part will be adequately addressed.

PART TWO

Considerations Against

4

The False Promise of Beneficent Killing

EDMUND D. PELLEGRINO

Several influential ethicists argue that, for reasons of compassion, mercy, respect for autonomy, and relief of pain, bringing about the death of a suffering person is a benefit, or at least brings about no harm or loss. This argument is advanced by secularists and by some professed Christians as well. It is also a theme in two recent circuit court decisions.[1]

The beneficence of helping patients to die has been most clearly argued by Beauchamp and Rachels, both of whom reject the distinction between killing and allowing to die. They differ, however, in the extent to which they would carry their logic when it comes to public policy.[2]

Beauchamp centers the moral justifiability of euthanasia and assisted suicide on the relief of suffering and a valid, voluntary request by the patient, particularly when pain management is inadequate, the patient's condition is overwhelmingly burdensome, and a physician is necessary to bring relief. He does not include involuntary or nonvoluntary euthanasia in his argument for justification. (Euthanasia is nonvoluntary if the patient lacks decision-making capacity and does not request euthanasia, and involuntary if the patient has decision-making capacity and does not request euthanasia.) He is also wary about legalization because he feels there is some truth in the slippery-slope argument, which in itself does not make assisted suicide wrong.[3]

Rachels is more radical. He characterizes his approach "not as a matter of faithfulness to abstract rules or divine laws, but as a matter of doing what is best for those who are affected by our conduct. If we should or should not kill, it is because in killing we are harming someone. That is the reason killing is wrong. The rule against killing has as its point the protection of the victim." Rachels carries his logic to its full conclusions. He deems killing beneficial for those who are alive but do not have a life, that is, those who lead "subnormal lives." This would apply to infants with multiple birth defects and patients with advanced Alzheimer's disease or in permanent vegetative states. For such persons, the benefits of assisted death are sufficient to justify nonvoluntary, and perhaps involuntary, euthanasia. Rachels sees no problem with legalization. Although he sees a "grain of truth" in the possibility that legalization might lead to involuntary euthanasia, he finds this concession "non-damaging." He is willing to run the risk of the slippery slope to gain the benefits of hastened death for those with subnormal lives.[4]

Both Rachels and Beauchamp deny a difference between killing and letting die. They shift the debate from questions of intrinsic evil and causation and intention in the act of killing to conditions under which killing would be beneficent. Thus, they leave room for rebuttal of their arguments if it can be shown that euthanasia and assisted suicide are, in fact, nonbeneficial, harmful, or wrongful. This rebuttal does not require engagement with their objections to the distinction between killing and letting die nor the significance of intentionality or causation.[5]

Two other conceptions of beneficence in killing should be mentioned, one moderate and one extreme. Brody and Miller represent a moderate and increasingly common view among physicians that there should be *prima facie* aversion to euthanasia and assisted suicide, but that in cases of extreme suffering, that obligation may be overridden out of compassion for the patient's suffering.[6] The extreme view is that of Dr. Kevorkian, who asserts that the right to kill oneself with assistance is an absolute liberty right with which no one, including government, should interfere. Kevorkian's argument leans less on beneficence than on absolute dominion of humans over their own lives. Even more extreme is the justification for euthanasia voiced in 1920 by Binding and Hoche in their description of the German program permitting the destruction of "unworthy life": "This is not an act of killing in the legal sense . . . In truth, it is a purely healing act."[7]

But however they locate themselves on this spectrum of opinions, most advocates justify euthanasia and assisted suicide as beneficent, compassionate, and respectful of human dignity and freedom, and thus as actions taken in the interest of the patient. It is this assertion of beneficence I wish to challenge by showing that euthanasia and assisted suicide are not necessary to relieve pain and suffering, not autonomous, not compassionate, not dignified, not private, and not a moral obligation of physicians. Moreover, they lead inevitably down a logical and psychological slippery slope.

Euthanasia and Assisted Suicide Are Not Necessary

Three reasons are usually advanced in answer to why a person might wish to end his or her life: (1) to end unbearable suffering or the anticipation of future suffering, (2) to prevent overtreatment at the end of life, or to control the way one dies, the better to live the last days of one's life as one sees fit, and (3) to exercise an inherent "right to die" whenever one judges life's quality to be unsatisfactory in any way one wishes to define "unsatisfactory."

Pain and suffering are separable experiences, each of which has its own genesis and each of which can be satisfactorily controlled by measures now available.[8] Pain is a physical response to any noxious stimulus, a bodily protective measure whose peripheral and central neurological mechanisms are becoming better understood. Much has been written in recent years about improved ways to control pain by a variety of measures with the proper use of analgesics, psychotropic drugs, and a variety of physical, pharmacological, surgical, and psychological adjuvants.[9] What is often diagnosed as untreatable pain is actually inadequately treated pain which can be relieved without rendering the patient unconscious. With the optimum and judicious use of those measures, there are virtually no patients whose pain cannot be relieved.

The protagonists of euthanasia and assisted suicide usually

cite some very moving cases in which, purportedly, all the requisite measures for pain relief were without benefit. Whether such cases exist, and in what number, is problematic at best. Critical details about how effectively optimum measures of pain control were employed in a particular case are usually wanting. Nor is it clear how much of the anguish was due to pain, how much to the non-nociceptive causes of suffering, and how much to the anguish of the caregiver. The way the physician approaches the treatment of pain can itself influence the judgment of "intractability."

But even if we were to assume that there are rare cases of truly untreatable pain and suffering, this would not be sufficient reason to justify moral approbation or legal sanction of euthanasia and assisted suicide. To do so would commit the fallacy of composition, that is, to attribute to the whole the characteristics of one of its parts. Such an extrapolation would weaken current protections against untimely death in the vastly greater number of persons and patients in whom pain and suffering are treatable. It would also erode the physician's obligation to deploy optimally all the measures available in comprehensive palliative care and to remove or ameliorate the circumstances impelling patients to ask for hastening of death. It would also invite, for the possible benefit of very few, broader deleterious societal consequences.

Generalizing from a few cases, especially in the media and popular press, tends to portray unbearable suffering as the inevitable outcome of any fatal or chronic illness or disability. As some of Dr. Kevorkian's cases attest, often it is the anticipation of future pain and suffering, or the fear of loss of "dignity" and "control," that leads to a request for life termination. The dangers of mistaken diagnosis and prognosis are obvious, as are the hazards of ending life even before it is clear that suffering will occur and to what degree.

Suffering is not synonymous with pain, as anyone knows who has sustained a pin-prick, a laceration, or even a fracture. These isolated nociceptive events are quickly recognized as painful, of course. But the facts that they are nonfatal and remediable, that the pain will be temporary, and that no significant alterations of either lifestyle or self-image are implied remove the element of suffering. Suffering, on the other hand, is the conscious response of a person to the meaning and implication of pain and to the unique predicament of the life within which pain, or other life disturbances, occur. The most intense suffering can occur in the absence of physical pain—for example, upon the death of a child, the news of a fatal but not painful illness, the sufferings of a loved one, rejection by one's peers, separation or divorce, loss of reputation, or a traumatic law suit. The range of possibilities of suffering without physical pain is as broad as the range of untoward events that may affect any human at any time.

Even when there is pain, suffering is a separable phenomenon which varies in its intensity, quality, and manifestation from one person to another.[10] Patients afflicted with a fatal illness that is not yet terminal suffer from the anticipation of pain. Patients who are terminally ill or dying suffer from fear of death and fear of the process of dying. They also suffer from a sense of guilt for being ill, for being a physical, fiscal, or emotional burden on others, or for causing loved ones to suffer on their behalf. Depression, an understandably frequent accompaniment of pain and fatal illness, is itself a cause of suffering. Patients also suffer from the pity, fear, or loathing they perceive in the well persons who come into their presence. Physicians, nurses, visitors, family, friends may unwittingly induce feelings of unworthiness, rejection, and alienation by the way they act in the presence of the sick and dying.

Suffering is unique for each person who suffers, and its treatment must be fitted to that uniqueness. To be sure, when pain accompanies the suffering, it must be relieved by the most effective means available. But relief of suffering requires much more. It must begin with an identification of its causes. Treatment requires removal of the cause. Skillful use of antidepressants and anxiety medication are indicated. But more important are emotional support, being present to the suffering person, and alleviating guilt or alienation. Pain relief and relief of suffering constitute the integrated approach of comprehensive palliative care.[11]

Most often, the request for euthanasia or assisted suicide is a plea for help in dealing with suffering as much as pain. The wish for death may be a desperate move to gain the caregiver's attention to the patient's experience of illness and suffering. It may also be an expression of disappointment at the lack of compassion of family and caregiver, or it may be an act of reluctant resignation when those around the patient fail to comprehend his predicament or the help he needs to confront it, or it may be a response to the fatigue, emotional and physical, the patient witnesses in family, physician, or nurse.[12]

The combined and integrated relief of pain and suffering shaped to suit the peculiarities of their manifestation in each person is the aim of comprehensive palliative care and the more sophisticated hospice regimens. Patients treated this way usually do not ask for termination of their lives; when they do ask for it, they tend to change their minds later. It is an injustice to offer these patients assisted suicide or euthanasia as options when so much more can be offered in the way of sophisticated treatment. Euthanasia and assisted suicide are easier options for the caregiver, since genuine palliative care demands much more on the caregiver's part. This is not to impute ill intent to those who conscientiously believe in the moral probity of assisted suicide but simply to recognize the emotional demands, the reality of fatigue and frustration, involved in the care of the terminally ill. Even the most beneficent among us must recognize these realities and the way they might alter our own approach to care if euthanasia or assisted suicide becomes a legal or moral option.[13]

A major factor in the move to legalize assisted suicide or euthanasia—even on the part of persons who might ordinarily oppose it—is the fear of being kept alive on tubes, wires, and machines when life is coming to an end through age or disease. There has been, and continues to be, justifiable cause for concerns about inappropriate overtreatment. Nonetheless, in the last two decades a sharp break has taken place in the medical tradition of treating until every last breath is exhausted. The turn to patient autonomy as a *prima facie* principle of medical ethics has led to better and earlier decisions to withdraw and withhold unnecessary or futile treatment. So much is this the case that the right to refuse treatment is now sometimes interpreted as a right to demand treatment even if it is medically futile.

Patients today have a variety of ways in which they can stay in control of their last days. The Patient Self-Determination Act requires that they be offered the options of a living will, a durable power of attorney, or designation of a surrogate when they enter the hospital.[14] Properly employed, these instruments should allay anxieties about overtreatment. To be sure, some physicians and caregivers ignore or by-pass these anticipatory declarations. Better public and professional education and oversight should change this. It is preferable to improve compliance with advance directives than to use the fact of noncompliance as a justification for euthanasia and assisted suicide.

As I shall show below, the decision to choose assisted suicide or euthanasia is questionably autonomous. At best an advance directive executed when one is well and distanced from illness, pain, suffering, or the actuality of death is, itself, a tenuous moral imperative. To be valid as well as safe, an advance directive requires full understanding between doctor, patient, and family—something difficult to achieve in this hurried age of fragmented care when a sustained relationship with a trusted physician is a fast-receding privilege.

In some quarters, the danger is now undertreatment rather than overtreatment. In their zeal to avoid the fate of "tubes and wires," patients and physicians may forego effective and beneficial treatment. It is very difficult to anticipate precisely all the intricate details of the reversible acute episodes that can occur in the natural history of an ultimately fatal disease. This is not to derogate advance directives but to warn about the difficulties in their application in concrete clinical decisions. If one really wants to "control" one's dying, one must be extremely careful to leave enough discretionary space for the physician to allow for the unforeseen episode remediable by a "tube" or a "wire." These may be in the patient's best interests even when death is inevitable and accepted. Patients who wish to be specific about "unnecessary" or "extraordinary" treatments must be helped to understand what these terms mean in modern medical technology.

Fears about overtreatment and loss of control are sure to be exacerbated by the results of a recent study (SUPPORT) that attempted to "improve" the care of terminally ill patients. Despite a plan of intervention based in providing physicians with computerized prognostic data and a cadre of nurses trained to work with patients, families, and physicians, little change in treatment occurred. In a significant number of patients, pain was not adequately relieved; moreover, physicians had misunderstood, had ignored, or had never apprised themselves of patients' preferences regarding resuscitation, either through direct communication or as expressed in advance directives such as living wills or durable power of attorney.[15]

Such studies could be seized upon by some as further justification for legalizing assisted suicide or euthanasia in order to protect patients against treatment abuse. But this is specious reasoning. The fact that physicians do not manage terminal illness well does not warrant sanctioning killing patients or assisting in their suicides. Indeed, the failure of the planned intervention in the SUPPORT study suggests that the restrictions the proponents of euthanasia and assisted suicide believe would prevent abuses would be equally ineffective. These restrictions would involve granting physicians even greater power to take control of the patient's dying, as has been demonstrated in the Netherlands' experience. If anything, the SUPPORT study shows how urgent it is to encourage and practice better pain and suffering control. This is a collective obligation the profession has not met adequately or energetically.

Interestingly, in another recent study of patients for whom life-sustaining decisions were not simply future possibilities but proximate probabilities, researchers found that undertreatment may be as much a concern as overtreatment.[16] Of the 421 nursing home patients interviewed, 60 percent said they would choose CPR, 80 percent would choose hospitalization, and 33 percent would choose a feeding tube. This does not mean that physicians are justified in ignoring patient wishes. It does indicate that substantial numbers of patients actually facing the decision would opt for treatment. It also suggests that, in terms of outcomes at least, many patients would agree with their physicians' decisions and would not be harmed by not being asked. The real harm is ignoring the patient's preferences, which is not morally acceptable.

Both studies show the need for better empirical data about preferences for treatment at the time when the decision immediately presents itself to populations at risk. Both studies underscore the need to better educate physicians to assure compliance with patient requests, participation in the preparation of advance directives, and better surveillance of the entire process.[17]

Those who favor euthanasia and assisted suicide often invoke a right to die, based in a right to privacy or a protected liberty. There is no basis in American jurisprudence, however, for limitation of the state's constitutional power to forbid assistance in suicide. The Fourteenth Amendment denies the state the power to "deprive any person of life, liberty, or property without due process of law." Assisted suicide is not a "liberty interest," since there is no constitutional interest in depriving someone of life or liberty. This demand has never been protected under the doctrine of personal liberty. To legalize assisted suicide contradicts both common law and Supreme Court precedent.[18]

Several recent court decisions have seriously muddied the legal issues. The Ninth Circuit Court in 1995 labeled the finding of a constitutional right to die an intervention "unknown to the past and antithetical to the defense of human life that has been a chief responsibility of constitutional government." It denied the relevance of *Cruzan* and *Casey*, distinguishing a right to refuse treatment from a right to an assisted suicide. That distinction was relevant also to several classic cases involving the right to refuse treatment.[19]

In a second opinion, the Ninth Circuit Court, now sitting *en banc,* reversed its first decision, finding violation of the prohibition of assisted suicide to be a violation of a constitutional liberty right. Almost simultaneously, the Second Circuit Court found the prohibition a violation of the Fourteenth Amendment's equal treatment clause.[20]

On June 26, 1997, the Supreme Court of the United States handed down its rulings on these two cases (*Washington v. Glucksberg* and *Quill v. Vacco*), unanimously upholding the ban on assisted suicide in the states of Washington and New York. However, further litigation built on specific cases remains a possibility, and a careful reading of the concurring opinions of the Justices provides some insight into the nature of these future legal possibilities. Despite the complex issues surrounding the Court's opinion, which is currently undergoing analysis by legal and ethics scholars, the ethical questions that are the concern of this chapter are not dependent upon legal approval or disapproval of assisted suicide.

Euthanasia and Assisted Suicide Are Not Autonomous, Compassionate, or Dignified

In our individualistic, rights-conscious society, one of the most powerful arguments favoring euthanasia and assisted suicide appeals to the right of autonomy. Autonomy is now a *prima facie* moral principle in medical ethics. Early in this century, the benign paternalism of the Hippocratic tradition yielded before the patient's legal right to refuse unwanted treatment. That right has been gradually extended—first to surrogates, then to living wills and durable powers of attorney, and then to a putative right to demand treatment.[21]

But if the moral and legal claim to autonomy is to be actualized in clinical decisions, the patient must, in fact, be able to exercise her autonomy. This means that both external and internal impediments to the exercise of the capacity to make self-determinations must not be such that they constitute a form of coercion in the direction of termination of life.[22] There are ample reasons, based in the phenomenology of the request for relief by death, to believe that the autonomy of such patients is dubious at best.

Legalization of euthanasia and assisted suicide would grant an enormous increment of power to that which the physician already possesses. The physician is even more fully in control once the decision to end life has been made. Physicians, like all other human beings, cannot entirely escape their own prejudices and biases about what constitutes quality of life, a good death, and whether suffering has meaning. In the end, physicians will be the key interpreters of any criteria established by law or society when applied to a particular patient. Their interpretations will vary tremendously and may well reflect their preferences rather than the patient's. This is not to ascribe to physicians a collective defect of character, but only to recognize the power of a physician's own values, beliefs, and fears when deciding about the lives of others.

S. H. Miles points to the medical literature which documents the hostility, anxiety, and inadequacy in dealing with suicidal patients, all of which can influence the physician's too-easy agreement with the suicide wish or delude him into thinking that he has a firmer grasp than is the case of the patient's rationality in choosing to die.[23] In the complex interpersonal interrelationships between physicians and dying patients, it is difficult, if not impossible, to discern who is influencing whom. One would be imprudent and questionably beneficent to end a life under such uncertainty. The complex and uncertain phenomenology of fatal illness, dying, and suffering make the exercise of genuine autonomy highly problematic.

Clinical depression is easily masked or misdiagnosed. It is often undertreated and may be a powerful impediment to the exercise of autonomy as well as being the reason for the patient's choice of death.[24] The patient's depression may well have its roots in the way others respond to them—the family with exhaustion and fatigue, the physician with his need to end a frustrating relationship with a patient whose treatment is difficult or unsatisfactory. The physician's response to his own fear of suffering or dying cannot fail to influence his attitude and his patient's response.

The person desperate enough to seek exit by suicide or euthanasia is beset with anxiety, despair, guilt, depression, and a sense of unworthiness. These, as much as pain, are at the root of the desperate plea for surcease through death. Often these feelings are exacerbated by the way family, friends, physicians, nurses, and others behave and respond to the patient's predicament. Any signs or semblances of insensitivity, indifference, revulsion, loathing, distancing, pity, or impatience to be about one's business are quickly transmitted to those in the grasp of a fatal illness. They can see either reassurance or confirmation of their worst fears in the way others approach them. Their feelings of alienation from the world of the well and their sense of a loss of dignity are easily reinforced. Unknowingly, physicians and family may add to a patient's depression or influence his choice of suicide.[25]

The decision to end one's life may appear to be freely chosen, but once such a decision is intimated or expressed definitively, the focus of everyone's attention shifts to the timing and circumstances of the act of exit. One person whose assisted suicide was described in detail in *The New York Times* put it this way: "I'm not afraid. I just feel as if everyone is ganging up on me, pressuring me. I just want some time."[26] At this patient's demise and that of another filmed for Dutch television, once the decisions were made in favor of a planned exit, control passed in many subtle ways to those around the patient. In both cases, the "assistants"—doctors, family, friends—began to suggest and manage when and how the event would occur. Their needs, rather than the patient's, subtly crept in, even with the best of intentions. Instead of gaining control, the patient loses control. The more vulnerable the patient, the more dangerous it is to vest control in others to whom vulnerability itself may be a sign of readiness to die.

After all, it is the physician, not the patient, who determines when the clinical situation is hopeless, when suffering is "intolerable," and when the patient is "ready" for suicide. All the proposed statutory conditions and regulations devised to prevent abuses designate the physicians as the determinants of futility of treatment, depression, or patient competence. The physician administers the lethal dose in euthanasia and the physician prescribes the lethal dose in assisted suicide. Benrubi would "safeguard" the process by involving three physicians—the personal physician, an anesthesiologist, and a psychiatrist. While the intent of this safeguard is sincere, it ends up medicalizing the decision almost completely. The patient must now make the decision three times with physicians unlikely even to participate in such a process unless they favor euthanasia and assisted suicide.[27]

If assisted suicide and euthanasia are legalized, the fatally ill—and even those chronically debilitated—will feel guilty if they do not take the expected route out of the world. They may even begin to "feel sorry" for those around them. When we add to this the physician's power to suggest assisted death as an available option, the momentum of the decision will be difficult to alter. Coercion need not be overt in its influence on a vulnerable, depressed patient when the immediate milieu and societal mores urge death. Freedom to choose under such circumstances is illusory and dubiously rational when depression is present. If pain and depression are treated, most patients abandon their desire for death.[28]

Equally as powerful as the argument from autonomy is the argument from compassion. Few of us can be in the presence of human suffering without feeling compassion—feeling something of the other person's experience and being moved to help. Despite the need for objectivity in their technical ministrations, health professionals must not, and cannot, lose their compassion if they are truly to be healers. But compassion is a powerful emotion that can take on a life of its own and, in distorted forms, can produce harm.

Compassion is not a self-justifying ethical principle. Even genuine compassion can be misdirected consciously or unconsciously. It is often very difficult even for conscientious observers to know whether the compassion they feel is directed to their own anguish or that of family or other caregivers rather than the patient. Those around the patient often become frustrated and emotionally exhausted and feel impelled to "do something"—"anything"—to relieve themselves or the patient.[29] The wish to get "it" over with can be as powerful a motive for those attending the patient as for the patient himself. Even genuine compassion is no guarantee against doing harm in the name of helping.

Compassion does not mean doing everything a person wants. True compassion demands co-feeling, entering into the unique predicament of the person suffering and sharing that whole experience. It means giving of oneself, not pitying the sufferer. Being present even when no easy solution is at hand may not be easy, but it is essential if the patient is to have a good death rather than one that satisfies and relieves the observer. The plea for assistance in suicide is a desperate plea for another kind of help—for support, reassurance of love, reaffirmation of one's humanity and dignity, for attachment, not detachment. To consider, offer, or suggest hastening of death is to detach oneself in an act of abandonment in a struggle that until that moment had been joined *together* with others.

Assisted suicide is a noncompassionate act of moral abandonment. It takes the desperate plea for extinction at face value. It denies that a "good" death may obtain even when suffering is present. How we die is our last act, our last gift to those we love. Those who are dying need the loving company of the living, not their farewell before a life has run its full course.

Another of the "humanistic" arguments for euthanasia and assisted suicide is that they are necessary to preserve human dignity. Indeed, "death with dignity" has become a slogan for the proponents of euthanasia and assisted suicide. Much depends here on the definition of dignity. Sickness and suffering do not—indeed, cannot—rob humans of their intrinsic and true dignity. Humans have dignity simply because they are human. This does not mean everyone we meet is dignified in appearance or behavior. It does mean that human persons have intrinsic worth and deserve respect, not by virtue of what they have or have not accomplished but because they share a common humanity with every other human. This is what entitles them to certain rights, and those rights are the basis for their moral claims upon others—claims to life, liberty, freedom from unjust aggression, and so on.

Humans, therefore, cannot lose dignity because they do not "control" everything that happens to them, or because they are in pain, are suffering, or are dying. The loss of "dignity" that the desperately ill person feels is loss of imputed, not intrinsic, dignity, a loss of worth they perceive in the way those about them see them.[30] Dying patients sense the pity, fear, and loathing their plight or changed appearance may induce in family and friend. They then impute this judgment to themselves as evidence for a loss of dignity. They become ashamed of their cachexia, disfigurement, and bodily and psychological metamorphosis. The mirror all too sadly confirms what they perceive others see in them. But the person behind the mask of illness remains a person entitled to the same respect she enjoyed before her illness began.

In a few extraordinary pages, *The New York Times* literary critic Anatole Broyard sketched how, when dying of prostate cancer, he responded to his physician. "Aesculapian power" is no myth. Like all power, it can help or harm. In the physician's hands, it can sustain or despoil the patient of his or her dignity.[31]

But the dignity of a death resides in how we face death, not in the way people respond to the way we look. We can die dignified deaths no matter how wan, wasted, or weak we may be. Dignity derives from the way we, ourselves, respond to what cannot be altered, to the challenge disease poses to our faith in ourselves. Dignity in dying is not in the eye of the beholder but in the way the suffering person chooses to die. Some choices are more dignified than others.

None of this is meant to deny the reality of the sense of loss of imputed dignity dying persons feel. Nor is it to depreciate the added suffering such loss invokes. Nor is it to castigate family, friends, and physicians who may feel genuine pity at the plight of the sufferer. It is to suggest, however, that there is another way to look at the question of a dignified death. It is to place much more responsibility on those who care for the patient to prevent the loss of dignity the sufferer experiences. It is also to suggest that efforts to restore a sense of dignity, rather than eliminating the suffering person, are more beneficent than regaining dignity by killing or assisting in suicide in the name of compassion.

Euthanasia and Assisted Suicide Are Not Ethical Obligations of Physicians

Despite the specific prohibition of any form of killing of patients in the Hippocratic Oath and tradition, some physicians today argue that terminating the lives of patients is consistent with the beneficent aims of medicine. At the one extreme is the position of Dr. Jack Kevorkian that medical ethics to this point has been a maleficent influence and that it must be altered radically to permit access to termination of life by physicians. Timothy Quill, though less brash, suggests the same, as do the physicians who prepared the Wanzer Reports, which sanction physician participation in assisting suicide in certain cases. All, with varying degrees of restriction to contain abuses, deem it morally praiseworthy to assist in the death of patients.[32]

Most recently, Miller and Brody have argued that euthanasia and assisted suicide are compatible with professional integrity. They propose that the prohibition against these practices must not be taken as an absolute but only as a *prima facie* obligation which can under "last resort" conditions be overridden, transforming them into acts of beneficence. As Miles has pointed out, this "signals a fundamental change in the moral boundaries and relationships between healers, patients, and society."[33] The societal implications of such a change are no less serious than the dangers to individual patients.

Although they try to distance themselves from Kevorkian's more sweeping condemnation of traditional medical ethics, Miller and Brody come to the same conclusion. The logical endpoint of their reasoning is not different from that of Kevorkian, the Dutch medical profession, or the Wanzer Committee, namely, that under certain conditions, to be determined by physicians, singly or in a troika á la Benrubi or in an oversight committee of some sort, patients may have their lives terminated at will.[34]

The prohibition against physician participation in euthanasia and assisted suicide has been elemental in the traditional ethics of medicine for a long time. Whether one subscribed to the Hippocratic Oath or not, and whether or not some physicians engaged in "mercy killing," no major professional organization has condoned euthanasia or assisted suicide. Today there are suggestions that the Hippocratic Oath and ethic should be dismantled or declared out of date.[35] But these attempts beg the central moral questions: Is the intentional, direct or assisted killing of patients consistent with the healing goals of medicine? At a minimum, it would have to be shown that such killing is a beneficent act in the patient's best interests. But this is exactly what is not the case.

Miller and Brody's contention that euthanasia and assisted suicide are consistent with the ethics of medicine is simply another step in the dismemberment of the traditional ethic of medicine that has gathered strength in the last quarter century. However one verbalizes the "traditional" ethic—in the Oath of Hippocrates, the Prayer of Maimonides, its variations administered at medical school commencements, or the Code of the American Medical Association—it is inconsistent with euthanasia and assisted suicide. These acts are far from being established morally or accepted professionally. The current fashion for deconstruction of the traditional ethic does not constitute a convincing moral argument for abandonment of a long-standing prohibition.[36]

Euthanasia and Assisted Suicide Are Not Private Matters

The proponents of euthanasia and assisted suicide argue that, like abortion, these practices are "private" choices. They defend the rights of others to disagree and not participate. On this view, it is an invasion of privacy for the state or the profession to intervene.[37] This position ignores the fact that none of us—even the most alienated—lives in complete isolation from other human beings and society. The very fact that physicians are called upon to "assist" belies the claim to privacy. Nothing so significant or dramatic as choosing to be killed or aided in suicide can occur without an impact on our fellow human beings. Family, friends, or communities may condone these practices, but they cannot escape its effects on them and the community of those linked in various relationships to the patient.

Justice deals not only with protection of the rights of individuals but also with the protection of the lives of others. Euthanasia and assisted suicide are built on the premise that some lives are not worth living. It is inevitable that lives so designated will be depreciated. These will usually be the lives not only of the sick and dying but of the handicapped, the disabled, the aged, and infants or those at the margins of society (the homeless, the aberrant, the retarded), that is, the candidates for "assistance" in dying. This is why the preservation of human life is, and has been, in the state's interest. To depreciate the state's interest in some of its citizens by sanctioning the deliberate ending of life is to give a message of unworthiness, despair, and abandonment to whole segments of our population. It is also to raise questions about their fitness for continued life when resources become scarce.[38] In a society as obsessed with the costs of health care and the principle of utility, the dangers of the slippery slope—both logical and psychological—are far from fantasy.

To see that the slippery slope is no fairy tale, one need only look at the living social laboratory of euthanasia in the Netherlands, where euthanasia has been socially sanctioned for some time. The clear guidelines designed to prevent abuse of the privilege have not been respected, nor have they prevented extensions beyond the original intent. In the Dutch government's own report of 1991, there were 1,000 cases of euthanasia without consent and 4,941 cases of excess medication, given without consent, which resulted in the patients' death.[39] The total of 5,941 cases of killing without consent was almost the same as the number with consent (5,495). In the latest report from the Netherlands, euthanasia has been progressively extended to infants, children, patients with psychiatric disorders, and patients with nonterminal illnesses. The empirical fact of the slippery slope is undeniable in the one country in which euthanasia has quasi-legal status.

Since the Remmelink Commission report, Dutch practice of euthanasia and assisted suicide has slipped further down the slippery slope it purported to avoid.[40] Three instances will suffice to establish the trend. First is the judgment of the Dutch Supreme Court in a case in which a psychiatrist assisted in the death of a severely depressed, nonterminal patient. The court faulted the psychiatrist only for a procedural failure in not getting a second opinion. However, it accepted psychic suffering as a category admissible for assistance in suicide. The court opinion judged the patient not to be psychotic and, therefore, capable of a valid request for death even though he was severely depressed. Will the next step be assisting the suicide of an adolescent unhappy with his life prospects or his cosmetic appearance, or afflicted with the transient angst of the precarious years of passage into adulthood? These forms of "psychic suffering" would be very difficult to disentangle. The fact is that if the patient is depressed, his "consent" could not be valid; if he is psychotic, he would not be allowed to dissent. In either case, assisted suicide or euthanasia would be a maleficent act.[41]

Another example is the opinion of the Dutch Pediatric Society and its ethicist, Heleen Dupuis, who defended nontreatment of an infant with duodenal atresia (Baby Ross) on grounds that if there is any doubt about the best interests of the child, there is no obligation to treat.[42] The decision is judged to be private, between parents and doctor and related to their values only. The ethicist states further that active euthanasia is indicated if the baby does not die right away. Dr. Dupuis did not think it wise a decade ago, but now, with the practice of voluntary euthanasia accepted, she believes expansion to handicapped infants is warranted. Dupuis also sanctions not reporting these cases in jurisdictions where the prosecutors have the wrong attitude, that is, will prosecute.

Finally, the same "attitudes" are at work in Dutch nursing homes. A survey indicated that requests for voluntary euthanasia are rare, but when requested, only in 40 percent of the cases were the state-mandated preconditions met. In the remainder, the time lapse between the request and the administration of euthanasia was very short. This was defended as "merciful." As in the pediatric cases, these cases too were reported as "natural" deaths so that the full extent of these practices are unknown.[43] The Netherlands social laboratory of euthanasia gives ample verification to Justice Cardozo's dictum that "any principle stands to expand itself to the limits of its logic." Fenigsen's case against Dutch euthanasia does not in retrospect appear exaggerated.[44]

A 25 percent rate of failure is expected in this form of assisted suicide, which makes active euthanasia a mandatory next step. In the eyes of its protagonists, once started, the physician or someone else must be prepared to kill the patient if the lethal dose is ineffective. Assisted suicide is a half-way house, a stop on the way to other forms of direct euthanasia, for example, for incompetent patients by advance directive or suicide in the elderly. So, too, is voluntary euthanasia a half-way house to involuntary and nonvoluntary euthanasia. If terminating life is a benefit, the reasoning goes, why should euthanasia be limited only to those who can give consent? Why need we ask for consent? Clearly, infants, the senile, the comatose, the feeble should not be denied this benefit even if they can't give consent.[45]

More subtle but equally compelling as the logical slippery slope is the psychological slope. Once the reluctance to overturn a long-standing moral barrier is overcome, what was previously wrong now appears to be right and good. The interplay of the doctor's behavior, his psychology, and his ethics is complex and difficult to discern clearly, but it is undeniable.[46] Killing and assisting in killing are emotionally charged activities of great intensity. To engage in killing for the first time involves the suppression of guilt and desensitization to an intuitively repugnant act. But desensitization does occur.

In a recent book, David Grossman shows how our soldiers were taught to kill and were successfully desensitized to it. As a result, the rate at which our troops actually fired on the enemy rose from a very low rate in World War II to a 90–95 percent rate in Vietnam. Very young people, most in their teens, were desensitized to their natural repugnance to killing, just as so many young people are being desensitized to killing and violence by the entertainment industry.[47]

In their training, physicians gradually become desensitized to the dismemberment of human bodies in anatomy and autopsy, to trauma, dying, and death. There is some evidence that participation in terminating life may discourage repetition.[48] But there is also the real possibility that the reverse is true. If we examine the pattern of behavior of physicians who have participated in violating other taboos—like participating in torture or genocide—we find that most of them were "ordinary" people.

Conclusions

Prominent medical ethicists have sought to justify euthanasia and assisted suicide by arguing that killing other human persons is not universally or absolutely prohibited. Rather, they assert, killing derives its moral status from whether it harms or wrongs others. They propose certain conditions and situations under which they believe killing by direct, voluntary euthanasia and assisted suicide are beneficent acts, that is, they protect the interests of others and produce effects that help, rather than harm, suffering persons.

But euthanasia and assisted suicide give an illusion of beneficence that is dissipated in the light of the clinical reality within which actual requests for termination, and that termination itself, occur. Thus, euthanasia and assisted suicide are unnecessary to end pain and suffering, very dubiously autonomous, noncompassionate, undignified for the subject, corrosive of the physician-patient relationship, and dangerous to the most vulnerable members of our society as well as to the community at large.

On inspection of the clinical context within which euthanasia and assisted suicide occur, the preponderance of evidence is decidedly in favor of maleficence, not beneficence. The magnitude and probability of these wrongs and harms are sufficient to vitiate any claim for the moral probity of these practices. Indeed, the beneficence which impels many to favor euthanasia and assisted suicide is illusory when examined in light of the realities of suffering and dying.

5

Facing Assisted Suicide and Euthanasia in Children and Adolescents

S U S A N   M.   W O L F

The recent surge in advocacy for legitimating active euthanasia and physician-assisted suicide in the United States[1] has largely ignored children and adolescents.[2] While an older literature exists examining infanticide and euthanasia (by which I will mean active euthanasia) in newborns, much of it aims to analyze the acceptability of abortion or termination of treatment.[3] In any case, current efforts to legitimate euthanasia and assisted suicide[4] generally avoid that literature. Moreover, there is virtually no advocacy for permitting these practices among older children and adolescents.[5] Instead, advocates have concentrated on competent adults. Support for assisted suicide and euthanasia thus rests on the assertion of competent patients' rights and physicians' duties of beneficence. By limiting proposals to competent adults, advocates brandish the sword of patient self-determination, while using voluntary choice as a shield against charges of abuse.

Relegating pediatric euthanasia and assisted suicide to the margins is reassuring. The intentional killing of children and adolescents, or assistance in their suicides, is surely more disquieting than the same practices among competent adult patients. Ignoring children may thus advantage those urging legitimation. Indeed, a prominent Dutch advocate recounts, "Being the spokesperson for a society advocating requested euthanasia, I certainly did not think it wise for me 10 years ago to begin this discussion of actively ending the life of newborns . . . when the discussion of euthanasia for adults was so new."[6]

But conducting the debate over assisted suicide and euthanasia without examining the consequences for minors ignores too much. It ignores reported cases of pediatric euthanasia in this country and elsewhere.[7] It also ignores the Dutch experience of initially permitting only adult euthanasia[8] but then discovering pediatric cases.[9] Now the Dutch pediatric and medical associations actually advocate pediatric euthanasia and assisted suicide,[10] and in two recent court cases physicians who performed pediatric euthanasia received no punishment.[11] Avoiding the pediatric issues ignores, too, the fact that minors may be more vulnerable to euthanasia and more apt to request assisted suicide than many others in the United States because of inferior pain relief,[12] the large number who are poor,[13] the substantial number who are uninsured,[14] the complex dynamics of parental decision making for ill or disabled minors,[15] and psychological differences between adults and those who are younger.[16] Finally, it ignores the difficulty of confining any right to these practices to adults, since rights to termination of treatment and abortion—the roots, many argue, of a right to assisted suicide and euthanasia[17]—have already been extended to minors.

Avoiding the pediatric issues is thus a mistake. It risks having the practices occur among children and adolescents with no applicable justification, no consideration of the special dangers, and no specific safeguards. This minimizes the rights and interests of minors. It obscures the dangers involved in taking the lives of some of the least powerful among us. And we never reach the question of how far legitimation of assisted suicide and euthanasia should really go.

The euthanasia and assisted-suicide debate has become one of the great contests of our time,[18] as we struggle with whether a profession traditionally committed to healing should now deliberately take life or assist suicide, especially in the only industrialized society that has thus far failed to guarantee health care coverage. So much is at stake in this life-and-death contest that it acts as a Rorschach test, revealing whose interests count. This debate becomes a test, then, of our commitment to children's rights and interests. This chapter explores the current neglect of pediatric issues in the United States and then the cautionary tale of the Dutch experience. That sets the stage for analyzing whether euthanasia and assisted suicide should be permitted for newborns, older children, or adolescents. I argue that pediatric application of these practices should be rejected.

Avoiding Pediatric Euthanasia

In the current U.S. debate, occasional attention to pediatric issues breaks a silence that otherwise prevails. In the litigation on whether the federal Constitution invalidates state bans on assisted suicide, for example, plaintiffs challenged these bans only as applied to competent persons and specifically competent adults.[19] Most advocates for legitimating the practices do not discuss pediatric application, whether scholars such as Ronald Dworkin,[20] reflective clinicians such as Timothy Quill,[21] or public figures such as Jack Kevorkian.[22] Even documents on end-of-life care that one might expect to touch on the topic do not.[23]

The prevailing silence about pediatric euthanasia and assisted suicide might stem from repugnance at the very idea of actively taking the lives of children. Yet there is evidence that repugnance may not be so widespread. The practice of pediatric euthanasia apparently exists in the United States. Newspapers have reported the euthanasia of a 9-year-old by a physician in San Francisco[24] and of a premature infant by a physician in Georgia.[25] Weir recounts a Connecticut case in which parents, in collaboration with a physician, "decided to kill . . . [an infant] by increasing the daily dose of anticonvulsive sedative and by stopping the [tube] feedings," a combination of active and passive means.[26]

Indeed, there is a long history of tolerating the practice in this country. Colonial America inherited from England the legal "doctrine that many defective newborns were 'monsters' . . . without a right to life."[27] Though the doctrine was in decline by the mid-1800s, authorities still regarded destruction of such infants as less serious than murder.[28] The early twentieth century saw calls to legalize euthanasia in order to control the costs of caring for these infants.[29] In a 1937 poll, 45 percent favored euthanizing them.[30] Proctor reports that American debate over euthanasia peaked in 1936–1941, but support abated in the early 1940s upon word of Nazi practices.[31]

Starting in the 1970s, a public discussion erupted over the acceptability of forgoing treatment for imperiled neonates.[32] That prompted renewed support for pediatric euthanasia in some quarters.[33] Some scholars argued that there was no real difference between forgoing treatment and active killing and that both could be applied to a newborn.[34] Others argued that very young infants failed to meet the criteria for personhood anyway, and so could permissibly be killed.[35] Increased debate over abortion in the 1970s similarly fueled support for euthanasia among scholars who maintained there was no principled distinction between ending the life of a fetus and a newborn, and that both interventions were acceptable.[36]

Thus there is a history of supporting pediatric euthanasia in the United States. Since the revelation of Nazi atrocities in World War II, support has been voiced mainly to bolster acceptance of other practices, termination of treatment and abortion. Yet now that the American public is directly debating euthanasia and assisted suicide, there is a notable silence on the pediatric applications. Still, cases occur, and the recurrent support for pediatric euthanasia in American history suggests this should come as no surprise. Both contemporaneous cases and the history compel more open discussion.

The Dutch Embrace of Pediatric Euthanasia

Explicit discussion of the pediatric issues is further compelled by the Dutch experience. The occurrence of pediatric euthanasia in the Netherlands despite rules requiring a patient's voluntary and competent choice, and the emerging Dutch defense of this departure, provide a cautionary tale for the United States.

Dutch advocacy of physician-assisted suicide and euthanasia, like American advocacy, has depicted the practices as exercises of patient autonomy and self-determination.[37] While making the Netherlands the first jurisdiction in the world[38] to tolerate the practices openly,[39] the Dutch have officially required that the patient voluntarily and competently request such a death.[40] The request of a surrogate will not suffice.[41] In keeping with this, the Dutch Medical Association has recently begun urging the superiority of physician-assisted suicide over euthanasia, precisely to assure patient control.[42] Against this background, the Dutch embrace of pediatric euthanasia—in which the patient makes no voluntary, competent choice—requires some explanation.

That explanation begins with a general slide toward nonvoluntary euthanasia. The formal rules requiring the patient's voluntary and contemporaneous request have failed to prevent euthanasia without it.[43] Dutch researchers[44] have documented a substantial number of deaths without explicit request. In a 1990–91 analysis, the government research team found that 0.8 percent of all deaths per year in one study, and 1.6 percent in another, resulted from "life-terminating acts without explicit and persistent request" or what they called "LAWER."[45] (A comparable analysis of 1995 data found the percentage of LAWER deaths to be 0.7 percent.)[46] These amounted to an estimated 1,000 cases per year[47] and included intentional death through administration of drugs, but not forgoing life-sustaining treatment.[48] In most LAWER cases the patient was reported to be incompetent, and in 41 percent of the cases there was neither prior discussion with the patient nor prior request (with similar results in 1995).[49]

Despite the fact that LAWER clearly violates the Dutch rules requiring a patient's voluntary and contemporaneous request, the government researchers were reluctant to condemn it. LAWER "is unlikely to disappear since there will always be some situations in which terrible suffering . . . arises when the patient cannot give a clear judgment. . . . Many doctors . . . feel that in such exceptional circumstances LAWER can be justified." The researchers concluded that with certain safeguards—"optimal palliative care[;] discussion with relatives, a colleague, and nurses[;] reporting[;] . . . absence of economic motives"; and consideration of the patient's best interests—LAWER would be acceptable.[50]

Nonvoluntary euthanasia has also occurred in cases in which the patient's competence to request euthanasia or assisted suicide was either questionable or absent. In June of 1994 the Dutch Supreme Court convicted but failed to punish a psychiatrist, Dr.

Chabot, for assisting the suicide of a physically healthy patient who developed a depressive disorder after her two sons died.[51]

Other kinds of cases raise questions about voluntariness as well. Gomez recounts cases of "[p]atients acting under coercion—either tacit or explicit—from . . . family members." He also describes patients acting without being adequately informed, who "[choose] euthanasia out of ignorance or misunderstanding of . . . [their] situation."[52]

Turning to pediatric euthanasia in particular, the government researchers reported relevant data in their 1990–91 analysis. They found 73 deaths by LAWER in which the patient was under 20 years old. Nearly half of those occurred in patients less than one year old. Another 15 were among those one to 11 years old. In the remaining 23, patients were thus 12 to 19 years old. Subsequently, the researchers analyzed deaths that occurred in 1995 among children less than one year old. They found that in 8 percent of cases a "decision to forgo life-sustaining treatment was combined with drugs given explicitly to hasten death." In another 1 percent of cases, there was a decision to give a drug to hasten death to a child who was not on life-sustaining treatment.[53]

Orlowski and colleagues asserted in 1992 that pediatric euthanasia was practiced in the Netherlands, though the exact numbers were unknown.[54] The researchers recounted that the Dutch Pediatric Society had published in 1989 a survey of the 8 major neonatal centers in the Netherlands, and found that "5 of the 8 actively terminated the lives of neonates with a predicted poor quality of life," while "3 of the 8 . . . openly terminated the life of older infants with severe birth defects."[55] Orlowski et al. also stated that "[p]ersonal communications with Dutch pediatricians . . . confirm that euthanasia of children is performed occasionally."[56] "In the Netherlands there are at least 10 . . . cases a year of active euthanasia of newborn infants . . ., according to official figures . . . [of] the Dutch Paediatric Association."[57] Fenigsen estimated in 1990 that the lives of 10 handicapped newborns "are actively terminated each year," although a study of 4 neonatal intensive care units reported one case of active and intentional termination of life in 1990 and none in 1993.[58]

Gomez reports one case involving a child among the 26 cases of euthanasia he studied. This was the case of an infant born with Down syndrome and duodenal atresia. Once a decision was made not to treat, the child was euthanized.[59] Other individual cases have been reported as well.[60] These include the case of a child born with congenital malformations, a limited life expectancy, and pain, who was euthanized by a Dutch gynecologist. The physician was convicted of murder, but without penalty.[61]

There are fewer reports of physician-assisted suicide for older minors. Orlowski et al. wrote that "[c]onversations with pediatricians . . . suggest that the other major pediatric group undergoing euthanasia [aside from newborns and infants] . . . is teenagers," though these are actually deaths by physician-assisted suicide. "One pediatric oncologist estimated that he used . . . [a certain technique to accomplish this] about eight times per year. . . . [P]ediatricians . . . suggest that assisted suicide is being employed . . . because of unfavorable publicity surrounding the previous use of active euthanasia in this patient population."[62]

Fenigsen recounts that a leading pediatric oncologist revealed his practice of assisting the suicide of children in his care approximately six times per year. Parents consented in some of these cases; in others they had no knowledge of what was happening.[63] Fenigsen further reports an opinion poll showing that almost 70 percent of the public were supportive of this practice.[64]

The Orlowski article and Fenigsen's writings have been controversial,[65] but not because of broad opposition to euthanasia and assisted suicide in minors. A committee of the Dutch Pediatric Association's Section on Perinatology reported in 1992 that "no consensus exists concerning the purposeful ending of life. . . . [T]here is, however, respect for different opinions."[66] Yet the Association's committee ultimately blessed pediatric euthanasia as long as the parents gave their permission.[67]

The Royal Dutch Medical Association has approved pediatric euthanasia as well. In 1995 the Association came out in favor of euthanasia in older minors, when they are capable of making a decision.[68] The Association asserted that the parents needed to be informed but could not override the child's choice.[69] The report relied to a great extent on the Patient Rights Act, effective in 1995. Under this Act, children under 12 have a right to information, but their parents must make medical decisions; from 12 to 16 a child may refuse treatment even over parental objection; and a minor 16 or over may decide independently. The Association suggested that these age limits be used as guidelines for euthanasia, "but the individual minor's capacity to assess his situation could well carry much more weight . . . in these cases."[70]

Individual commentators have supported these practices as well. While Orlowski et al. regard euthanasia for children younger than 7 as a "major step down 'the slippery slope'" because such a child lacks decisional capacity and so cannot make a voluntary request, they support it under certain circumstances for older children.[71] They argue that children 7 to 14 are usually capable of assent to treatment, and so may elect euthanasia as long as their parents agree. They further argue that adolescents 14 and older can give voluntary consent, and so should be able to choose euthanasia even over parental objection.

Visser et al. maintain that a decision for nonvoluntary active euthanasia in children "may be made when nontreatment is not followed by death and untreatable pain and suffering continue."[72] Leenen and Ciesielski-Carlucci agree, at least for "a severely handicapped baby."[73] Dupuis agrees for a severely handicapped child.[74]

All of this support for pediatric euthanasia and assisted suicide clearly departs from the Dutch rules. Indeed, because the Dutch reserve the term "euthanasia" for voluntarily requested death, supporters of pediatric application often do not even use the term. The 1992 report from the Dutch Pediatric Association, for example, says "[t]he term 'euthanasia' is not used because, in neonatology, requests cannot come from the patients themselves—a prerequisite in the legal definition of euthanasia."[75]

This review of the Dutch situation suggests several lessons. First, formal commitment to limiting euthanasia and assisted suicide to those patients making a competent and voluntary request will not necessarily prevent the practices in children. Yet pediatric euthanasia and assisted suicide may not be treated as a challenge to the usual autonomy justification for these practices. The requests of adolescents and even children as young as 7 may be deemed autonomous enough. And for younger children and newborns, parental choice may be deemed sufficient. Thus the pediatric practices may be tolerated with little further justification and consideration of their particular dangers. In effect, children may be smuggled into practices designed for adults without careful attention to the separate problems involved.

Bringing Pediatric Practices Out of the Shadows

Whether one approves of or deplores assisted suicide and euthanasia for adults, permitting these practices on children and adolescents without adequate justification or consideration of the dangers is difficult to defend. Indeed, there are compelling reasons to demand separate scrutiny for pediatric euthanasia and assisted suicide.

First, the usual autonomy and self-determination justifications do not apply to most children. Unless a patient is competent to make her own treatment decisions, or left instructions while previously competent, decisions about treatment are not simply a matter of respecting patient autonomy and self-determination. Decision-making about termination of treatment is instructive. In the case of younger children—newborns and those too young to articulate binding treatment preferences—the dominant approach is that parents or other guardians must decide in the patient's best interests. Even in the case of children and adolescents old enough to participate in decision-making and to assent to parental choices, we still customarily turn to parents or guardians for effective consent.[76] And whenever a surrogate is making treatment choices without binding instructions from a previously competent patient, the decisional process can no longer be described as patient self-determination. Thus pediatric euthanasia and assisted suicide cannot rest on an autonomy justification, particularly for younger children. A separate justification is required.

Second, the other primary justification for assisted suicide and euthanasia—on grounds of beneficence—is especially problematic in the case of children. Decisions about pediatric assisted suicide and euthanasia in children unable to decide for themselves will usually rest with the parents or guardian. A substantial literature discusses the problems of parental decision-making.[77] Work on termination of treatment issues illuminates the understandable problem of parents deciding a child would be better off dead, based not so much on the child's discomfort and experience as on the parents' anxiety and psychological discomfort, a highly controversial basis on which to choose death for another.[78] And lengthy debate about surrogate decision-making has revealed still unresolved problems, such as relying on stereotypes about disability and projections of discomfort onto the patient, rather than attempting analysis of what this particular patient is experiencing.[79] So counting on parents or guardians to authorize euthanasia or assisted suicide using the best interests or substituted judgment standards would allow the unresolved problems with those standards and the known complexities of parental decision-making in pediatric cases to be played out in still more fatal circumstances than we currently allow.

Relying on beneficence from physicians is equally questionable considering how children with medical problems historically have been treated. There is a long history of undertreating pediatric pain, certainly in newborns and even in older children.[80] Thus there is a real danger that medical personnel moved to consider euthanasia or assisted suicide because of a child's apparent pain and discomfort may be overlooking the less fatal alternative of adequately treating the child's symptoms.

This history of inadequate pediatric pain relief may be related to a longer history of viewing children as the "other," beings with whom we adults have difficulty identifying. Scholars studying how children have been regarded at different times in different cultures find a range of views, of course.[81] Yet there is a recurrent tendency to see children as something other than full members of the community. This is particularly evident in the case of sick and disabled children, who have been subjected to infanticide and abandonment in many eras and cultures.[82] Infanticide "is made easier by cultural belief that a child is not fully human until accepted as a member of the social group."[83] Permitting pediatric euthanasia and assisted suicide in the United States would allow this historically recurrent pattern full flower in our culture and time with the officially sanctioned deaths of children.

Indeed, modern European history suggests special cautions. The only governmentally permitted pediatric euthanasia in this century has been the Nazi euthanasia program. And that program began by euthanizing ill and disabled children.[84] Use of the Nazi analogy requires care.[85] The primary disanalogy between present-day calls for the legitimization of euthanasia and Nazi euthanasia is that Nazi euthanasia was involuntary (to say the least), while present-day calls are for voluntary euthanasia. But the disanalogy begins to break down and the analogy starts to strengthen in focusing on pediatric cases. Annas and Grodin recount in their book on Nazi physicians that "[h]ospital archives are full of letters from parents requesting their children be granted euthanasia."[86] Clearly the Nazis also euthanized children without parental request, and indeed over horrified objection. But the point is that when present-day proponents of pediatric euthanasia focus on parental request to show how present-day practice would be distinguishable from Nazi practice, they overstate the difference. Parents may request the practice in both contexts. Moreover, in both contexts parentally requested euthanasia is not voluntary from the child's point of view. The only way pediatric euthanasia or assisted suicide could be characterized as voluntary from the child's standpoint would be by awaiting the child's development of and exercise of the capacity for voluntary choice. In fact, the Dutch experience, with reports of young children euthanized when incapable of voluntary choice and with the Dutch Pediatric Association advocating pediatric euthanasia as long as the parents agree, suggests that the lessons of Nazi pediatric euthanasia have some applicability to current practice.

Even very recent U.S. events counsel caution. In the United States societal commitment to meeting the health needs of children has been marked by ambivalence. At the federal level, the Medicaid program (a key source of health care coverage for poor children) has been vulnerable to cuts in the past, and recent welfare reform has in fact cut support for poor and disabled children, while new federal legislation promises to extend health insurance to at least some of the millions of children uninsured.[87] With the commitment to children waxing and waning, many wonder what ever happened to earlier calls for children's rights?[88] Against this background it is hard to see pediatric euthanasia as an act of beneficence.

The one category of minors in which euthanasia and assisted suicide might be defended on grounds akin to those used for adults is adolescents. Many of them may seem able to make a competent and voluntary choice. There is disagreement, however, about the age at which an adolescent might make such a choice. As noted above, Orlowski et al. suggest that children can give effective consent starting at 14, but a number of authors argue that true competence requires cognitive capacity plus maturity of judgment, which sets in later.[89] Holder also hesitates to draw the line at 14. She concedes that, "Most literature on the subject of the dying child indicates that prior to fourteen or fifteen years of age most children do not understand the real implications of death."[90] Yet even when an adolescent older than 14 opts for death, Holder argues that the physician should instead follow the directions of objecting parents.

There are two special groups of adolescents who probably should be analyzed as adults: emancipated minors and those found to be mature minors. Emancipated minors are those treated as adults under state law, often because they are not living at home and are self-supporting. Mature minors are those found able to make decisions for themselves. Holder's position is conservative: she still urges caution, at least in the former case, in the absence of parental consent.[91] However, the argument for treating these two groups as adult decision-makers is strong.

Apart from emancipated and mature minors, there are problems with simply applying the justifications for adult euthanasia and assisted suicide to adolescents. First, adolescents' autonomy and self-determination are in a state of coming-to-be. One cannot know that at any particular moment in adolescence the minor has reached the developmental point of being able to reflect on death in keeping with her settled values and to make a choice that is authentically her own. Doing that requires not only the cognitive capacity to understand information, but also a maturity and sense of self. Of course, one also cannot be sure that people have reached this developmental point just because they reach 18 or 21, when the law deems them to have done so. But the age of majority reflects a social judgment that by then a great many people have achieved the capacity for competent choice and, indeed, are making choices for which they should be held accountable.

Second, adolescents who remain economically and otherwise dependent on their parents may not make fully voluntary choices. Certainly, adults too may have economic and emotional dependencies. Yet in both adults and adolescents, pronounced dependency may reach the point of compromising voluntariness. This is one reason that health care professionals are often urged to check whether an adult Jehovah's Witness really wants to refuse blood by consulting the patient alone, apart from family and religious authorities. In an adolescent, who may never have known independence, who may not yet have had the chance to choose (through marriage or otherwise) those on whom to be dependent, and who may not yet have separated physically or psychologically from parents, dependence is surely pronounced. Thus the adult justification of voluntary choice cannot simply be applied.

Confronting the Normative Questions

Pediatric euthanasia and assisted suicide thus require their own analysis to see whether they can be justified and their dangers defused. But because the pediatric population is heterogeneous—ranging from the neonate to the adolescent capable of extensive participation in treatment decisions—the analysis must proceed in three parts.

First, euthanasia and assisted suicide with the request or agreement of adolescents who can participate quite fully in the decisional process requires an analysis that treats these individuals' preferences with respect. This is the clear trend in approaching decisions about forgoing life-sustaining treatment.[92] As noted above, scholars frequently assert that adolescents starting at age 14 have the capacity to make health care decisions as an adult would.[93] Though I discuss below dispute on that point, and the law does not treat the choices of such adolescents as strictly equivalent to the choices of competent adults (at least when the adolescent is not an emancipated or mature minor under state law), analyzing whether the minor's wish authorizes assisted suicide or euthanasia requires proceeding initially by analogy to the competent adult. Yet ultimately, it also requires attending to research on adolescent decision-making and the advantages of delaying the age at which the patient may authorize assisted suicide or euthanasia. It also demands analysis of whether the state's interest in preventing assisted suicide and euthanasia among adolescents is stronger than among competent adults.

The second part of the analysis applies to children at an earlier developmental stage. These are children old enough to communicate thoughtfully but clearly not yet able to decide as an adult would. They can often participate in decision-making, but not fully. Commentators frequently assert that 7 is the age at which children can give meaningful assent,[94] though there are some who claim the age is younger.[95] The key problem in this age group is that children cannot be assumed to decide competently and voluntarily. Claims that they have a right to assisted suicide or euthanasia are thereby weakened. And the state's interest in preventing euthanasia and assisted suicide—practices even less voluntary and less competently chosen than among adolescents—is commensurately stronger. Once the ability of these children to decide for themselves is dismissed, we are left with the question of whether the decisions of others (the parents or guardians and medical personnel) should authorize euthanasia and assisted suicide. This leads into discussion of the third age group, for whom that question is central.

The third and final age group includes newborns, infants, and children younger than 7. This is the pediatric population in which euthanasia has most often been advocated. Here the child does not meaningfully participate at all in decision-making. For this population, euthanasia is nonvoluntary, with no element of consent or even effective assent from the child. Problems with empowering parents and others to authorize euthanasia come to the fore, as does the state's interest in preventing euthanasia when there is no trace of individual choice.

We turn first, then, to the case of adolescents, individuals approaching the age of majority but still minors. The age of majority is, of course, an arbitrary line. It has some correlation with increased maturity, but individual variations are enormous; some people are more mature at 15 than others at 20. The law compensates for this to some degree by recognizing the intermediate categories of emancipated and mature minors. Yet even many adolescents who do not qualify for these categories can participate quite fully in decisions about their treatment. They may request assisted suicide or euthanasia, or may agree with the suggestion of parents or others that assisted suicide or euthanasia is the proper course.

What advocacy there is for legitimating assisted suicide or euthanasia at the election of such adolescents rests on the argument that starting around age 14 they can make such choices as competently and voluntarily as adults. Orlowski et al. argue that "The Dutch practice of euthanasia for adolescent patients with an adequate degree of decisional capacity . . . can be viewed as an expanded and consistent application . . . of proposals for voluntary active euthanasia." They maintain that "it would be inappropriate to rule out their ability, based on age alone." Thus these adolescents should be treated as adults: "[their] wishes for euthanasia should be honored even over parental objections."[96]

Whether euthanasia or assisted suicide should be allowed in these cases thus depends first on whether these practices should be legitimated for competent adults. That debate is far more familiar than the specifically pediatric analysis attempted in this chapter. Authors have written at length on the nonpediatric issues,[97] and many of us have suggested that euthanasia and assisted suicide should not be legitimated, even for competent adults.

Advocacy for assisted suicide or euthanasia for competent adults hinges on two claims: that physician duties of beneficence authorize involvement in these practices, and that respect for patient self-determination creates a right to them. Yet several arguments cast doubt on these propositions.

First, the beneficence claim is highly problematic. The fight over assisted suicide and euthanasia is not about the right of patients—be they adults or children—to kill themselves; suicide has been decriminalized in the United States.[98] Instead, the question is what physicians may do, whether they may assist suicide or perform euthanasia. It is clear that legitimating these practices would fundamentally change the traditional core commitment of physicians to "give no deadly drug, even if asked."[99] Many, including myself, have cautioned against this change, arguing that its effects on medical education, the patient-physician relationship, and the interaction at the bedside would be calamitous.[100] The rule against physicians killing stands as a safeguard against abuse of the nearly unique powers society already grants doctors over life and death. For an individual physician, managing those powers means dealing with ambivalence at the bedside of an extremely ill or disabled patient. Burt describes the urge both to rescue and to obliterate from sight.[101] The prohibition on assisted suicide and euthanasia keeps the physician from enacting the negative side of that ambivalence.

Some proponents nonetheless argue that traditional duties of physician beneficence and nonabandonment permit assisted suicide and euthanasia.[102] Yet it is a strange view that counts intentionally ending the life of a patient as fulfillment of these duties; the physician eradicates the patient's problem—be it depression or uncontrolled pain, for example—by intentionally eradicating the patient.[103] The view is particularly strange given the option of fulfilling those duties by instead rendering good care, including expert pain relief, palliative care, and termination of life-sustaining treatment if requested.

In fact, these less fatal alternatives have not been effectively tried as yet. Patients currently cannot count on getting expert pain relief and palliative care.[104] And although rights to refuse treatment and use advance directives have been much proclaimed, a gap persists between this rhetoric and clinical realities.[105] Thus we do not really know whether we need assisted suicide and euthanasia. Nor do we know how many patients and which ones would seriously request these practices if pain relief, palliative care, and terminal care were as good as they should be.

Once analysis exposes these problems with claims of beneficence, arguments based on patients' rights come to the fore. In ethical terms, these arguments are framed in the language of patient autonomy or self-determination; in legal terms, advocates have claimed a constitutionally protected liberty interest[106] or relied on the Constitution's guarantee of equal protection.[107] But talk of patients' rights does not succeed in legitimizing assisted suicide and euthanasia either.[108] While law and ethics clearly recognize a right to be free of unwanted bodily invasion even if the predicted consequence is death, there is no established right to a third party's assistance with bodily invasion for the purpose of ending one's own life.[109] The latter exists nowhere in the text of the Constitution or the traditions of this country. The Supreme Court found a clear difference between the right to refuse treatment and assisted suicide in *Vacco v. Quill* and *Washington v. Glucksberg*; indeed, the Justices recognized the difference repeatedly in *Cruzan* by framing the constitutional right there narrowly as a right to be free of bodily invasion, thus excluding more active practices.[110] Nor should the states' decriminalization of suicide be misconstrued as creation of a right to suicide, much less to assistance.[111]

Thus both beneficence and rights arguments are shaky grounds on which to legitimate assisted suicide and euthanasia. But both have a further defect: they tend to ignore social context and how these practices would likely play out in the United States.[112] Were euthanasia and assisted suicide to be legitimated, we would have to worry about how they would work not only for those well off but also for the more than 40 million who lack health insurance and thus the resources to cope with serious disease.[113] The United States remains the only developed country that fails to guarantee health coverage for all.[114] It seems easier to grant a right to assisted suicide and euthanasia than a right to health care and coverage, but this is a rights strategy that differentially benefits the well off. For those without ready access to options at the end of life, instead securing access to assisted suicide and euthanasia is hardly a net gain.

One response might be that the rights and practices could be carefully tailored so that patients must be contemporaneously competent and voluntarily requesting the practice, must be evaluated to see if less fatal options should be offered, and must in fact be offered those options. But the Dutch data on physicians failing to report the practices for monitoring,[115] and on the practice slipping beyond the competent,[116] give empirical fuel to long-standing concerns that we could not contain these practices, once they were legitimated for a subgroup. And arguments that termination of treatment and abortion jurisprudence ground a constitutional right to assisted suicide further fuel the concern, since neither termination of treatment nor abortion has been confined to competent adults.

Moreover, the supposed rules governing termination of treatment and good terminal care are not yet consistently observed in clinical practice. We have a long way to go in the United States before good pain relief and palliative care are routinely offered, established rights to refuse treatment and use advance directives are reliably honored, and the "art" of caring for the dying is widely applied. So there is little reason to believe that best-case conditions would apply to euthanasia and assisted suicide.

All of these arguments, which have been developed elsewhere with regard to adult patients, apply as well to assisted suicide and euthanasia in adolescents who are "near-adults," even when not emancipated or found to be mature minors. Indeed, those arguments acquire greater force. Whatever problems adults have had in getting good pain relief, respect for treatment refusals, and sensitive terminal care, there are reasons to believe minors have had more difficulty. As noted above, pain relief, for example, is notoriously bad for minors. And minors will in most cases have fewer economic resources and less bargaining power than adults. If terminal care requires even more improvement for adolescents than for adults, it is commensurately harder to argue that beneficence commands the drastic step of assisting suicide or euthanasia.

Moreover, the rights argument applied to adolescents is flawed by the fact that we cannot count on adolescents' choices about assisted suicide and euthanasia to be competent enough, to exhibit enough stability of values and preferences, and to be voluntary enough to merit the deference we arguably should pay to comparable adult decisions. On competence, Weithorn and Scherer review the data on adolescents' capacity to make decisions to participate in research. They describe a division in the literature, with "[s]ome authors [concluding] that the cognitive capacities required for consent to . . . treatment or research typically mature to adult or near-adult levels by . . . ages fourteen or fifteen," but "[o]thers [urging] greater caution in reaching conclusions as to adolescents' competency."[117] They discuss a study frequently cited for the proposition that adolescents start at 14 to reason as adults do. But they note that some adolescents in the study did reason differently than adults on one of the four dilemmas presented, involving the prospect of changes in physical appearance. Though Weithorn and Scherer end up arguing that adolescents 14 and older are competent to consent to research and treatment, others such as Scott and colleagues disagree with this categorical conclusion, arguing that the research in this area is too thin, and that it emphasizes cognitive skills to the exclusion of maturity of judgment.[118]

Adolescent choices to die carry more serious and irrevocable consequences than nonfatal treatment and research decisions, of course, and so one would expect a stricter standard of competence to be applied.[119] Moreover, the standard should be stricter for choosing suicide or euthanasia than choosing to refuse life-sustaining treatment; the former choices make death certain and swift, because once the act is initiated there is no opportunity for a change of mind or correcting error. It is not clear that the research to date can support the conclusion that adolescents 14 and over can ponder future options and choose certain death with the competence of an adult. While the occasional adolescent might, creating a rule that would extend a right to assisted suicide or euthanasia to this entire class seems untenable.

The finality and swiftness of suicide and euthanasia similarly raise the question of whether adolescents exhibit the same stability of relevant values and preferences as adults. This, again, is an empirical question. Certainly, descriptions of adolescence as a time of rapid change, including in values and perspective, are commonplace. They counsel caution before treating adolescent choices for suicide or euthanasia as sufficiently fixed to merit irrevocable, fatal action.

Related to this is the question of whether these adolescent choices are made with the degree of voluntariness we would demand of adults. If adolescent choices are influenced considerably by external circumstances over which the adolescent lacks control, and if those choices are quite changeable in response to changes in circumstances, voluntariness is compromised. Voluntary choice requires a certain degree of independence from the demands of others and the constraints of the moment. Volumes have been written, of course, on what constitutes free choice. But reviewing the data on adolescents, Weithorn and Scherer are more troubled by the question of whether they act with the requisite degree of volition than by the capacity question discussed above. "Not until . . . [mid- to late-adolescence] are minors more self-reliant than are younger adolescents and less responsive to the pressure of social factors."[120] The authors cite research "indicat[ing] that adolescents may exercise less voluntariness than do young adults."[121] And adolescents are likely to be more constrained by relevant circumstances than adults, less able to dispute insurance limits, for instance, or to marshall needed financial resources. This, too, counsels caution before regarding adolescent choices for assisted suicide or euthanasia as sufficiently voluntary.

Yet even if adolescents were regarded as making such choices in a sufficiently competent, stable, and voluntary way, the state has stronger interests in banning assisted suicide and euthanasia for adolescents than for adults. So even if a future court were to conclude that adults have a constitutionally protected interest in assisted suicide that is not overcome by countervailing state interests (a court revisiting the federal Constitution after *Washington v. Glucksberg* and *Vacco v. Quill,* or perhaps construing a state constitution), any such interest of adolescents may well be overcome. One state interest traditionally recognized is an interest, indeed a duty, to protect the vulnerable, especially from death. Even the Ninth Circuit opinion finding a constitutional right to assisted suicide in *Compassion in Dying* (later reversed by the Supreme Court) recognized this state interest. The court found the interest weak when an adult is terminally ill and competently electing the procedure. Yet language in the opinion suggested the state interest would not be weak in the case of an adolescent. The state had cited suicide statistics among the young. The court, after acknowledging that the state had an interest in preventing suicide, conceded that "suicide by teenagers and young adults is especially tragic."[122] And the judges went on to conclude that it was among competent adults who were terminally ill that the state's interest in preserving life was diminished. The court further said that the state could permissibly regulate assisted suicide to make sure patients were "truly competent."[123]

Hoberman suggests that the state may have an additional interest. He argues that allowing assisted suicide among adolescents would convey state approval of adolescent suicide itself. He fears a contagion effect in this age group. Moreover, "no adolescent should possess the right to take his or her own life; they are not equipped mentally, emotionally, or experientially to make . . . [that] decision."[124] Thus the state has a strong interest in maintaining the value of adolescent life, especially among adolescents themselves.

One might respond that the state has the same countervailing interest when patients forgo life-sustaining treatment, yet those interests have not been regarded as overcoming patients' rights and parents' authority to refuse in adolescents' cases. But state approval of a right to refuse treatment merely communicates that individuals have a strong interest in being free of unwanted treatment. It does not bless an adolescent's taking active steps to end her own life, or have another do so.

Thus there are ample grounds on which to reject empowering adolescents to opt for assisted suicide or euthanasia, certainly when the adolescent is neither emancipated nor found to be a mature minor. The arguments against legitimating the practices for adults apply with even greater force to adolescents. Yet even if the right were recognized for competent adults, there are strong reasons to hesitate before extending the right to adolescents. And there are stronger state interests to justify a ban.

We next turn away from adolescents to children younger than 14 but able to give assent, those roughly 7 to 14. Children in this age group clearly are not competent to give adequate consent. Thus, debate about this group must focus on whether parental consent combined with the child's assent can justify assisted suicide or euthanasia. This is because that combination of consent and assent is the recommended approach to decisions about life-sustaining treatment.[125]

This combination approach, however, abandons a commitment to the necessity of voluntary and competent patient choice to an even greater extent than adolescent decision-making would. The younger child is likely to be extremely influenced by the parental choice. Weithorn and Scherer maintain that "[c]hildren and young adolescents typically exercise less autonomy and less resistance to social influence than do adults. . . . They are . . . more vulnerable to . . . [manipulation] and are less likely to view themselves as being in control of their destiny. Therefore, they are unlikely to be capable of giving voluntary consent."[126]

In keeping with the Dutch emphasis on voluntariness, the Dutch Medical Association argues that the euthanasia decision is such a personal one that only the child herself can decide.[127] Yet this overlooks problems with the competence of children younger than 14. Data indicate, for example, that 9-year-olds understand less information, or understand it less fully, than do adults.[128] Younger children may be competent to assent, but competent assent demands less decisional skill than legally valid consent.[129]

The problems involved in recognizing a right of adolescents to assisted suicide or euthanasia are thus even more serious when considering younger children. Moreover, the state's interest in protecting the lives of these children is at least as strong as among adolescents, given that younger children are more vulnerable and less self-determining than adolescents. Finally, the state's entitlement to regulate so as to confine the practices to the truly competent would exclude these younger children even more certainly.

What remains by way of argument for assisted suicide and euthanasia in this age group is the claim that the parents or guardian should be able to make the choice for these patients. Yet this claim raises a host of problems. They are problems that have been most often examined in considering neonatal and infant euthanasia.

We finally turn, then, to newborns, infants, and children younger than 7. In this category, claims of patient self-determination fall away. The parents or guardian, working with the medical caregiver, make the treatment decisions. Most children this young are probably incapable of suicide, leaving euthanasia as the primary practice in question. Yet were euthanasia to be legitimated for this category of children, the practices could not be described as chosen by the patient or voluntary. Instead, a third party is deciding.

Euthanasia in this category of children thus cannot be justified by relying on autonomy or self-determination. That entire branch of argumentation for legitimizing assisted suicide and euthanasia simply does not apply. The remaining question is whether nonvoluntary euthanasia can be justified. A lengthy debate has already concluded that forgoing life-sustaining treatment can be justified and assigned to parental discretion within certain limits, as long as the practice is in the best interests of the child. Analysis of euthanasia must proceed from that starting point.

Indeed, the two practices are factually linked in a number of cases in which treatment was foregone but the adults then felt the child did not die quickly enough.[130] We see further cases in which the child for whom treatment was foregone was not dying imminently, but life was felt to be of poor quality, painful, and perhaps limited in duration.[131] Cases such as this starkly raise the question of whether permitting treatment withdrawal should now lead us to permit euthanasia. Some have in fact argued that there is no principled distinction between the two.[132]

But that flies in the face of the distinction long drawn between stopping treatment to allow disease to take its course and intentionally, directly taking the life of a child.[133] The latter, a form of infanticide,[134] provokes widespread abhorrence, at least in this era and culture. Kuhse and Singer survey the history of infanticide in various cultures to argue that our current prohibition is deviant and the practice should be permitted.[135] But Post challenges their history.[136] Moreover, their argument would homogenize all cultures. Indeed, the United States *is* deviant in cultural respects: we live in a two-centuries-old constitutional democracy that defends individual freedoms. We no longer tolerate slavery, women are not chattel, and children are not property. In fact, the problem for much of our history has been that we were not deviant enough; it took much of our history to eradicate slavery, secure property rights and the vote for women, and embrace child-centered standards in custody disputes and other matters directly affecting children. Our "deviant" respect for even incompetent individuals should continue to make us wary of authorizing others to kill them.

Some find this inconsistent with permitting abortion; they argue that we do, in fact, permit infanticide before birth.[137] Yet balking at killing beings who by all accounts are full persons is not inconsistent with permitting abortion.[138] There is no agreement and recognition in law that fetuses are full persons.[139] Thus a prohibition against killing full persons by euthanasia does not clearly apply to fetuses. Second, even if the fetus late in gestation becomes "like a baby,"[140] states are permitted to restrict postviability abortions to those in which the pregnant women's health or life is at stake.[141] The rules governing abortion thus are consistent with a postbirth prohibition of infanticide; as birth approaches, we permit greater restrictions on abortion. Finally, abortion is permitted because the person in whose body the fetus resides retains rights of liberty, privacy, and equal treatment. As technology now stands, the only way she can be free of an unwanted or health-threatening pregnancy is through abortion.[142] But once the child is born, no right of the parents requires their killing the child. And postbirth, the child is a being with full rights in a society that does not permit citizens to kill one another, even in familial relationships.

Thus there is a coherent basis for the abhorrence widely felt at infanticide, and that abhorrence can be reconciled with abortion jurisprudence. Instinctively, many have drawn a line between forgoing treatment to allow disease to take its course and intentionally, directly causing death through euthanasia in newborns and other children unable to participate in treatment decisions. We have drawn a line, but should we continue to do so?

In fact, the troubled experience with forgoing treatment in this category of children may be the strongest argument for not permitting euthanasia. The many "Baby Doe" cases, associated legislation, and extensive commentary[143] evidence the controversy that has surrounded parental refusal of life-sustaining treatment. A parent's reaction to the birth and burden of an extremely ill or disabled child is often complex and may be ambivalent.[144] Thus great effort has been devoted to limiting and channeling parental decision-making so that parents do not favor their own interests over the child's best interests.[145] It seems clear that parents deciding in the child's best interests might forgo treatment whose burdens to the child appear to exceed its benefits. They might also apply that decisional standard to opt for effective pain relief and palliative care, even if that requires sedating the child to unconsciousness. Yet given these options, it is hard to see how the child's best interests might dictate going further to euthanasia. Once the child is receiving aggressive pain relief and palliative care, and perhaps is fully sedated, no interest of the child commands direct steps to end life. The only argument for those steps is based on the parents' or medical caregiver's sensibilities. But in the realm of forgoing treatment, we have generally rejected those sensibilities as justifiable grounds on which to make a life-and-death decision for the child; the child's own interests must dictate the outcome. The rule for euthanasia cannot be laxer; if anything, direct killing should demand more strictly child-centered standards. Yet a truly child-centered standard cannot be formulated that rationalizes euthanasia in this category of children.

Even if a child is permanently unconscious, it is hard to justify euthanasia. Despite claims that these children lack interests entirely, such children are not objects to be used and abused at will. They are live human beings to whom we owe respectful decisions focused on their own circumstances. Remaining child-centered in these cases would permit forgoing treatment, as the child would never experience the benefits of treatment. Forgoing treatment will then generally lead to death. There is no child-centered argument for speeding the process of dying through euthanasia. A permanently unconscious child experiences no pain, suffering, or other harms in the interim.

To permit euthanasia rather than insisting on and relying upon good pain relief, palliative care, and terminal care for young children is thus to give up on a child-centered standard. And it gives up not only in particularly hard cases but also as a matter of explicit decision rules. It returns us to an era in which parents could consign a child to death for their own convenience. It flies in the face of the decision rules we have already developed, such as forgoing treatment based on the child's best interests and refusing to allow parents to forgo such treatment based on their own religious convictions.[146]

Giving up on a child-centered standard would have implications beyond the pediatric realm. After all, insistence on a child-centered approach is the pediatric application of a broader insistence that treatment decisions be patient-centered, whatever the patient's age or level of decisional capacity. This insistence is fundamental to the U.S. law and ethics of medical treatment.[147] Thus treatment decisions are governed by patients' preferences or, when those cannot be ascertained or extrapolated, patients' best interests.[148] It is this devotion to serving the individual patient that now causes quandaries in considering rationing, allocation schemes, and managed care approaches in which beneficial care is sometimes deliberately withheld. As Callahan has argued, such efforts to limit resources make this a particularly inauspicious time to abandon a patient-centered commitment by accepting active killing, especially of the most vulnerable patients among us.[149]

Performing euthanasia cannot be seen as serving the child; it only succeeds in granting the parents' wish. Professional ethics are transformed, and physicians abandon the commitment to serve the patient above all. And they do that precisely at a time when their commitment to serving individual patients is being tested by resource scarcity and the conflicts of interest intrinsic to managed care. Physicians thereby also abandon progress toward seeing the child as fully human, able to experience pain and discomfort, and deserving of adequate pain relief and palliative care—a being with interests in her own right, separate from parental interests.[150]

Empowering parents and guardians to authorize nonvoluntary euthanasia in children thus cannot be justified by analogy to forgoing life-sustaining treatment. Nor is there any plausible argument that these young children are rights bearers voluntarily and competently exercising their rights. Finally, state interests in protecting the vulnerable from being killed at the direction of others reach their zenith in this population. Those Dutch authors who insist on a patient's voluntary choice and thus object to euthanasia and assisted suicide in young patients who cannot provide it are surely right.[151]

Toward an Honest Debate

Reasonable people will differ on the question of whether to legitimate assisted suicide and euthanasia for competent adults. I have argued, here and elsewhere, that at least for now we should be reluctant to legitimate them in the United States.[152] We have millions of citizens who are uninsured; a history of deficient health care for minorities, children, the poor, and women;[153] and documented deficiencies in pain relief, palliative care, and social support for the ill and disabled.[154] Were we to correct even some of these problems, it is not clear what demand for assisted suicide and euthanasia would remain.

But the reasons for rejecting assisted suicide and euthanasia for children and adolescents are more compelling. There is a long history of taking children's lives to serve others' ends. Even parental decisions may be born of ambivalence toward an ill or disabled child. And pain relief, palliative care, and social supports for children have been particularly poor. Finally, permitting euthanasia of incompetents evokes some of the worst horrors of twentieth-century history; it is a path we properly fear to go down again.

Thus one might expect contemporary advocates of assisted suicide and euthanasia to emphasize that only competent adults are candidates, while children and adolescents are not. After all, advocacy based on respect for patient autonomy and self-determination does not apply to younger children, and applies only problematically to adolescents. And state interests in protecting these populations and preventing nonvoluntary killing are undoubtedly strong. But in fact, advocates have been slow to condemn pediatric euthanasia and assisted suicide. Even as the Dutch begin to perform and defend the practices, the U.S. debate about assisted suicide and euthanasia largely ignores the pediatric issues. Children remain at the margin.

This failure to speak openly about the pediatric side allows the debate about assisted suicide and euthanasia to continue as if these practices only applied to competent adults and always rested on patient choice. Yet the Dutch experience and cases from the United States show that this is a fiction. It is a fiction that unfortunately rests on our historical willingness to regard children as less than full people, their medical care as less important than adults', and their interests to be a function of their parents'.

Debating assisted suicide and euthanasia now requires abandoning this fiction. If assisted suicide and euthanasia are to be legitimated in the United States, advocates must say whether minors will be included. If so, those advocates bear the extraordinary burden of demonstrating how that can be reconciled with American law and physician ethics. And if minors are *not* to be included, someone must persuasively explain how we will avoid proceeding down the path the Dutch now tread, allowing the deliberate killing of children.

6

Religious Viewpoints

JAMES F. CHILDRESS

Powerful arguments for assisted suicide and voluntary active euthanasia invoke two major constellations of moral ideas: on the one hand, the values of personal autonomy (self-determination or self-rule) and respect for personal autonomy; on the other hand, the disvalue of human suffering and the value of compassionate responses to that suffering. The slogan "death with dignity" often combines these values, with "dignity" representing both patients' control over their dying and their freedom from pain and suffering. The vision of "death with dignity" sustains vigorous efforts to legalize assisted suicide and active euthanasia. However, major religious traditions strongly defend "medical pacifism" and oppose a "culture of death" that justifies these modes of selective killing.[1]

It is not surprising that religious communities have regularly formulated principles and rules for physicians and patients and their families—after all, medicine deals with birth, illness, suffering, and death, all matters that typically fall under religious systems of belief, ritual, and practice. Some of these principles and rules, also unsurprisingly, indicate what should and may be done when a patient is terminally ill and experiences extreme and uncontrollable pain and suffering.

Religious perspectives appear in particular communities and traditions. I will focus primarily on Judaism, Roman Catholicism, and Protestantism as major Western theistic traditions, with only a few observations about other traditions—among other religions, Islam is close to these three traditions on suicide, assisted suicide, and active euthanasia, while Buddhism and Hinduism display more ambiguity about these actions; for example, they have historically accepted some acts of suicide, such as those of holy men.[2]

Despite important differences, Judaism, Roman Catholicism, and Protestantism share certain major outlooks and norms that bear on biomedical ethics. The common language of "Judaeo-Christian tradition" is not wholly satisfactory because it masks much that is distinctive about each one. Nevertheless, decisions about life and death within these traditions are structured in part by a shared perspective on God's sovereignty: God is directly or indirectly in control of life and death—He giveth life and He taketh it away—and His will, whether expressed through revelation or through natural law, should be respected. In general, then, a "good death" occurs within the broad context set by this perspective, including its significant moral limits. This fundamental belief in God's sovereignty is only the first of several religious beliefs that challenge secular (and some religious) arguments in support of suicide, assisted suicide, and euthanasia.

These three traditions all view the Hebrew Bible, what Christians call the Old Testament, as scripture, and it at least partially shapes their conception of God and God's relation to the world as well as the meaning and significance of human life and death. It is not their only authority, however: Christianity recognizes another scripture, the New Testament, and both Christianity and Judaism include traditions of interpretation along with appeals to reason, to philosophical approaches, and to experience as other important sources of authority.

The general opposition within these traditions to suicide, assisted suicide, and active euthanasia, as three closely related acts, rests finally on religious-moral arguments against suicide. After all, "voluntary euthanasia is actually a form of suicide; it is taking one's own life, albeit with the assistance *(assisted suicide)* or the intervention *(intervention)* of another. Suicide requires that an individual (1) *intend his or her own death* and (2) *act in such a way as to bring it about.*"[3] The moral wrongness of assisted suicide and voluntary active euthanasia stems from the wrongness of suicide itself. If suicide itself is not justifiable, then assisted suicide and voluntary active euthanasia are not justifiable. Both assisted suicide and voluntary active euthanasia involve agents other than the one whose life is ended; they differ only in their final agency, that is, who performs the final act, the one whose death is brought about (assisted suicide) or someone else (voluntary active euthanasia). I will only mention here and there *non*voluntary euthanasia (without a patient's will) or *in*voluntary euthanasia (against a patient's will).[4] If suicide, assisted suicide, and voluntary active euthanasia cannot be justified within a particular tradition, then it is highly unlikely that nonvoluntary and involuntary euthanasia can be justified.

Even though these three traditions articulate a broad consensus that suicide, assisted suicide, and voluntary active euthanasia are generally wrong, we must state this consensus carefully and with appropriate qualifications. More specifically, we cannot fully understand any tradition's position on such actions until we grasp two dimensions or aspects of their religious-moral norms: (1) their meaning, range, or scope, and (2) their weight or stringency (as absolute, prima facie, or relative).

Not all religious thinkers, to take one example, absolutely oppose suicide and voluntary active euthanasia. Some defend prima facie or presumptively binding rules that leave open the possibility of selectively justified acts. To take another example, even an apparently absolute moral rule against suicide may incorporate what others would consider "exceptions," but it may do so as a *specification* of its meaning rather than as an actual *exception*. Hence, without ever justifying acts of suicide, a religious tradition may specify the meaning, range, and scope of its rules so as to accommodate acts that another tradition would oppose as acts of suicide. Thus, it is important to note just how these three traditions distinguish some refusals of life-sustaining medical treatments from suicide and some types of passive euthanasia, that is, letting die, from active euthanasia, that is, killing. Some "exceptional" cases may appear under these other categories.

Other factors also qualify generalizations about religious opposition to suicide and related acts. First, differences in the structure and authority of religious organizations are clearly relevant—some traditions, for instance, stress the authority of the local religious community, while others stress hierarchical institutional authority.

Second, not all the participants in a particular religious community accept its official positions on suicide, euthanasia, and other matters. Some participants silently object, while others explicitly dissent. Silent opposition or explicit dissent may appeal to an alternative strand of interpretation of scripture or tradition, or it may appeal to reason (for example, by arguing that traditional distinctions between killing and letting die or between ordinary and extraordinary means of treatment are not rationally defensible) or to experience (for example, by stressing the extreme pain and suffering patients sometimes experience while dying).

Third, official religious communities often recognize differences between what we might term moral and pastoral responses to acts—for instance, apparent acts of suicide or attempted suicide or active euthanasia may actually be *excused* in some circumstances because of judgments about the agents' lack of responsibility, even though these acts remain *unjustified*. In particular, religious communities do not usually deny customary burial practices to those who apparently committed suicide on the grounds that they were not fully responsible for their actions, perhaps because they were temporarily insane as a result of extreme pain and suffering.

Shared Religious Perspectives

In addition to the broad theme of divine sovereignty already noted, Jewish, Roman Catholic, and Protestant traditions share the theme of *covenant* as expressed, for instance, in God's covenant with humanity following the flood, with Israel, and, specifically for Christians, in Christ. Sometimes covenant is used as a general category for various relationships with God as creator, provider or orderer, and redeemer, as well as with human creatures who also image God. Human covenants, such as medicine, can mirror and reflect God's covenants, and such covenants share several features: They are rooted in events or actions; they engender moral community; they endure over time; and, in contrast to contracts, their terms cannot be fully specified. One of the most influential Protestant works in modern medical ethics, Paul Ramsey's *The Patient as Person,* takes covenant faithfulness as the primary category for understanding medicine and its responsibilities in light of the Christian faith, and, for him, it supports a strong condemnation of active euthanasia.[5]

God's covenantal action, Christianity and Judaism agree, begins with his creation of human beings in his own *image,* and this conviction has important implications for decisions about life and death. In *Evangelium Vitae* (The Gospel of Life), Pope John Paul II stresses that "in the biblical narrative, the difference between man and other creatures is shown above all by the fact that only the creation of man is presented as the result of a special decision on the part of God . . . to establish a *particular and specific bond* with the Creator . . . The life which God offers to man is a gift by which God shares something of himself with his creature" (emphasis added). According to the biblical account, "Then God said, 'Let us make man in our image, after our likeness; and let them have dominion . . .' So God created man in his own image, in the image of God he created him; male and female he created them. And God blessed them, and God said to them, 'Be fruitful and multiply, and fill the earth and subdue it; and have dominion over . . . every living thing that moves upon the earth'" (Gen. 1:26ff; cf. 5:1 and 9:6; see also 1 Cor. 11:7 and James 3:9).

Although the image of God has been variously interpreted as reason, free will, and spiritual capacities, including the capacity for self-transcendence, major strands of both Judaism and Christianity view the human person as an animated body or embodied soul or spirit, and as relational rather than atomistic. No doubt religious convictions about the creation of human beings in God's image partially overlap or converge with secular views of autonomy and respect for autonomy, but, for Judaism and Christianity, both embodiment and relationality prevent easy identification with such secular views.[6] For example, one Protestant theologian criticizes modern secular views of autonomy for holding that "when it comes to life and death, therefore, each individual is moral sovereign over his or her own existence. Of course, the Christian community would judge unacceptable such an elevation of human autonomy," in part because it implies that individuals own their bodies and have unlimited dispositional authority over them.[7] By contrast, Judaism and Christianity hold that divine ownership and dispositional authority set the context for human trusteeship or stewardship.

As Genesis 1:26ff indicates, scriptural directions for agents to image or to obey God also include human dominion, which is most often conceived as trusteeship or stewardship rather than unlimited control. According to *Evangelium Vitae,* "Man's lordship . . . is not absolute, but ministerial: It is a real reflection of the unique and infinite lordship of God" (#52). The divine authorization of human dominion, which presupposes that human beings are in but also distinguished from the rest of nature, is critically important, for instance, in debates about human responsibility in developing and using biomedical technologies to extend human life, to enhance its quality, and to meet various human needs and desires.

Human agents, created in God's image, have a *negative* obligation to refrain from killing themselves or others who are also created in God's image. This obligation is stated not only in the Decalogue, or Ten Commandments ("Thou shalt not kill") but also in the covenant with Noah after the flood: "Whoever sheds the blood of man, by man shall his blood be shed; for God made man in his own image" (Gen. 9:6). Although the phrase "sanctity of life" often appears in modern religious discussions, it is not biblical, and there is some debate about its appropriateness. Nevertheless, it provides one way to express the intrinsic value of human life, as an implication of God's creation. It is usually held to be knowable outside religious contexts as part of the Noahide covenant or the natural law. Despite the widespread affirmation of the sanctity of life, human life does not have an *absolute* value in mainstream Judaism and Christianity—for example, these traditions permit and even encourage martyrdom in some contexts, usually accept killing in war and in self-defense, often admit capital punishment, and authorize letting terminally ill patients die under some circumstances.

In addition to the obligation not to kill, there are *positive* obligations to neighbors. Both the Hebrew Bible/Old Testament and the New Testament stress the positive obligation of neighbor-love (for example, Lev. 19:18; Luke 10:27–28). This religious-moral norm could support assistance in suicide or voluntary active euthanasia *if* suicide itself were acceptable. Hence, part of the modern debate concerns not only whether death is in a person's best interests (and may, for instance, be prayed for) but whether it may ever be brought about by direct killing rather than merely by letting die (under carefully defined circumstances).

Creation in God's image could provide a positive warrant for "playing God" in a fitting way.[8] However, we commonly hear the charge that physicians and others "play God" by usurping God's sovereignty and power over life and death, for example, through genetic interventions or measures to end life. In general this charge identifies two features of divine activity that should not be imitated: God's unlimited power to decide and to act. Thus, critics of "playing God" usually demand accountability along with respect for substantive limits, such as not killing others. But human agents also sometimes inappropriately "play God" by extending the dying process. Another common charge is that those who inappropriately extend the dying process, rather than letting God's will or nature take its course, deny human finitude and mortality, make an idol of mere biological life, and so forth. How these lines are drawn and limits set is crucial to understanding these religious traditions.

As the language of "playing God," image of God, trusteeship, and stewardship suggests, many religious arguments against suicide and euthanasia draw on metaphors and analogies, usually between ordinary human relationships and activities, on the one hand, and relationships between God and human life, on the other hand. Many of the metaphors and analogies central to theistic debates about suicide involve, as Margaret Pabst Battin notes, property relationships (for example, life is a "loan" or "trust" from God or is God's "temple," "handiwork," or "image") and personal or role relationships (for example, human beings are God's "children," "sentinels," "servants," or "trustees").[9] Construing life as a "gift" invokes both types of metaphors and analogies. Hence, the obligation to protect human life, including one's own, grows out of God's gracious gift of life. According to *Evangelium Vitae,* "Man's life comes from God; it is his gift, his image and imprint, a sharing in his breath of life. God therefore is the sole Lord of this life: Man cannot do with it as he wills . . . the sacredness of life has its foundation in God and in his creative activity: 'For God made man in his own image'" (#39).

Debates about suicide and euthanasia often probe these metaphors and analogies: Are there limits on what a recipient may do with a gift? If the gift is faulty—for example, there are serious genetic defects—may it be returned or destroyed? Or is the gift, which may involve considerable suffering on the recipient's part, then viewed as a way for God to test or educate the recipient? Efforts to challenge traditional religious conclusions regarding suicide and euthanasia often reinterpret or reevaluate the human relationships and activities invoked in the metaphors and analogies (for example, what exactly are the moral implications of gifts?) or challenge their extension to the divine-human relationship. Centrally important are the evaluation of human suffering—whether it is valued, merely tolerated, or always opposed—and the implications of "quality of life" for responses to God's "gift of life."

Roman Catholicism

To examine these themes, we turn first to Roman Catholicism. The Roman Catholic moral tradition has strongly opposed suicide, assisted suicide, and active euthanasia, while formulating several distinctions that allow patients to refuse, and family members and health care professionals to withhold or withdraw, life-prolonging treatment under some circumstances. The U.S. Catholic bishops recently summarized this position in their revised *Ethical and Religious Directives for Catholic Health Care Services:* "The truth that life is a precious gift from God has profound implications for the question of stewardship over human life. We are not the owners of our lives and hence do not have absolute power over life. We have a duty to preserve our life and to use it for the glory of God; but the duty to preserve life is not absolute, for we may reject life-prolonging procedures that are insufficiently beneficial or excessively burdensome. Suicide and euthanasia are never morally acceptable options."[10]

According to *Evangelium Vitae,* a recent encyclical in which Pope John Paul II opposes what he calls the "culture of death," the Christian tradition "has always consistently taught the absolute and unchanging value of the commandment 'you shall not kill'" because it is a very serious sin to kill a human being who bears the image of God and because only God is the master of life (#54, #55). Nevertheless, difficult situations emerge "in which values proposed by God's law seem to involve a genuine paradox" and the Church had to think further, for example, about killing in self-defense, in warfare, and in capital punishment (#55). This reflection involved specification, in the sense of seeking the precept's deeper meaning: "Yet from the beginning, faced with the many and often tragic cases which occur in the life of individuals and society, Christian reflection has sought a *fuller and deeper understanding* of what God's commandment [not to kill] prohibits and prescribes" (#55).

It thus became implausible to view the biblical prohibition of killing as absolute, unconditional, or exceptionless in light of conflicting values behind the precept, including the positive protection of life itself. Hence, the Church over time sought to specify this precept in light of these values.[11] And this specification further determined the precept's meaning by restricting its range and scope of application in at least two ways: first, to innocent persons, and, second, to direct actions (the second specification emerged later). According to *Evangelium Vitae* (#57), "The commandment 'you shall not kill' has *absolute value* when it refers to the innocent person," and "the direct and voluntary killing of an innocent human being is always gravely immoral," whether as an end or as a means. The moral rule against directly and voluntarily killing an innocent human being covers suicide, as well as assisted suicide and active euthanasia.

The prohibition of suicide is justified not only as a specification of or deduction from the rule against directly killing the innocent. Other reasons also appear. In a passage that largely reflects St. Thomas Aquinas's discussion of suicide, the *Catechism of the Catholic Church* notes that "suicide contradicts the natural inclination of the human being to preserve and perpetuate his life. It is gravely contrary to the just love of self. It likewise offends love of neighbor because it unjustly breaks the ties of solidarity with family, nation, and other human societies to which we continue to have obligations. Suicide is contrary to love for the living God."[12]

The distinction between direct killing and indirect killing is crucial in distinguishing unacceptable acts of suicide, assisted suicide, and active euthanasia from acceptable acts of forgoing life-prolonging treatment and of using medications that may hasten death. It is wrong directly to kill a suffering patient even at his or her request, but it may be permissible to relieve that patient's suffering through medications that will probably, but indirectly, hasten his or her death. In addition to consent from the appropriate parties, the rule of double effect requires that the action causing death be good in itself or at least indifferent; that the agent intend only the good effect, not the bad effect; that the bad effect not be a means to the good effect; and that the good effect outweigh the bad effect.[13] Through such categories, the Roman Catholic moral tradition can even praise some voluntary acts that foreseeably result in the individual's death—for example, falling on a hand grenade in order to save one's comrades. Such acts are not considered acts of suicide.

Roman Catholic moral theology further distinguishes ordinary from extraordinary or—in more recent language—proportionate from disproportionate means of treatment. If patients forgo *ordinary* or *proportionate* treatments, their actions constitute suicide, or if families and clinicians withhold or withdraw such treatments, their actions constitute homicide. However, if patients forgo, or families and clinicians withhold or withdraw, *extraordinary* or *disproportionate* treatments, which are sometimes called "heroic" or "aggressive," their actions do not constitute suicide or homicide. And they may be morally justifiable. "To forgo extraordinary or disproportionate means is not the equivalent of suicide or euthanasia; it rather expresses acceptance of the human condition in the face of death" (*Evangelium Vitae* #65).

In general, treatments with no reasonable chance of benefit or with burdens to the patient and others that outweigh their benefits may be considered extraordinary or disproportionate and thus may be forgone, withheld, or withdrawn without incurring a moral judgment of suicide or euthanasia. Nevertheless, controversies continue about the criteria for drawing these distinctions. On the one hand, there is debate about whether the criteria include judgments about quality of life, or only about the quality of treatments—differential judgments about quality of life could greatly extend the range of application of the distinction between ordinary and extraordinary. On the other hand, it is difficult to assess the use of such medical technologies as artificial means of nutrition and hydration, especially for certain groups of patients. Accordingly, the U.S. Catholic bishops identify a consensus that "nutrition and hydration are not morally obligatory" when they bring no comfort or cannot be assimilated. Despite such settled judgments, other questions require "further reflection, as, for example, the morality of withdrawing medically assisted hydration and nutrition from a person who is in . . . [a] 'persistent vegetative state.'"[14]

In view of the important distinctions between direct and indirect and between ordinary and extraordinary, not all letting die is acceptable. Euthanasia can occur by omission—*Evangelium Vitae* defines euthanasia as "an action or an omission which of itself and by intention causes death, with the purpose of eliminating all suffering" (#65). Furthermore, euthanasia involves the "malice proper to suicide or murder," depending on the circumstances, and "suicide is always as morally objectionable as murder" even though important distinctions exist between assisted suicide and voluntary active euthanasia, on the one hand, and nonvoluntary and involuntary euthanasia, on the other (#66).

The Church recognizes that a person who commits or attempts to commit suicide, an objectively immoral act, may not be subjectively responsible, perhaps in part because of the widespread "culture of death," which attempts to legitimate such acts (#66, and passim). In addition, "grave psychological disturbances, anguish, or grave fear of hardship, suffering, or torture can diminish the responsibility of the one committing suicide."[15] Even though Catholics who commit suicide are not supposed to receive an ecclesial burial, most in fact do receive one because of one or two suppositions: (1) They were at least temporarily deranged and hence not responsible for their actions, or (2) they may have re-pented at the last moment.[16] Thus, pastoral responses to suicide, including suicide to avoid intense pain and suffering, are more complex than merely condemning the (objective) act itself.

The methodological debate between the Roman Catholic hierar-chy and the so-called proportionalists—a debate that concerns how to define particular acts in moral evaluation—bears signifi-cantly on substantive debates about suicide, assisted suicide, and euthanasia. Proportionalists insist that moral species terms, which identify the moral nature of acts, do include or should include more than the mere physical, material event; they do or should include the whole set of morally relevant circumstances, as the prohibition of murder does but the prohibition of homicide does not. Only where these circumstances are included can a prohibition be considered absolute. Hence, proportionalists, such as Richard McCormick, S.J., Joseph Fuchs, S.J., and others, insist that we must look at all the morally relevant circumstances "be-fore we know what the action is and whether it should be said to be 'contrary to the commands of the divine and natural law.'" According to the proportionalists, we know that killing is gener-ally wrong, but the exceptions are also important. The magis-terium has strongly rejected this methodological approach, in part because it appears to open the door to exceptions to absolute moral norms.[17]

Finally, Roman Catholic piety has often praised the acceptance of physical suffering as a way God sometimes tests and educates his children, but not to the extent of making it obligatory or disavowing medications to relieve pain. According to the *Declara-tion on Euthanasia,* "Suffering, especially suffering during the last moments of life, has a special place in God's saving plan; it is in fact a sharing in Christ's passion and a union with the redeem-ing sacrifice which he offered in obedience to the Father's will. Therefore one must not be surprised if some Christians prefer to moderate their use of painkillers, in order to accept voluntarily at least a part of their sufferings and thus associate themselves in a conscious way with the suffering of Christ crucified." Neverthe-less, the *Declaration* continues, "it would be imprudent to impose a heroic way of acting as a general rule," and for the majority of sick people, it recommends "the use of medicines capable of alleviating or suppressing pain, even though these may cause as a secondary effect semiconsciousness and reduced lucidity" (or, as noted earlier, even hasten death). Still the *Declaration* expresses some concern about the phenomenon of habituation and about the loss of consciousness that may prevent the patient from discharging moral and familial obligations and from preparing himself or herself "with full consciousness for meeting Christ."[18]

Protestant Traditions

Even though Roman Catholicism is more diverse than it was prior to Vatican II, it is still more uniform, at least in its official teachings, than Protestantism (or, for that matter, Judaism). It is rarely possible to identify *the* Protestant position on any matter of significance, mainly because Protestantism encompasses so many different denominations (over two hundred in the United States) and perspectives (ranging from fundamentalist and evangelical to liberal). Protestants are by and large more individualistic in decisions about life and death because they lack Roman Catholicism's hierarchical institutional structure and instructional authority and Judaism's rabbinical authority in interpreting the law.

Some Protestants contend that suicide is wrong because it violates biblical rules against killing, while others hold that it is wrong because it displays a lack of gratitude toward, trust in, and faithfulness toward God as creator, preserver, and redeemer. And, of course, these arguments may be combined. However, even Protestants who emphasize a revealed morality, with rules drawn from scripture, are often suspicious of the detailed casuistry they see in Roman Catholicism or Judaism. Hence, with some exceptions such as Paul Ramsey, they are less likely to develop highly detailed casuistical distinctions, even when they try to mark off acceptable from unacceptable acts.[19]

Two prolific and influential earlier writers in biomedical ethics—Paul Ramsey and Joseph Fletcher—represent the two ends of the spectrum of Protestant positions regarding the weight or strength of the prohibition of suicide and euthanasia. In general Ramsey views the moral rules against suicide and active euthanasia as absolute, and brings "exceptional" cases under a refined or deepened understanding of these rules, while Fletcher views those rules, at most, as mere guidelines based on previous experience. Fletcher defended suicide and active euthanasia in some situations, based on a personalistic philosophy, on an identification of *agape* or neighbor-love with the principle of utility (doing the greatest good for the greatest number), and on an understanding of agape/utility as unconstrained by other principles and rules.[20] By contrast, Ramsey rejected both suicide and active euthanasia on grounds of "in-principled love," understood as covenant faithfulness, while he accepted a wide range of treatment refusals limited by the kinds of considerations that mark Roman Catholic distinctions between direct and indirect effects and between ordinary and extraordinary means of treatment.

Another Protestant theologian, Arthur Dyck, also rejects euthanasia on the grounds that mercy or kindness requires both not harming (including not killing) and benefiting others, and that not harming others takes priority over benefiting others. Against arguments for beneficent euthanasia (or assisted suicide), Dyck proposes an ethic of "benemortasia," which would extend the following kinds of care to patients whose death is imminent: relief of pain and suffering, respect for the right to refuse treatment, and provision of health care without regard to ability to pay.[21] Critics of such an approach contend that death is not always a net harm, even if it is always a harm, and that killing or assistance in suicide may express mercy, kindness, and care (neighbor-love) in particular circumstances.

Critics have similar objections to another Protestant position that rejects both suicide and active euthanasia because of what they symbolize and express about the Christian agent's character or about the Christian narrative. The Methodist theologian Stanley Hauerwas, who has drawn heavily from the Mennonite and Roman Catholic traditions, has helped many Protestant ethicists focus on virtue and narrative rather than on principles and rules in explicating Christian morality. In reflecting on suicide and euthanasia, he highlights both virtue and narrative in providing reasons for living. One of his arguments holds that "our unwillingness to kill ourselves even under pain is an affirmation that the trust that has sustained us in health is also the trust that sustains us in illness and distress; that our existence is a gift ultimately bounded by a hope that gives us a way to go on; that the full, present memory of our Christian story is a source of strength and consolation for ourselves and our community."[22]

Echoing the importance of narrative, Allen Verhey who, in taking a Calvinist evangelical (but not fundamentalist) approach to the Bible, notes that scripture does not explicitly condemn suicide, but that it "states, if indirectly, much more powerfully than simple prohibition, why suicide, assisted suicide, and euthanasia are forbidden. They do not fit the story of God's grace and faithful human response. They cohere rather with the story of betrayal and denial." Furthermore, with particular attention to virtue, Hauerwas stresses that suicide and euthanasia undermine our convictions about "what it is to live bravely in the face of suffering," including being a burden to others.[23]

Lutheran Gilbert Meilaender, who also attends to virtue and narrative as well as to rules, holds that an agent acting out of the *motive* of neighbor-love can never *aim* at or intend the suffering neighbor's death, even if death would be a good *result* (and acceptable if it occurred through letting die rather than killing). Against critics who contend that letting the patient die, rather than killing the patient, will only prolong the patient's suffering and will thus contradict the agent's merciful motive, Meilaender argues that in the Christian worldview, "in which death and suffering are great evils but not the greatest evil, love can never include in its meaning hastening a fellow human being toward (the evil of) death, nor can it mean a refusal to acknowledge death when it comes (as an evil but not the greatest evil)." Hence, it is important to keep in view the Christian background assumptions for the operation of neighbor-love, rather than reducing it to a form of humanitarian action. In the Christian vision of the world, Meileander continues, "love could never euthanatize."[24]

Conceptual and normative problems sometimes arise when absolutist positions confront new situations occasioned by technological developments. A good example is the debate about withholding or withdrawing artificial nutrition and hydration. While some Protestant absolutists have been able to accept these acts for certain groups of patients—sometimes even extending, as Ramsey did, the category of the dying patient to include the patient in a persistent vegetative state—others argue that it is not possible to withhold or withdraw artificial nutrition and hydration, in contrast to the respirator, without intending to kill the patient and thus without violating the obligation of neighbor-love.[25]

In contrast to Ramsey's and others' absolutist positions, some Protestant communities and individual thinkers hold that the moral norms against suicide and active euthanasia, while more than mere maxims or rules of thumb (as in Joseph Fletcher's "situation ethics"), are presumptively or prima facie binding, that is, binding when all other things are equal, rather than absolute. Such norms can be overridden, outweighed, or rebutted under some circumstances, and acts of suicide and euthanasia can thus sometimes be justified from a Christian standpoint even if they always remain tragic, mournful, and so on.

For example, in light of the debate about the joint suicides of Dr. Henry Pitney Van Dusen, former president of Union Theological Seminary, and his wife, the Presbytery of New York City's 1976 pastoral letter concluded that "it is clear that for some Christians, as a last resort in the gravest of situations, suicide may be an act of their Christian conscience." Taking a similar approach, James M. Gustafson holds that "suicide is always a tragic moral choice; it is sometimes a misguided choice. But it can be, I believe, a conscientious choice . . . Life is a gift, and is to be received with gratitude, but if life becomes an unbearable burden there is reason for enmity toward God."[26]

It is naively anthropocentric, Gustafson insists, to assume as some do that God's activity will always, at least in the long run, promote the individual's welfare. Such an assumption appears in the arguments against suicide made by Darrel Amundsen, an evangelical: Christian "attitudes and responses to suffering and dying must be molded by the reality that their Creator and Sovereign will cause all things to work together for their good and that their Lord has called them into a fellowship of His suffering in which they are sustained by dependence upon Him. Hence, for Christians to take their lives in order to escape from the trials and testings ordained by Him would be a failure of love and a breach of trust." This assumption is challenged on two grounds in an extensive argument which, in a legal framework that permits but regulates voluntary euthanasia, it would be entirely appropriate for a believing and practicing Christian patient to request and for a believing and practicing Christian doctor to provide euthanasia. According to Paul Badham, this assumption does not correspond to human experience, because there is evidence that much human suffering is not ennobling, and it is not followed with rational consistency, because Christians are not prepared to accept its implication and refrain from analgesics.[27]

Lonnie D. Kliever, writing within the Wesleyan tradition, further argues that euthanasia in some circumstances can support "the sanctity and solidarity of human life." He notes that the "religious case [for euthanasia] is based on natural rather than revealed theology," but that it provides a distinctive alternative to a narrow philosophical justification based on individual autonomy and to a dogmatic theological opposition based on sanctity of life. Still another Protestant, who also operates with a strong presumption against assisted suicide and active euthanasia, concedes with greater reluctance: "I believe that some extreme and rare circumstances do justify euthanasia. As stewards of the Master's resources we are called to use our God-given capacities to serve human needs, and those needs might include escape from a life that is worse than death." However, justifying an act in extreme cases does not necessarily imply justifying a public policy that condones assisted suicide or active euthanasia.[28]

The Anglican moral tradition, represented in the United States by the Episcopal Church, is often viewed as a third way between Roman Catholicism and Protestantism, even though its central moral categories often overlap the Roman Catholic tradition. In early 1996 a vigorous debate erupted about the morality of assisted suicide and active euthanasia when the Episcopal Diocese of Newark adopted the Report of a Task Force on Assisted Suicide, which held that "there are circumstances where involuntarily prolonged biological existence is a less ethical alternative than a conscientiously chosen and merciful termination of earthly life."[29] This report stresses reverence for God's creation, but notes that some destruction is "inevitable and necessary" in creation and that "the wilful taking of life . . . can be morally justified only if the good desired outweighs the potential evil and only if that good cannot be achieved in a less destructive manner." In accord with God's saving action in freeing people from the bondage of suffering (for example, in the Exodus from the land of Egypt), it seeks to liberate those "who might otherwise feel enslaved to a biblically driven mandate to suffer virtuously and without release. Such a mandate is not theologically defensible, and is thus in force for no faithful Christian."

In response, the Committee on Health, Human Values, and Ethics of the Episcopal Diocese of Southern Ohio (February 23, 1996) agrees that "there may be circumstances in which it could be morally permissible to take one's own life or to assist another in doing this." However, it opposes efforts to develop an Episcopal Church "policy of supporting persons in their decisions for assisted suicide" as well as any "suggestion that medically assisted death is morally equivalent to withholding or withdrawing medical treatment necessary for sustaining life." An act of assisted suicide would need "close and prayerful consideration to the circumstances of each individual case." While such an act should not be rejected out of hand, it should be the "exception and not the rule."[30] These Episcopal groups share a presumption against assisted suicide but then admit that it can sometimes be justified on religious-moral grounds. However, they differ about where to draw the lines and set the limits—particularly about whether the justifying circumstances are broad or narrow—and about whether there should be a church (and a state) policy accepting and supporting such decisions. Critics of a liberal church (or state) policy worry that the truly exceptional would then become routine, especially in view of social pressures.[31]

Jewish Traditions

For Judaism, which, like Christianity, is not monolithic, the discussion of suicide and euthanasia, as well as conceptions of a good life and a good death, must be placed in the context of a willing, active deity's relation to the world and to the human beings within it. Through its rejection of suicide, Judaism "affirms its high valuation of life and its belief in the sovereignty of the Creator."[32]

The Talmud (the authoritative body of Jewish tradition, including *halakhah,* that is, law) holds that the duty to protect human life takes priority except where murder, sexual immorality (such as incest or adultery), or idolatry would be required in order to discharge it. According to some rabbinical sources, Saul's suicide was undertaken in order to avoid profaning God.[33] Similarly, martyrdom is acceptable under some circumstances, as a way to affirm rather than to deny God.

Judaism presumes that no one would willfully commit suicide and deny God's sovereignty, and it thus sets a high burden of proof to establish that an act of self-caused death was actually willful. The rules for rituals of mourning and internment exclude the person who has committed suicide. However, as in other traditions, a critical question concerns which acts count as acts of suicide. Identifying the key criterion as *willfulness,* the Jewish tradition has developed such detailed rules of evidence for willfulness "that for all practical purposes almost all suicides are treated as individuals who destroyed themselves 'unwillfully,'" and they are accorded the usual rites for the dead. In effect, some self-caused deaths that would otherwise be counted as suicides are removed from that category because of the lack of sufficient evidence of willfulness. Even the fear of suffering, for example, may be sufficient to undermine willfulness and thus *excuse* the agent by removing the condemnatory label of suicide; by contrast, avoidance of murder, sexual immorality, or idolatry could *justify* allowing and even bringing about one's own death.[34]

The Jewish tradition rules out euthanasia on the same grounds as suicide—human life as created in the image of God. It requires that the dying person be treated as a living person in all respects and that nothing be done that might cause or hasten death—for example, closing the patient's eyes or removing a feather pillow from under the patient's head. While excluding euthanasia, an important text notes: "We do not put salt on his [the dying patient's] tongue to prevent his death." Also excluding actions that cause the dying to die quickly, another important text holds: "But if there is something that delays his death, such as a nearby woodchopper making a noise, or there is salt on his tongue, and these prevent his speedy death, one can remove them, for this does not involve any action at all, but rather the removal of the preventive agent." The important distinction is between actively hastening death, which is prohibited, and removing impediments or hindrances to death, which is permitted, but only for the person who is in his or her death-throes.[35]

In contrast to the Roman Catholic rule of double effect, Rabbi Solomon Freehof, a Reform rabbi, responds to the question whether a patient who is terminally ill, and who suffers from severe pain, can ask for medications that will relieve his pain but also hasten his death, by saying that "for a man to ask that his life be ended sooner is equivalent to his committing suicide. Suicide is definitely forbidden by Jewish Law."[36]

Much of the debate hinges on the conception of the dying person *(goses)*, whose death is considered imminent (within three days, according to some authorities). Only a patient whose death is imminent and irreversible may be allowed to die under some carefully drawn circumstances. Judaism thus recognizes a more extensive obligation to use technologies to prolong life than does either Roman Catholicism or Protestantism, in part because of its belief in the equal value of each moment of life. However, even the Orthodox branch of Judaism allows withholding "any additional non-routine medical services, so as to permit the natural ebbing of the life forces" for the *goses*.[37]

Methodological differences are important within Judaism, just as they are in Roman Catholicism and Protestantism. The Orthodox, Conservative, and Reform Jewish branches differ in part according to their approach to tradition, particularly as embodied in halakhic rules. The Orthodox branch concentrates on these rules, the Conservative branch emphasizes that the proper interpretation of these rules depends on attention to the principles or values back of the rules, and the Reform branch stresses the principles or values themselves rather than the rules. Reconstructionist Judaism concurs with the Reform branch that traditional Jewish law is not binding, but it tends to emphasize community more than the Reform branch, which tends to stress personal autonomy.[38]

David Ellenson also draws a significant distinction between halakhic formalism and a covenantal method, both of which cut across traditional boundaries in Judaism. The latter puts a higher value on autonomy, while downplaying rabbinical authority. "The person's autonomy as a covenantal creature standing in relationship to God would ultimately be affirmed as the highest value in the system." Obviously this methodological dispute could have important implications for debates about suicide and euthanasia; at the very least, for instance, the covenantal approach would increase the range of considerations and possible actions.[39]

A more traditional legal approach encounters several obstacles in extending Jewish principles or values into contemporary debates, because it must (1) identify precedents, (2) adduce principles from these precedents, and (3) apply these principles to new sets of facts. Regarding the first point, Louis Newman notes that it is not always easy to determine the appropriate precedents in the debates about euthanasia. For instance, traditional sources permit prayers for the speedy death of a dying individual who is experiencing great pain.[40] One important question concerns whether there is a significant difference between praying to God to hasten an individual's death and actively trying to hasten it oneself. At least the former is easier to view as letting God's will be done.

In the second place, it may not be clear exactly which principle or rule can be drawn from a precedent. For instance, which principle or rule operates in the precedents regarding *goses?* Rabbi J. David Bleich argues that "any patient who may reasonably be deemed capable of potential survival for a period of seventy-two hours cannot be considered as *goses.*" By contrast, Ronald Green suggests that modern medical technologies may have destroyed the traditional category of the *goses,* as defined in terms of temporal limits, and that *goses* may need to be redefined in terms of the hopelessness of the patient's condition or continued quality of life.[41]

Debates center on what kinds of impediments to death may be removed (the woodchopper problem) as well as the circumstances under which they may be removed (the *goses* problem). Even if it is clear that the woodchopper constitutes an impediment to dying, it may be unclear how this impediment should be construed—

as something physically removed from the person, as something which has no therapeutic value, as something not placed there by the patient or those caring for that person, or simply as anything whatsoever that prevents a person from dying. Similar questions can be raised about the circumstances under which an impediment to death, of whatever sort, can be removed. Shall we restrict the principle that impediments may be removed to individuals who are in severe pain, to those who are irreversibly comatose and so feel no pain at all, or to those in neither of these categories who are terminally ill for whom medical technology can offer only palliative care but no cure.[42]

And some suggest that woodchopping may be stopped and salt may be removed because they are not part of "the therapeutic armamentarium employed in the medical management of this patient. For this reason, these impediments may be removed. However, the discontinuation of instrumentation and machinery which is specifically designed and utilized in the treatment of incurably ill patients might only be permissible if one is certain that in doing so one is shortening the act of dying and not interrupting life."[43]

Third, beyond determining precedents and extracting principles (even broad ones such as the value of human life, because of problems of scope and range of applicability), the final interpretive step, according to Newman, applies these general principles to contemporary cases by determining "whether a new fact pattern does or does not correspond to the facts underlying previous rulings." This third step includes what James Gustafson calls an "evaluative description" of the fact patterns of acts and their circumstances. Consider, for instance, a wide range of acts and circumstances, including the patient's circumstances (whether terminally ill, whether in pain, whether he or she has prepared an advance directive, whether the treatment will be extremely costly), the technologies (respirators, feeding tubes), and the acts involved (not starting versus stopping, withholding cardiopulmonary resuscitation versus pulling the plug). "Evaluative descriptions" of different circumstances, technologies, and acts will obviously shape the way traditional principles and rules are employed in particular cases and types of cases. Regarding different medical technologies, for example, the tradition appears to give strong support to viewing respirators as "heroic" under some circumstances, while debates continue about artificial nutrition and hydration.[44]

Obviously debates about evaluative descriptions include whether the label euthanasia is used at all, and, if it is, whether the more specific label active euthanasia or passive euthanasia is used. A few Jewish commentators attempt to justify active euthanasia on grounds found in the tradition. And Baruch Brody argues that the tradition is more flexible than many recognize because rabbinical authorities have always engaged in casuistry; that is, they have always balanced several values, including the "great" but not absolute value of preserving human life, the "nearly absolute prohibition against taking the life of the innocent," even if that person is dying, along with other values, such as adherence to God's law and "avoiding cruel and painful deaths."[45]

Finally, Judaism tends to view suffering as something to be avoided or removed whenever possible, but not at the expense of life itself. It is not tempted to glorify suffering the way Christianity sometimes does. While stressing that the practical differences between the traditions are minimal at this point, Rabbi Immanuel Jakobovits notes, however, that "in general, Christianity is distinctly more panegyrical in its commendation of physical suffering than is Judaism."[46]

Conclusions

The three traditions I have examined in this analysis generally and strongly oppose suicide, assisted suicide, and euthanasia. However, as I have suggested, we cannot understand a particular tradition's views about such actions until we grasp (1) the meaning, range, and scope, and (2) the weight and strength of its relevant moral norms. The debates within these traditions often, but by no means always (especially in Protestant thought), focus on the meaning, range, or scope of the prohibition of suicide or active euthanasia, rather than on its weight or strength. Religious

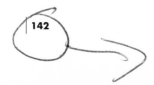

traditions often maintain coherence over time by expanding, deepening, or specifying a norm's meaning, range, or scope, rather than by overturning it, particularly if they previously considered it to be absolute. Such a change does not appear to threaten the religious tradition's authority as dramatically as overturning a norm. However, as I noted, some religious thinkers, particularly in Protestant traditions, argue for a conception of norms as prima facie or presumptively binding and then for balancing those norms in particular circumstances. Where that conception operates, orderly change can occur through the expansion of the conditions that justify overriding or outweighing the norm.

Whichever approach is taken, these traditions are not static; they represent change as well as continuity. And a religious community's further reflection, in relation to both scripture and tradition, may be occasioned by experience, such as the experience of suffering in the use of new technologies to prolong life.[47] Over the last twenty-five years, these traditions have had to face questions about how to define and refine their categories of moral analysis, such as ordinary and extraordinary and *goses,* in a way that would maintain coherence, integrity, or fidelity and yet also fit contemporary moral experience. To take just one example, they had to consider whether artificial nutrition and hydration could be morally withheld or withdrawn: Could withholding or withdrawing artificial nutrition and hydration meet the conditions recognized in each tradition for legitimate decisions to withhold or withdraw life-prolonging medical treatment, or did it represent an instance of forbidden suicide, assisted suicide, or active euthanasia? The religious communities' answers are not complete, uniform, or final, and ambiguities and ambivalence remain, but at least significant parts have accepted the legitimacy of forgoing artificial nutrition and hydration under some circumstances.

Recent studies suggest that liberals (or conservatives) in Protestantism, Roman Catholicism, and Judaism may share more with liberals (or conservatives) in the other traditions than with their own religious colleagues who do not share that liberal (or conservative) orientation.[48] Nevertheless, the debates between liberals and conservatives within and across these traditions often turn on interpretations of perspectives and norms from scripture and tradition, such as God's creation of human beings in his own image and the prohibition of suicide. Even though in general all three traditions strongly oppose suicide, assisted suicide, and euthanasia, liberals on these matters do not totally lack resources within their own traditions to support their positions. But they also frequently appeal to experience and to reason to demonstrate the inadequacy of some traditional categories—thus, they might stress the suffering patients now endure because of new medical technologies, or they might argue that traditional distinctions, such as between killing and letting die, are not rationally defensible. Furthermore, in each tradition, debates about methods of religious-moral reasoning have significant implications for substantive arguments about these problems—for example, the debate about intrinsic evil and proportionate reason in Roman Catholicism, about the weight or strength of moral norms in Protestantism, and about halakhic formalism and covenantal method in Judaism.

I have concentrated on the norms and judgments regarding *acts* of suicide, assisted suicide, and voluntary active euthanasia, but much of the debate in the United States now concerns whether public laws and institutional and professional policies should accept such acts as legitimate. Formal religious opposition to acts of assisted suicide and active euthanasia does not always translate into opposition to liberal laws and policies, especially in the context of religious-moral pluralism, just as acceptance of some acts of assisted suicide and active euthanasia as morally justifiable does not always imply acceptance of liberal laws and policies. While there is, of course, a rough correlation between moral judgments about such acts and moral judgments about laws and policies, judgments about laws and policies are more complex than merely the acts they prohibit, permit, or regulate.[49]

Formal religious communities and individuals within the three traditions I have examined do not universally oppose the legalization of assisted suicide (particularly physician-assisted suicide) and active euthanasia. For instance, in the November 1991 public referendum in Washington State on Initiative 119, the legalization of "aid-in-dying" for terminally ill patients—which was defeated by 54 to 46 percent—the Unitarian Universalist Association, the

Pacific Northwest Council of the United Methodist Church, and the Interfaith Clergy Council strongly supported the initiative, while the Washington State Catholic Conference and the Evangelical Lutheran Church strongly opposed the initiative. Furthermore, according to Andrew Greeley's analysis of the National Opinion Research Center's annual General Social Survey, there was a substantial increase over the decade of the 1980s in support among religious believers for the legalization of physician assistance in ending life. Even most Protestant fundamentalists came to agree that "doctors should be allowed by law to end the patient's life by some painless means if the patient and his family request it," and higher percentages of members of other groups agreed with that statement. However, it is notoriously difficult to validate such responses because of different understandings of key categories, and they may not lead to action or even support for specific legislation.[50]

Some religious communities and individuals, while continuing to view assisted suicide and active euthanasia as prima facie or presumptively wrong, may simply accept the movement to liberal laws and policies in light of powerful secular appeals to respect individual autonomy and the desire to avoid pain and suffering as part of different conceptions of a "good death." After all, they might conclude, suicide itself has been decriminalized, and decriminalization of assisted suicide and voluntary active euthanasia might not be so detrimental to the public interest as long as these acts are subject to public regulation. Nevertheless, if physician-assisted suicide is legalized in the United States, religious communities will undoubtedly press to protect the conscientious refusals of individuals, including medical and health care professionals, and of religious communities and institutions, such as religious hospitals, as well as to establish state and professional regulation in order to protect individuals' moral rights and interests.[51]

Not all Christian and Jewish arguments to retain the legal prohibition of assisted suicide or active euthanasia—or to establish strong regulations if they are legalized—are themselves religious in nature. Quite often they invoke general moral principles or values, usually embedded in the social-cultural ethos, and they frequently appeal to the probable negative consequences of liberal laws and policies, rather than to the intrinsic wrongness of acts of assisted suicide or euthanasia. Even though religious communities may judge particular *acts* of suicide, assisted suicide, and euthanasia to be intrinsically wrong on religious-moral grounds, often they also use secular arguments to oppose liberal *rules* of practice. They may hold—and many who believe that some acts of assisted suicide or active euthanasia are morally right also concur—that it is crucial to retain legal prohibitions of assisted suicide and active euthanasia in order to restrain potentially misguided angels of mercy and to limit efforts to dispose of individuals who, for one reason or the other, are considered socially undesirable, and they may doubt that legal regulation would be as effective as legal prohibition.

Quite common is some version of the slippery-slope argument—for instance, "society should remain intolerant of the practice of mercy killing because [of the] fear the moral erosion that tolerance of it could cause." Even religious ethicists who hold that some acts of suicide, assisted suicide, and active euthanasia are justifiable may also believe that it would be "a mistake at this time in history to establish a public policy condoning active euthanasia," because of the dangers just mentioned as well as the difficulties of capturing in law all the complexities of particular cases.[52]

In short, whether religious or nonreligious, many critics of the legalization of assisted suicide (and active euthanasia) point to the difficulty of drawing and maintaining defensible lines and limits in law, to the dangers of abuse, especially because of society's devaluation of the elderly and its failure to provide universal access to health care, and to the horrors of the holocaust in Nazi Germany as important reasons to oppose liberal laws and policies regarding assisted suicide and active euthanasia. And many doubt that public or professional regulation would be as effective in protecting the weak and vulnerable. Furthermore, whether laws and policies permit or regulate assisted suicide or active euthanasia, opponents often contend that they will contribute to what the Vatican calls a "culture of death" or a "climate of death" which legitimates such acts and may even over time make them socially and culturally, if not legally obligatory. One version of this criticism contends that legalizing and professionalizing assisted suicide, which many believe will increase options, will in fact "effectively eliminate an option, namely, the option of staying alive without having to justify one's existence."[53]

Such arguments may not reflect a religious community's distinctive moral discourse, but they are quite common and important in both religious and secular debates. And, for some religious communities and individual participants, they may also reflect certain religious convictions—for example, beliefs about human sinfulness may increase the plausibility of slippery-slope arguments.[54]

PART THREE

Perspectives

7

Factual Findings

PAUL VAN DER MAAS AND LINDA L. EMANUEL

Euthanasia and physician-assisted suicide stand among a core of subjects, along with capital punishment and abortion, that have aroused controversy through the ages. The circumstances of societies differ, but the arguments pro and con have remained to a great extent the same. They have generally relied on logical or religious reasoning, balancing competing principles to establish or disprove a patient's right to assistance in dying. But dealing with ethical questions requires both principled reasoning and an assessment of the facts and context of the question.

So, current contributions from empirical or observational research to the otherwise ancient debate are important to illuminate the context in which different principles and their limits are applied. Findings from the behavioral and social sciences and ethnology, among other fields, can help us to assess the contextual factors involved in physician-assisted suicide and euthanasia. Many questions remain to be answered, but some data are available, especially from the Netherlands and the United States.

Some questions that arise concern prevalence or outcome, and these are best addressed through epidemiological studies. For instance, what is the prevalence of various types of physician-assisted suicide and euthanasia? How frequently do circumstances arise when physician-assisted suicide and euthanasia might be considered and justified? What is the prevalence of other types of death—among patients in intensive care, palliative care, or no medical care, and so on? Regarding outcome, epidemiological questions might include: How often are patients' assisted or unassisted suicides botched? And among these, how many attempts are repeated? How long is the interval between terminal diagnosis and death in physician-assisted suicide and euthanasia versus other types of death?

Important empirical contributions from the social and behavioral sciences can be found in opinion surveys among physicians, other medical professional groups, patients, and the general public. These encompass a range of questions. Would legalization of physician-assisted suicide and euthanasia undermine trust in the profession? Would legalization potentially reduce patients' need to resort to suicide? What are the emotional states of patients who request assisted death? How do patients, families, or professionals who have planned for, or engaged in, physician-assisted suicide or euthanasia feel about it in retrospect? In addition to opinion surveys, psychometric scales have been developed to measure specific patient characteristics, ranging from degree of social interaction to depth of depression. These can help answer a number of relevant questions: What types of suffering beyond physical pain, such as depression, do dying patients experience? How often are those who express interest in physician-assisted suicide competent to make such a decision? How much care and support are they enjoying in their personal and community life?

Some of the issues in the euthanasia debate relate to differences in traditions, beliefs, social structure, or other ethnocultural variations, and all can be of profound importance. While survey methodology can get at some of these issues, observational studies, focus groups, in-depth interviews, and narrative analyses are more flexible tools for probing the meaning of cultural and ethnic-related concerns. Typical questions to be explored include the following: How do religions influence people's approach to suffering and terminal illness? Do family traditions regarding communication, respect, or interdependence influence a person's inclination to request physician-assisted suicide or euthanasia? How do community rituals regarding illness and dying affect the behavior of individuals facing death?

Just how much of a contribution empirical data can make to deliberation depends on the type of arguments being addressed. Some arguments in the ethical debate presuppose empirical information. Examples include the argument that hospice care is always sufficient to alleviate suffering, and the slippery-slope argument that euthanasia, if permitted in a few cases, will be abused in many cases. Both of these arguments could be settled to a great extent by empirical facts, at least for specific cultures and times. Other types of ethical arguments are, however, by definition valid only within a theoretical or highly specific set of cases. For example, the argument that active and passive euthanasia are morally identical is often supported by specific paired examples. In theory, the two situations may appear to be morally identical, but empirical studies of real contexts point to some clear moral differences. Here identification of the prevalence of the different types of contexts can be helpful.

Some *a priori* ethical arguments that flow from a higher moral claim can never be empirically refuted or confirmed. For instance, a well known sanctity-of-life argument states that human life is sacred and therefore should not be snuffed out under any circumstances. A counter-argument states that life's very sacredness means that it should not be allowed to linger in suffering or indignity, that physician-assisted suicide and euthanasia can be a greater form of respect for human life's sanctity. Polling data can measure how many people agree with either of the opposing positions, but the individual adherent to either position will be able to say that even if the entire world takes the opposite view, his or her own position is morally superior. Thus, empirical data can make only a very limited contribution to this type of moral question.

Another limitation of empirical data is the tendency for either side of a debate to use selected data to support its position. This can be seen quite clearly in the uses made of the first nationwide study on end-of-life decision-making in the Netherlands (the Remmelink Commission study).[1] Nonetheless, this selective use of data is not altogether negative, insofar as it provides a vehicle for sane and honest engagement with the issues.

We will now turn to various arguments for and against physician-assisted suicide and euthanasia and will try to determine the contribution that empirical studies have made, or may make in the future, to the ongoing debate.

Arguments Where Empirical Work Can Help

PALLIATIVE CARE   The question of whether palliative care to control suffering is, or could be, a sufficient alternative to suicide or euthanasia is mainly an empirical issue. The two most important questions are: What kind of suffering can be alleviated by palliative care, and to what extent? And what kinds of suffering prompt patients to request physician-assisted suicide and euthanasia?

Few question that, in practice, the availability of high-quality palliative care is currently limited in the United States as well as in the Netherlands and probably most other countries. Treatable pain often goes untreated, and depression and anxiety are common but also often insufficiently addressed. Treatment of the multiple other symptoms that afflict the dying are often ignored in standard textbooks of medicine, and few physicians have been trained in palliative care, either in medical school or in postgraduate programs. Therefore, it is not surprising that, in practice, suffering is incompletely alleviated. Even when palliative care is available, both patients and their families are frequently dissatisfied; according to several key outcome measures, satisfaction with palliative care is sometimes no greater than that with conventional care.[2]

The more difficult question is whether *ideal* palliative care could sufficiently eliminate unbearable suffering. We are not aware of the existence of any trial directed at answering this question. Some data on physicians' opinions are available, however. In Holland, 55 percent of physicians disagree with the statement that "adequate alleviation of pain and/or symptoms and personal care of the dying patient make euthanasia unnecessary." Of nursing home physicians (who provide much of palliative care in the Netherlands), 41 percent strongly disagree with the statement (although the majority of these never have performed physician-assisted suicide and euthanasia, it being extremely rare in Dutch nursing homes). In 1986 the World Health Organization (WHO) stated that in less than 10 percent of cancer patients even optimal pain management could not give sufficient relief.

The fact that almost 48 percent of U.S. oncologists said that they themselves would, under some circumstances, ask for euthanasia or physician-assisted suicide may suggest that they think palliative care cannot reliably make suffering bearable in all circumstances. On the other hand, limits to pain medication use are often set by the patient or family, a fact that underscores the difficulty of defining, except perhaps on a case-by-case basis, what constitutes unbearable suffering and what qualifies as sufficient comfort.[3]

The most common justification offered for physician-assisted suicide and euthanasia is unbearable physical suffering. Given two scenarios involving a terminal cancer patient that differ in the severity of physical suffering, the proportion of U.S. physicians who consider physician-assisted suicide justified is 26 percent for physical and nonphysical suffering and 6.5 percent for nonphysical suffering alone. Comparable differences were found among cancer patients and in the general public.[4]

This finding stands in marked contrast with the fact that physical pain or other suffering is not the dominant factor that prompts patients to think about or turn to physician-assisted suicide and euthanasia. Although pain is one of the reasons cited in 46 percent of Dutch patients requesting assistance in dying, only 3 percent of requesting patients cited pain as the only reason. Current loss of dignity was cited by 57 percent, and anticipated loss of dignity by 46 percent. Findings from the United States support those from the Netherlands. In the state of Washington, 70 percent of patients requesting physician-assisted suicide were experiencing less than severe pain. Among those requesting active euthanasia rather than physician-assisted suicide, more were experiencing severe pain, but almost half were not. Reasons cited for their requests were concern over future loss of control (77 percent), being a burden (75 percent), being dependent (74 percent), and loss of dignity (72 percent). Further, and of critical importance, patients with depression or emotional distress were more likely than patients with pain to incline toward discussion of physician-assisted suicide or euthanasia with their physicians.[5]

Thus, empirical research indicates that traditional palliative care is probably not a full solution to the problem of unbearable physical suffering, although in most cases it may be sufficient. But it also questions the assumption that physical suffering is the relevant and justifying form of suffering for most patients who request assistance in dying. Furthermore, the findings point to the importance of depression as a potential motivator. Because the forms of suffering that prompt patients to consider physician-assisted suicide and euthanasia are often emotional or social rather than physical, and often involve anticipatory rather than current suffering, it is critical to the debate over end-of-life decisions to understand the different conceptions of dignity, dependence, and burden that dying patients hold and to appreciate the social context in which those concepts operate.

The debate over palliative care would benefit if, in future empirical research, requests for physician-assisted suicide and euthanasia prompted by physical suffering were distinguished from requests intended to avoid personally or socially undesirable states. Each of the above should also be separated from depression-related requests. The moral defensibility of each differs, as should the medical evaluation, the decision-making process, and the management of symptoms.

In-depth studies about the major forms of suffering from severe or terminal disease and the conditions under which this suffering leads to requests for assistance in dying are needed. And intervention studies directed at alleviating nonphysical forms of suffering, such as depression, social isolation, fear of indignity, fear of loss of control, and fear of being a burden, would add an important dimension to the debate over palliative care as an alternative to suicide or euthanasia in suffering patients.

THE SLIPPERY SLOPE The slippery-slope argument supposes that there might be some justifiable cases of physician-assisted suicide and euthanasia, but its legalization is not worth the detrimental consequences. Although balancing the suffering of dying patients against social benefits for the living is difficult, this kind of balancing must be faced on a regular basis in matters of public policy. Therefore, it is relevant to know how many people would, in the view of those concerned, benefit from physician-assisted suicide and euthanasia. This number might be viewed as an estimate of an ideal minimal rate.

With this ideal minimal rate in hand, researchers could then address at least two questions: Is physician-assisted suicide and euthanasia occurring at a higher rate than the ideal minimum, under either legal or illegal conditions? And in localities where physician-assisted suicide and euthanasia are permitted, has there been an increase of sloppy, undocumented, or unwanted types of life-ending acts, such as active euthanasia in the absence of a competent patient's request? A third question might be added: Once physician-assisted suicide and euthanasia are permitted, is there an increase in the types of social thought that proponents of the slippery-slope argument fear, such as the notion that certain categories of people are unworthy of living?

At present the data available are insufficient to establish an ideal minimal rate that would be justifiable on grounds of untreatable suffering. Such an estimate would assume situations where quality palliative care is available for every relevant patient and where all other necessary safeguards against misuse are in place. Since these conditions do not routinely pertain, the estimate is hard to come by. Nevertheless, an approach to estimation is possible.

WHO estimates that less than 10 percent of cancer cases involve untreatable pain.[6] For noncancer deaths this percentage would be much lower, due to the lower frequency of untreatable pain and the high proportion of deaths (31 percent) that are rapid, without time for end-of-life decisions. Further, the ideal minimal rate for physician-assisted suicide and euthanasia would be less than the total rate of untreatable pain, since not all patients in this situation will request such assistance in securing death. Unfortunately, a firm estimate of how many would request physician-assisted suicide or euthanasia and be eligible by established criteria is not available. It is clear, however, that not all who suffer will seriously request physician-assisted suicide and euthanasia, and of these, only some are eligible in the sense of being competent adults, fully informed of the alternatives, persistent in their request, uncoerced by family members or others, free of depression, and terminal.

The ideal minimal rate would certainly be augmented if additional types of cases were considered justifiable—for instance, if physician-assisted suicide and euthanasia were considered justified by being a burden or by fear of future indignity. It is unclear by how much these cases would change the rate. If terminality were not included as a criterion, justifiable rates would go even higher. The dilemma of the slippery-slope argument is illustrated by the difficulty of deciding which cases to draw the estimates from. How much and what kind of suffering counts as unbearable depends on assumptions that are greatly determined by the context of social thought.

If we assume that the ideal minimal rate would fall somewhere well below 10 percent of cancer cases, how do actual rates of physician-assisted suicide and euthanasia compare? In the Netherlands, physician-assisted suicide and euthanasia on explicit request of the patient occurred in 7.0 percent of all cancer deaths. In about half of these cases, pain was one of the reasons patients asked for assistance in dying, but in only 4 percent of these cancer cases was pain the only reason. For noncancer deaths these figures are much lower: physician-assisted suicide and euthanasia on the patients' explicit request occurred in only 0.7 percent of all noncancer deaths. Pain was one of the reasons for the request in 16 percent of these cases and it was the only reason in 1 percent. In the Netherlands 2.7 percent of all deaths involve physician-assisted suicide and euthanasia on the patient's explicit request. About 37 percent of all serious and persistent requests will lead to physician-assisted suicide and euthanasia being performed. Nearly half of the serious and persistent requests are refused because alternatives are still available, the request is not well considered, the patient does not have a proper understanding of the disease, or the physician has objections either in this specific case or as a matter of general principle.[7]

Estimates of rates in the United States are more uncertain due to the likely legal repercussions for reported acts. Participation in surveys is low, and even in confidential surveys, reporting is probably less accurate than usual. Consequently, the proportion of U.S. deaths that involve physician-assisted suicide and euthanasia is unknown. We do know that 12 percent of oncology patients and 16 percent of the general public report that they have given serious consideration to assisted suicide. Actual rates of request and follow-through are less clear; 13 percent of physicians report one or more patient requests within a year; and 14 percent of oncologists report that they have participated in physician-assisted suicide and euthanasia at some point in their career. Given the large number of patients seen by physicians annually and the number of deaths that oncologists oversee in a career, the proportion of deaths in the United States that involve physician-assisted suicide and euthanasia is likely to be small. Available estimates of the rate at which U.S. physicians refuse to comply with patient requests are comparable with rates in the Netherlands. So for instance, in one study of 156 patients requesting physician-assisted suicide 73 percent were declined. U.S. physicians' reasons for declining the request included (in order of declining frequency) that they were morally opposed to assisting suicide, the patient's symptoms were treatable, depression was involved, the illness was not terminal, they feared legal consequences, the patient's suffering was insufficient, or they did not know the patient well enough. A possible interpretation of these findings is that there are some safeguards against misuse in the U.S. as well as in the Dutch medical profession.[8]

To determine whether there is nevertheless a slippery slope to be avoided, we must have at a minimum measurements from two or more different time points. At present, such data are available only from the Netherlands, where identical surveys were held in 1990 and 1995.[9] During this period, physician-assisted suicide and euthanasia on explicit request of patients rose from 2.1 to 2.7 percent of all deaths. At the same time, rates of euthanasia in patients who were unable to make a current explicit request barely changed, going from 0.8 to 0.7 percent of all deaths. The number of explicit requests for physician-assisted suicide and euthanasia increased by 9 percent, from 8,900 to 9,700 cases. In 1990, 30 percent of the requests were granted, as compared with 37 percent of requests in 1995.

There are several indications that the quality of decision-making improved during the interval between these two surveys. Consultation with one or more colleagues occurred more frequently, and written reports documenting the decision-making process and its outcome were more prevalent. Also, in 1995 about 41 percent of all cases of euthanasia and physician-assisted suicide were reported, against 18 percent in 1990.

Thus, although there was a significant increase in physician-assisted suicide and euthanasia on explicit request of the patient, at the same time the quality of the decision-making, the documentation of cases, and public scrutiny improved. This illustrates that the slippery slope debate has had no simple yes/no outcome but that continuous careful monitoring of facts and circumstances is a necessary condition for a relevant discussion.

The 0.8 percent of deaths in the Netherlands in 1990 that physicians initiated without the patient's explicit request has been used as evidence of the slippery slope of abuse. Proponents of euthanasia argue instead that the number would be larger in the absence of the kinds of open regulation that is now in place. Prior to the 1995 survey, this 0.8 percent rate was not conclusive of any trend or cause but only indicated the existence of this category of cases.[10] The 1995 survey has now shown that the number has remained almost constant at 0.7 percent of all cases. Thus, neither the argument that such cases increase in number over time, nor the argument that open regulation lowers the rate, is well supported by the data.

Dutch physicians themselves, when surveyed, show only moderate concern about the possibility of a slippery slope. A minority feels that physician-assisted suicide and euthanasia would rise in times of economic stress (13 percent) or if physician-assisted suicide and euthanasia were no longer punishable (32 percent). (At present in Holland it is illegal but not prosecuted if the requirements of careful practice are followed.) When asked, "Have your own opinions about euthanasia changed during the whole period that you have been practicing medicine?" 61 percent of Dutch physicians said that they had not changed their opinion, 25 percent said that they had become more permissive, and 14 percent said that they had become more restrictive. Both groups mention their own experience, the increased societal discussion, and the development of guidelines and explicit legal policy as reasons for their shifting opinions, often toward the middle ground. Of those who had become more permissive, only 44 percent had performed euthanasia; of those who had become more restrictive, 66 percent had direct experience with the practice. Of those who had been practicing medicine over 20 years, 39 percent said they had become more permissive, while 9 percent had become more restrictive.[11]

Whether or not there is a slippery slope in effect in Holland, extrapolation from one country to another is of limited validity. For instance, a survey among Australian doctors, using the same questionnaire as was used in Holland, estimated the occurrence of euthanasia without the patient's explicit request at 3.5 percent of all deaths, which is considerably larger than Holland's 0.7 percent. By contrast, the estimated frequency of physician-assisted suicide and euthanasia in Australia was 1.9 percent, lower than Holland's rate of 2.7 percent. Different cultures may have different types of potential for misuse. In the United States one study indicated that physicians, nurses, and social workers who approve of physician-assisted suicide and euthanasia tend to have less empathic personality profiles and lower clinical skills in symptom alleviation, and tend to spend less time with their patients. Another U.S. study indicated that families may be more interested in physician-assisted suicide and euthanasia than patients.[12]

These data raise the possibility, although they do not settle the issue, that trends in Australia or the United States would follow a different path from trends in the Netherlands. Certainly that has been the case with abortion. The Netherlands' abortion rate is the lowest for any Western country, and unwanted teenage pregnancies are virtually absent, perhaps partly due to the open discussion of contraception and teenage sexual relationships. The legalization of abortion apparently did not put Holland on a slippery slope, and may have been a factor in preventing much physical and mental suffering. But it is unclear that similar conclusions would be reasonable for the United States.

In conclusion, empirical research indicates that the ideal minimum rate of physician-assisted suicide and euthanasia for terminal patients who are suffering unbearably is quite low. The slippery slope argument that actual rates would rise much higher owing to misuse or abuse could theoretically be settled with relevant data, but so far the data available are insufficient. What we do know from the Netherlands for the period 1990–1995 suggests that open regulation neither leads inevitably to a slippery slope nor provides a sure restraint on misuse. Further, the presence or absence of a trend cannot readily be generalized to other cultures.

There is clear need for reliable prevalence and time series studies of current physician-assisted suicide and euthanasia and other end-of-life decisions. Comparisons are needed between societies which take into account relevant cultural, legal, and health service characteristics. Attempts to define the efficacy of types of legislation and types of safeguards would be better guided if such studies were available.

CULTURAL COMPARISONS What can we learn from other cultures about end-of-life decision-making? It is well documented that different cultures hold very different opinions toward assisted suicide and euthanasia. Monotheistic cultures tend toward a total ban on suicide in general, including physician-assisted suicide, and on euthanasia. Other cultures, however, condone assisted suicide and euthanasia. Often it is relatives of the patient or clan members who assist; in many cultures, in fact, there is no separate medical profession. Euthanasia and assisted suicide have been extensively documented among the Inuit and among the Dinka tribe in the Sudan. But examples can be found from Siberia, Melanesia, the Fiji Islands, North and South American Indians, Africa, ancient Greece and Rome, Hindu cultures, and pre-Christian Europe. The motivations for these practices appear to differ widely among cultures, ranging from economic pressure (food scarcity in the case of the Inuit), to honor and dignity (in Japan), to the loss of the capacity for responsible leadership (among the Dinka).[13] It seems that generally the conditions for acceptable assisted suicide and euthanasia and the procedures involved are well defined in each of these societies.

Two additional conclusions may be drawn, very cautiously, from the anthropological literature. First, respect for other persons' lives probably forms the basis of any stable society, but in some cultures this respect does not exclude the option of assisted suicide and euthanasia under well-defined circumstances and with established procedures. Second, the person who assists needs to be trusted by the person who is going to die, as well as by other members of society.

The relevance of information from non-Western countries for public policy in Western societies is, and probably will remain, limited. Within the West, however, the high life expectancy and standards of medical care that Western societies share lead to many common problems as well as possible solutions, despite large cultural differences that also exist. Many culturally situated studies and cross-cultural comparisons are essential to the debate over end-of-life decisions, even if the studies are not entirely generalizable.

Smaller-scale social and interpersonal dynamics are also relevant aspects of culture, and there is an extensive literature available in psychology and the social sciences. Social attitudes toward death and dying, the response of families to their ill and burdensome members, and the dynamics of shame and dignity are among the topics that have been addressed, but very little of this work is directly applicable to the question of physician-assisted suicide and euthanasia. One also finds scattered commentaries on the interpersonal dynamics between physicians and their dying patients, in particular the phenomena of transference and countertransference, but more empirical approaches to this area are lacking. Although studies of smaller-scale interpersonal dynamics within a culture will be in many ways unique, they can be helpful if inferences are drawn and applied carefully.[14]

Arguments Where Empirical Work Has Some Limited Relevance

THE MORAL DISTINCTION BETWEEN ACTS AND OMISSIONS
Recent biomedical philosophers have argued that the distinction between act and omission need not carry moral weight.[15] How often do circumstances occur when there would appear to be no moral difference between act and omission in end-of-life decisions?

Decisions to withhold or withdraw life-prolonging treatment have been made for 20 percent of all patients who die in the Netherlands and are more common than decisions to actively assist death, which altogether make up 3.4 percent of deaths. Physicians in the United Kingdom and Australia are also much less opposed to making nontreatment decisions than to assisting with suicide or performing euthanasia.[16]

When physicians make a decision not to treat, in many cases they think of this omission decision as not prolonging life, rather than as shortening life. This was reported by many Dutch clinicians, especially nursing home physicians. The most common reason cited for nontreatment was the burden of treatment as described by the patient (43 percent of patient cases). Loss of dignity (31 percent) and dependence (24 percent) were cited less often than among patients requesting physician-assisted suicide and euthanasia (57 and 33 percent respectively). The distinction between nontreatment and euthanasia is apparently especially important for physicians in neonatology. This has been pointed out in the official position paper of the Dutch Pediatric Society and is supported by the observation that at least half of all neonatal deaths are preceded by a decision to withhold or withdraw life-prolonging treatment, while the administration of lethal doses of drugs is extremely rare.[17]

The manner of dying also differs between the two types of decisions. The time between a decision not to treat and the death of the patient is usually more prolonged, because the most common nontreatment decisions involve withholding antibiotics and other therapeutic drugs. Nontreatment decisions with more immediate death such as removing mechanical ventilation are less frequent, but even in these cases death is slower than with standard methods of physician-assisted suicide and euthanasia.[18]

Thus, in some circumstances the intention and the outcome may be the same whether a nontreatment decision is made or an act to shorten life is taken. In most circumstances, however, the intention and the outcome differ. At some points and for some people the distinction between act and omission is immaterial, but in most instances and for most people the distinction remains.

Before an end-of-life decision is made, at least four questions should be addressed: What is the intent of the action taken, or not taken? Which agents are involved in the decision (patient, physician, or another)? What is the patient's remaining life expectancy? Is the patient able to judge his situation and to make an adequate decision? Unfortunately, there are few empirical data on the way in which any of these criteria play out in reality. For instance, physician, patient, and family intentions in their end-of-life decision-making are not well described or quantified in empirical reports. It would be helpful to know the epidemiology of intent to shorten versus the intent not to prolong life, and to understand how intents relate to the different categories of actions and outcomes for dying patients.

Further, some quantification of different conceptions of natural, expectable, and desirable life span would also be helpful, along with the relationship of medical intervention to each of the concepts. In a technically advanced society, conceptions of what a natural life span is probably assume considerable medical treatment. In a less technical or wealthy society this may be much less the case, since the techniques available to prolong life are quite limited. Such studies could help elucidate how people decide whether a certain nontreatment or intervention decision shortens the patient's "natural life," or artificially prolongs it.

PATIENT AUTONOMY A key issue that can be approached in part empirically is the degree to which a request for physician-assisted suicide or euthanasia is made of a patient's own free will. In the Netherlands and the United States, there is general respect for the autonomy of a patient's personal decision, at least in principle. In the Netherlands, 52 percent of physicians believe that everyone is entitled to make decisions about their own life and death. Among U.S. doctors the wider acceptance of physician-assisted suicide than of euthanasia perhaps represents a perceived difference in patient autonomy with these two types of intervention. In the Netherlands this difference in acceptability is smaller. Dutch culture generally considers it the physician's responsibility to check whether a physician-assisted suicide has succeeded and, if necessary, to give a final injection, so that physician-assisted suicide is potentially not so very different from euthanasia. Dutch physicians generally see both acts as warranted obligations to the patient's autonomous wishes.[19]

How often are patients' requests for physician-assisted suicide and euthanasia actually confused pleas for some other kind of help, and how often are they overly determined by wishes other than the patient's? In the United States, 39 percent of prescriptions for lethal doses of medicine remained unfilled, and about two-thirds of requests for physician-assisted suicide and euthanasia are refused by physicians. This would support the likelihood that many requests for death are not deeply genuine or persistent.

Currently, the data are insufficient to allow us to distinguish disguised requests for different kinds of help from genuine requests for physician-assisted suicide or euthanasia. Anecdotal evidence, however, supports the view that such requests can pose for different needs. For instance, the requests can go away when these different needs are met, for instance by providing reassurance that the patient will not be abandoned, education about alternatives, help with advance planning, and assistance in their social and personal support.

Psychological studies document in many ways the influence of others on patients' ostensibly free choices, including unacknowledged coercion and countertransference. Cases reported in the media echo this concern. Further, the disability literature underscores how profoundly the social environment's support or nonsupport influences patients' ability to make autonomous choices. Indeed, physicians' own feelings and beliefs can be powerful, and it is unlikely that in every situation they will suppress their personal opinion for the sake of patient autonomy.[20]

Sociodemographic data that might confirm or deny coercion of vulnerable members of society are, unfortunately, limited. The data available raise no great suspicion of systematic social coercion in Holland or the United States. Compared with all deaths, physician-assisted suicide and euthanasia occur more often in younger patients, which is partly explained by the fact that about three quarters of all physician-assisted suicide and euthanasia occur in people dying of cancer. Also in the United States, a higher proportion of requests come from young patients (46 percent of patients under 65 years); in the AIDS population especially, a high proportion of deaths are assisted. Because many AIDS patients are relatively young, well educated, and well aware of the expected course of their disease, these data might be interpreted as having a generational and possibly cultural explanation. In the United States, one public advocate of physician-assisted suicide and euthanasia has personally provided it to approximately twice as many women as men, but there are no studies that indicate whether or not his actions reflect systematic U.S. trends.[21]

Thus, respect for patient autonomy seems to be important in principle, and safeguards of process may help guarantee that the patients' wishes are primary, even though conditions for perfectly free decisions rarely pertain. At present there is little or no evidence that vulnerable social groups are receiving coerced physician-assisted suicide and euthanasia.

More data are desirable on sociodemographics, refusal rates, reasons for refusal, and psychological dynamics among people involved with suffering and dying patients. Data on the social setting and process of decisions, for instance, the prevalence of and correlates of second opinions, would help researchers assess the influence of others and the ability of due process to restrain misuse. Follow-up studies in individual cases, starting with the patient's request and documenting the contributions of all parties involved, would help answer many questions, including which physician-assisted suicide and euthanasia requests pose for different needs.

PHYSICIANS' OBLIGATIONS Can empirical research help us answer the question, Should the medical profession ever assist death? There can be no doubt that the medical profession holds among its primary values the support of life and the alleviation of suffering. But whether medical professional values prohibit or occasionally demand physician-assisted suicide and euthanasia has been a hotly debated question in more than one era and culture. The contribution of empirical research to this debate is largely limited to opinion data and tallies of published position statements.

At present the Royal Dutch Medical Association is the only medical association that supports the possibility of physician-assisted suicide and euthanasia as a professional responsibility. Many Dutch health care institutions also have explicitly documented policies on end-of-life decision making. In the Netherlands, 54 percent of physicians believe that in certain situations it is the physician's professional duty to raise euthanasia as a possibility with the patient, and 91 percent believe that euthanasia should be performed only by a physician. Many physicians in Holland also believe that at times the physician has a responsibility to administer an injection in cases of physician-assisted suicide when the drugs taken do not result in death.[22]

Physicians from other countries currently appear to be split on whether or not physician-assisted suicide and euthanasia are sometimes acceptable, or whether or not performing them is conceivable. The American Medical Association and 45 or more other professional medical organizations oppose physician-assisted suicide and euthanasia, while the American College of Physicians has adopted a neutral position, and some other organizations have endorsed physician-assisted suicide and euthanasia. Individual physicians' opinions are divided (see table).[23] As is often the case, survey data provide important but limited insight. For instance, the possibility of justifying or assisting in rare cases of physician-assisted suicide and euthanasia is not the same as being willing to actually partake in them. Following the recent legalization of assisted suicide in Australia, so many physicians expressed their unwillingness to assist that patients traveling to Australia for the purpose were unable to obtain physician assistance in suicide.

Professional opinion appears to differ from public opinion in the United States. Whereas a small percentage of patients and the general public report that trust in their physicians would be undermined by their involvement in euthanasia or physician-assisted suicide, the vast majority of physicians (80 percent) believe that trust would be undermined in this way. In a similar pattern, only 35 percent of oncologists, as compared with 66 percent of the public, supports legalization of euthanasia. In the Netherlands there is no such gap, with 88 percent of physicians and 89 percent of the public finding physician-assisted suicide and euthanasia occasionally acceptable; the majority of both groups is in favor of some form of legalization.[24]

Physicians' opinions on end-of-life decisions in different countries

Active euthanasia sometimes acceptable

	Yes (%)	No (%)	Not sure (%)
United States[a]	23 (45)		
Netherlands	97	4	
Canada	44	46	10
Australia	44	55	
Denmark	34		

Law should permit euthanasia

	Yes (%)	No (%)	Not sure (%)
United States[b]	35 (43)		
Netherlands	92	1	7
Canada	51	40	9
Australia	45	39	
United Kingdom	47	33	19
Denmark	29		

Performing euthanasia conceivable

	Yes (%)	No (%)	Not sure (%)
Netherlands	88	12	
Canada	28	51	20
United Kingdom	46	32	21

Ever performed euthanasia or assisted in suicide

	Yes (%)	No (%)	Not sure (%)
United States	14		
Netherlands	53	46	
Australia	19	73	9
United Kingdom	14	86	
Denmark	5		

Ever received request for euthanasia or physician-assisted suicide

	Yes (%)
United States	57
Netherlands	77
Australia	33
United Kingdom	45
Denmark	30

a. Approve of euthanasia in situations with incurable cancer patients having unremitting physical pain. (In parentheses: Approve of physician-assisted suicide in situations with incurable cancer patients having unremitting physical pain.) See note 23 for explanation of wording and sources of data for each country.

b. Would vote to legalize euthanasia on a referendum. (In parentheses: Would vote to legalize physician-assisted suicide on a referendum.)

Thus, there is general acceptance that the primary values of the medical profession are to support life and to alleviate suffering. Whether or not that may sometimes include euthanasia and physician-assisted suicide can in itself not be empirically decided. Attitude studies from several countries document that part of the profession thinks that physician-assisted suicide and euthanasia are acceptable and should be permitted by law, while the other part finds them unacceptable or at least not suitable for legalization.

A thorough study of the attitudes of physicians toward physician-assisted suicide and euthanasia across cultures and over time is indicated. Uniform or at least comparable and unambiguously worded questions are indispensable for these comparative studies. Further exploration of the relationship between individuals' terminal care experience and opinions on physician-assisted suicide and euthanasia in the medical profession, as well as in the public, would be helpful. Studies on the efficacy of palliative-care techniques may also be relevant to the way in which professionals implement their professional duty to alleviate suffering.

PRIVATE VERSUS PUBLIC ACTS The question, Are decisions for physician-assisted suicide and euthanasia a purely private or a public matter? cannot be empirically settled. Information about directly or indirectly expressed opinions, however, is useful here. In the Netherlands, where all physician-assisted suicide and euthanasia cases should be reported to the coroner, an estimated 41 percent are in fact being reported. Most physicians (92 percent) think that some form of legal regulation is desirable, although 79 percent of Dutch physicians also believe that euthanasia has become too much of a politically charged topic. Among the Dutch medical profession, physician-assisted suicide and euthanasia are not viewed as simply one person's decision. Physicians refuse large numbers of patient requests, and there are often long periods for decision-making after a request. This illustrates that the Dutch medical profession, while it considers physician-assisted suicide and euthanasia to be very intimate issues between patient and doctor, sees them as an issue of public importance.

Surveys are needed on physicians', patients', and the public's opinion regarding the optimal forms of control for the society in question. These should be specifically directed at the different types of decisions and decision situations as well as at the balance between private control (free choice), professional control (in the form of documented second-opinion procedures or of policy or ethics committees), and public control (legislation).

Arguments Where Empirical Data Are of Little Help

LEGALITY The merits of legalization or prohibition of physician-assisted suicide and euthanasia are partly a matter of legal and political theory and partly a matter of public and professional opinion. Dutch law accepts that in exceptional cases the physician may decide to comply with the patient's request for physician-assisted suicide or euthanasia. The accepted argument is that there can be situations where the duties of prolonging life and alleviating suffering are in conflict, because only death will end the patients' suffering. Although euthanasia is a criminal act in Dutch law, in the vast majority of cases the public prosecutor decides not to prosecute. Of the 6,324 cases reported from 1991 through 1995, inquests were conducted in 34 cases; 21 of these were dismissed, while in other cases physicians were prosecuted.[25]

In the absence of a constitutional right to physician-assisted suicide owing to the recent decision of the U.S. Supreme Court, the question of state prohibition or legalization remains. The deliberations of legislative bodies may draw on many of the diverse arguments laid out here.

On a separate question, some state commissions, institutional review boards, and others have argued that the very illegality of physician-assisted suicide and euthanasia inhibits the study of these practices. This erroneous argument should be discarded, since other illegal acts, both criminal (murder and rape, for example) and civil (tax evasion, traffic violations), are extensively studied. The quality of debate could be improved by empirical study.

SANCTITY OF LIFE The sanctity-of-life concept is a moral, *a priori* assertion, which in itself cannot be supported or refuted by empirical data. Attitudinal data may contribute to the debate, however.

Public opinion on the validity of the view that all human life is sacred and therefore all acts to end it are wrong has been exhaustively investigated. In the Netherlands and also in countries with generally less tolerant views on physician-assisted suicide and euthanasia, a sizeable proportion of physicians and the public consider euthanasia conceivable or are even in favor of legalizing it. In the Netherlands, 1 percent of physicians believe that physician-assisted suicide and euthanasia should always be punishable, while 20 percent think that they should be punishable with rare exceptions, and 72 percent think that they should not be punishable provided a set of strict criteria is met.[26]

What can we learn from the attitudes of physicians and families who have had actual experience with physician-assisted suicide and euthanasia? Do they support or oppose them? In Holland, as physicians spent more time in practice, 25 percent became more permissive, while 14 percent became more restrictive toward assisted dying. But those becoming more permissive had, overall, less experience with physician-assisted suicide and euthanasia.[27] Culture-wide trends, however, are difficult to separate from physicians' experience-driven changes in attitude, so this data will not securely settle the question.

Thus, empirical data have little bearing on the sanctity-of-life debate. Even if there were a marked change in opinion with experience, it is unclear what inference would be valid. Whether or not the sanctity of human life prohibits physician-assisted suicide and euthanasia is a matter of moral, religious, legal, or social reasoning that is little affected by empirical data. Nevertheless, tracking opinion on the connotations and arguments involved may be helpful in facilitating respectful discussion and evidencing trends in thought.

DIGNITY Is physician-assisted suicide and euthanasia more dignified than natural death? Dignity is a function of personal and social context. Otherwise identical circumstances can be dignified or undignified depending on the attitudes of the person suffering and of the other people involved. Objective measures do not determine what is dignified and what is not. Empirical data may, however, be helpful in addressing questions such as: For a specific culture, what are the optimal conditions that would make dying a dignified stage of life? The reasons for physician-assisted suicide and euthanasia requests and refusals may become relevant in such studies.

The most frequent reasons for requesting physician-assisted suicide and euthanasia are the patient's present loss of dignity or the fear of having to die in an undignified way (57 percent).[28] The conceptions of dignity in suffering and dying in different societies can be studied empirically. The conditions under which suffering can be perceived as meaningful and under which patients can retain their dignity can also be investigated, as well as the ways to maximize those conditions.

Conclusions

To summarize, for at least nine arguments for and against physician-assisted suicide and euthanasia, we have at present some relevant data. We have tried to sort the ethical arguments into three major categories: those which hinge on empirical data; those which are very case-dependent and where the occurrence of the different contexts should be studied; and moral, *a priori* assertions, where useful empirical studies tend to be limited to surveys on the distribution of opinions.

One main conclusion that should alter the direction of the physician-assisted suicide and euthanasia debate is that pain is not the most important motivator of patients or families who request physician-assisted suicide or euthanasia. This stands in contrast with the most widely supported justification for physician-assisted suicide and euthanasia, namely, mercy for intolerable pain. Rather than pain, fear of lost dignity and of being a burden drive most requests for assistance in dying. Yet, in the United States, indignity and burdensomeness are not seen by most members of the public, by the majority of physicians, or by the vast majority of bioethicists as being a justification for physician-assisted suicide and euthanasia. The significant role of social context in defining indignity and burdensomeness would make these arguments less defensible under the usual justification of a person's right to autonomy. Thus, the debate needs to come to grips with this surprising fact and settle whether, and if so when, indignity or burdensomeness could justify physician-assisted suicide and euthanasia.

A second main conclusion is that the quality of the debate would be vastly improved by further serious research into a wide range of issues surrounding the practice of physician-assisted suicide and euthanasia. By far the most important contribution would be reliable epidemiological studies about the practice of end-of-life decision-making in different countries. Such studies should not only collect information about physician-assisted suicide and euthanasia but also about other end-of-life decisions, including pain alleviation with high dosages of opiates and decisions to withhold or withdraw life-prolonging treatment. These and many other studies proposed above would clarify and guide the dialogue, both in asking the right questions and in applying the principled arguments in a known context.

End-of-life decision-making will probably become increasingly important in our society, both quantitatively and qualitatively. The aging of our society, the rate at which cancer deaths (with their associated pain and suffering) are replacing cardiovascular deaths (where life often ends suddenly), and the increasing sophistication of medical technology will likely enlarge the proportion of deaths that occur under medical care. And as the public's awareness of these changes grows, patients will expect to be more and more involved in all decision-making about their medical care. An open, fruitful discussion can start from the premise that end-of-life decisions are being made, and that these decisions should be informed by a wide range of empirical data, if they are to be consistent with high standards of medical care and with an involved medical profession.

It is our belief that new empirical studies will greatly improve the quality of the ethical debate both in society generally and in the profession, will assist in the formulation of responsible public regulations, will promote and guide the quality of medical training, and, most importantly, will help improve the quality of care for the dying.

8

Why Now?

EZEKIEL J. EMANUEL

Why have euthanasia and physician-assisted suicide become such prominent issues in the 1990s? In 1988 the landmark article, "It's over, Debbie," appeared in the *Journal of the American Medical Association (JAMA).*[1] Since that time, *Final Exit,* the Hemlock Society's suicide manual, has spent seventeen weeks on the *New York Times* best-seller list and sold over half a million copies; Dr. Kevorkian has helped more than thirty people end their lives and has been acquitted by three juries; Oregon has enacted an assisted suicide referendum; a federal appellate court has permitted physicians to assist suicide, and another federal appellate court has even recognized a constitutional right to euthanasia and assisted suicide;[2] more than twenty states have considered legislation on euthanasia and assisted suicide; and the U.S. Supreme Court and the Florida Supreme Court have both ruled that there is no right to physician-assisted suicide.

This heightened interest in euthanasia and physician-assisted suicide is not restricted to the United States. In Canada the Sue Rodriguez case, involving a woman with amyotrophic lateral sclerosis (Lou Gehrig's disease) who requested euthanasia, was heard by the Canadian Supreme Court. In 1995 the Northern Territory in Australia legalized euthanasia and assisted suicide. Dutch courts have also recently ruled on euthanasia cases involving infants and patients with mental illness. And interest in euthanasia in Britain has included several important legal cases as well as a major report by the House of Lords.[3]

There have been numerous explanations for this sudden interest in euthanasia and physician-assisted suicide. In declaring euthanasia a constitutional right, the Ninth Circuit Court argued that "the emergent right to receive medical assistance in hastening one's death [is the] inevitable consequence of changes in the causes of death, medical advances, and development of new technologies." Others claim that physicians' indifference to dying patients and the inept and insensitive care these patients often receive have stimulated interest in euthanasia. Still others see euthanasia and physician-assisted suicide as the ultimate triumph of the growing movement for autonomy and patients' rights to control their lives, specifically to control the manner and timing of the end of their lives.[4]

But this is not the first time in history, even modern history, that euthanasia and physician-assisted suicide have become prominent public issues. One way to begin to understand the current interest—to understand its causes, significance, and possibly how we should approach it—is to consider the history of euthanasia and physician-assisted suicide.

A History of Euthanasia and Physician-Assisted Suicide

Debates over the ethics of euthanasia and physician-assisted suicide are as old as medicine itself. In ancient Greece and Rome, there was no censure for suicide. Consequently, physician assistance, either through euthanasia or physician-assisted suicide, was widely accepted and practiced. As the great historian of ancient medicine Ludwig Edelstein has written: "Many people preferred voluntary death to endless agony. This form of 'euthanasia' was an everyday reality . . . many physicians actually gave their patients the poison for which they were asked."[5] Indeed, most of the prominent Greek philosophical schools—the Platonists, Cynics, and Stoics—endorsed physician-assisted suicide to escape the pains of disease, public humiliation, and other problems. The Romans also accepted the Stoic view of euthanasia and physician-assisted suicide. Seneca, for instance, expressed the prevailing view: "Against all the injuries of life I have the refuge of death. If I can choose between a death of torture and one that is simple and easy, why should I not select the latter? . . . Why should I endure the agonies of disease when I can emancipate myself from all my torments?"

In the first century A.D., Pliny the Younger, whose letters recorded the details of everyday life in Rome, described the typical case of Titius Aristo, "who has been seriously ill for a long time . . . he fights against pain, resists thirst, and endures the unbelievable heat of his fever without moving or throwing off his coverings. A few days ago, he sent for me and some of his intimate friends, and told us to ask the doctors what the outcome of his illness would be, so that if it was to be fatal, he could deliberately put an end to his life."[6]

Some ancient writers even went so far as to enumerate the conditions, both social and medical, for which euthanasia and physician-assisted suicide should be deemed acceptable. Pliny the Elder suggested suicide for bladder stones, stomach disorders, and headaches. He remarked that "the Stoic founder, Zeno, committed suicide in his old age prompted by the agonizing pain of a foot injury." Other writers explored the various procedures for euthanasia and physician-assisted suicide, ranging from phlebotomy to poisons.

But this widespread acceptance and practice of euthanasia and physician-assisted suicide was not without its critics. The Hippocratic school of medicine was most prominent in its refusal to participate in euthanasia and physician-assisted suicide. The most renowned statement of this position is in the Hippocratic Oath, which requires physicians to pledge "never [to] give a deadly drug to anybody if asked for it, nor . . . make a suggestion to this effect."

Beginning in the second or third century A.D., attitudes began to shift, mostly because of the increasing importance of Christianity and the growing opposition of Christianity to suicide. As Christianity spread, its opposition to euthanasia and physician-assisted suicide also spread. While the paucity of historical records limits the ability to precisely document this change in attitudes and practices, at least some historians claim that sometime between the twelfth and fifteenth centuries, European physicians became consistently opposed to euthanasia.

With the rise of the Renaissance and the rediscovery of ancient Greek and Roman writers, some early modern European intellectuals began advocating suicide, physician-assisted suicide, and euthanasia. Among the most vocal and prominent were Thomas More and Francis Bacon. In 1516 Sir Thomas More has Raphael Hythloday tell of the practice of euthanasia in *Utopia:* "They console the incurably ill by sitting and talking with them and by alleviating whatever pain they can. Should life become unbearable for these incurables the magistrates and priests do not hesitate to prescribe euthanasia . . . When the sick have been persuaded of this, they end their lives willingly either by starvation or drugs, that dissolve their lives without any sensation of death. Still, the Utopians do not do away with anyone without his permission, nor lessen any of their duties to him."[7]

In the seventeenth century, Francis Bacon argued that physicians were overly aggressive in prolonging life and that they should instead perform what we consider euthanasia. In *Advancement of Learning* Bacon wrote: "I esteem it the office of a physician not only to restore the health, but to mitigate pains and dolors; and not only when such mitigation may conduce to recovery, but when it may serve to make a fair and easy passage . . . Augustus Caesar was wont to wish to himself . . . that same *Euthanasia.*"

As part of a general attack on religious authority, many writers, including John Donne, Montesquieu, and other English and French philosophers, attacked Church-based prohibitions against suicide. While they did not explicitly advocate euthanasia, their arguments could also justify it. Most clear and unflinching in this regard was David Hume, whose essay "On Suicide" argued "that Suicide may often be consistent with interest and with our duty to ourselves, no one can question, who allows that age, sickness, or misfortune, may render life a burden, and make it worse even than annihilation."[8]

Rousseau and most of the great German philosophers, including Kant, Hegel, Schopenhauer, and Nietzsche, opposed suicide and euthanasia. Kant, for instance, argued:

The man who contemplates suicide will ask "Can my action be compatible with the Idea of humanity *as an end in itself?*" If he does away with himself in order to escape from a painful situation he is making use of a person merely as a *means* to maintain a tolerable state of affairs till the end of his life. But man is not a thing—not something to be used *merely* as a means; he must always in all his actions be regarded as an end in himself. Hence I cannot dispose of man in my person by maiming, spoiling, or killing.

Nietzsche, himself afflicted by severe pains, thought it more noble to will life despite pain.

None of this intellectual interest in suicide and euthanasia seems to have had any major effect on the way medicine was practiced or to have provoked a broader, sustained public interest.[9] Things began to change in the early part of the nineteenth century due to advances in medical therapeutics and changes in attitudes. In the early nineteenth century, morphine was isolated, providing an effective mechanism to alleviate pain. Simultaneously, physicians in Germany began advocating "euthanasia," but they meant by this comfort and support of the dying patient, avoidance of heroic measures that so often made death miserable, and use of medications like morphine to ease the symptoms associated with dying. These German physicians never advocated what we now view as euthanasia, that is, the intentional and active termination of life.

Most notable in this regard is a thesis by a German medical student from Jena, Carl F. H. Marx, entitled *Medical Euthanasia:*

It is easily apparent what can be accomplished by administration of medicines where there is no room for the preservation of life or for the restitution of health. What good will it do the incurable patient to apply dangerous and dubious therapeutic measures? The entire plan of treatment will here confine itself within "symptomatic and palliative indication" . . . Soothing, soporific, sedative, analgesic, and antispasmodic medicines will answer such a purpose . . . To end the patient's pitiful condition by purposely and deliberately hastening death, how can it be permitted that he who is by law required to preserve life be the origination of, or partner in, its destruction? This would be both against religion and against utterances of the wisest men.[10]

This perspective also gained credence in the Anglo-American world in the mid-nineteenth century. In 1846 John Warren performed the first operation with anesthesia at the Massachusetts General Hospital. In 1848 he published a book, *Etherization: With Surgical Remarks* in which he described providing ether to ease the death of a 90-year-old-woman.[11] Ether was used, he wrote, to treat the "pain of mortification . . . [and pain] of the abdomen with convulsive twitchings of the limbs . . . with perfect relief." More generally, he suggested that ether might be used "in mitigating the agonies of death." During the Civil War, American physicians became more experienced in using hypodermic morphine to relieve pain, and its use spread after the war.

In 1866 Joseph Bullar reported in the *British Medical Journal* using chloroform for the "palliation" of excruciating pain during the death of four patients.[12] In urging chloroform and narcotics for the dying, Bullar, a physician at the Royal South Hant Infirmary, argued that "where disease can only be palliated, that palliation becomes a very important part of our duties." He also addressed what he called the ethical question, arguing against those who invoked religious reasons to object to using chloroform for palliation claiming that pain was part of God's plan. Warren and Bullar never recommend using ether, chloroform, or morphine to end a patient's life but only to relieve "the pains of death."

In 1870 interest began to shift from easing the dying process to euthanasia and physician-assisted suicide as we currently understand those terms. It was in that year that an Englishman, Samuel D. Williams, a nonphysician, addressed the Birmingham Speculative Club on the topic of euthanasia. Going beyond the suggestions of Warren and Bullar, Williams advocated using chloroform or other medications not just to relieve the pain of dying but to end intentionally a patient's life. Williams argued:

> The main object of the present essay being merely to establish the reasonableness of the following proposal:—*That in all cases of hopeless and painful illness, it should be the recognized duty of*

the medical attendant, whenever so desired by the patient, to administer chloroform or such other anaesthetic as may by-and-by supersede chloroform—so as to destroy consciousness at once, and put the sufferer to a quick and painless death; all needful precautions being adopted . . . to establish, beyond the possibility of doubt or question, that the remedy was applied at the express wish of the patient [emphasis in the original].[13]

Such an isolated speech, before a provincial club by a relatively obscure person, might have vanished from the public arena unnoticed. Williams's speech, however, was not ignored. It was printed in a collection of essays of the Birmingham Speculative Club and was widely reviewed in the most prominent British literary and political journals of the day—including *The Spectator* and *The Saturday Review*—which praised his ideas as "remarkable" and for their "considerable ingenuity" and "plausibility." His speech was reprinted as a book in 1872 and favorably reviewed, with lengthy quotes, in the widely circulated *Popular Science Monthly*.[14] In 1873 Lionel Tollemache published an article entitled "The New Cure for Incurables" in the *Fortnightly Review*. His aim was to popularize Williams's position and to bolster the justification for letting physicians assist patients with "cancer, creeping paralysis, or something equally unpleasant" to die and avoid the "ingenious cruelty [of being] kept suffering against nature and against his own will."

Williams's proposal seemed to express a deep but unarticulated view. The latter third of the nineteenth century in Britain and the United States was characterized by an individualistic conservatism which praised *laissez faire* economics, scientific method, and rationalism, in opposition to reverence for authority, tradition, and sentimental attachments. This Gilded Age was also a time of industrialization, intense corporate competition, and unprecedented strikes and clashes between unions and the corporations trying to crush them. It was a time in which free market economics caused wild oscillations, with major depressions sparked by the panic of 1873, the droughts of the 1880s, and the stock market crash of 1893.

This raw individualism, economic competition, and rationalism were reinforced and sanctioned by appeals to Darwinism. After publication of *The Origin of Species* in 1859, intellectuals rushed to incorporate Darwinism into their theories; it gave the imprimatur of rigorous science to sociology, economics, and other disciplines. Through the work of Herbert Spencer in Britain, William Graham Sumner in the United States, and others, the concepts of "survival of the fittest" and "struggle for existence" became, according to Richard Hofstadter, "the store of ideas to which solid and conservative men appealed when they wished to reconcile their fellows" to the practices and hardships associated with the era's individualism and laissez faire economic policies.[15] Social Darwinism "serves students of the American mind as a fossil specimen from which the intellectual body of the period [1870–1900] can be reconstructed."[16]

Williams's ideas quickly became the subject of intense debate within the medical profession. The *Medical and Surgical Reporter* ran an article in 1873 that asked "whether, when a patient is past all hope, a victim to a fatal disease, entailing great agony . . . [and] he and the family alike beseech us to 'put an end to his misery,' we ought to do so?" The conclusion was that "it would be no benefit to the race, even if public sentiment and our own conscience justified us in invoking Death to relieve suffering." The article ended with the hope that new substances would be able to relieve pain "while the intellect and special senses will continue in their unimpeded activity."

In April 1879 the South Carolina Medical Association heard a report from its Committee on Ethics regarding active euthanasia and vigorously debated the issue, as well as whether to keep its discussion secret from the public.[17] The committee argued that "it is the physician's duty to make death as easy as possible when it is inevitably soon to occur" but argued that the taking of human life was unethical. It also feared the abuses that might arise if euthanasia were permitted.

Over the next few years, other medical societies debated euthanasia. For instance, in May 1884 Dr. Henry Leffmann addressed the Third Meeting of the Medical Jurisprudence Society of Philadelphia with a talk entitled "Euthanasia: a consideration of the permissibility of terminating life in cases of hopeless and painful illness." In 1889 Dr. Frank Hitchcock presented the annual oration before the Maine Medical Society on euthanasia. He lamented the paucity of information in the "medical literature on the management of the dying, or on the treatment best adapted to the relief of sufferings incident to that condition." But he concluded by quoting the ex-Chief Justice of the Supreme Court of New York to the effect: "To be justified by law, the [physician's] motive must be simply to relieve the pain of dissolution. The doctor has no right to administer anything with the intention of terminating life." Similarly, during the 1880s British and American medical journals wrote editorials on euthanasia, often referring back to Williams's speech as the original formulation of the idea.[18]

Yet while becoming acclimated to using narcotics for pain relief, most physicians and medical societies rejected Williams's suggestion and rigorously distinguished active and passive euthanasia. Dr. Wilhite of South Carolina was typical in arguing that "physicians might soften suffering, but not hasten death." The *Boston Medical and Surgical Journal* wrote an editorial noting some musings by "the Poet at the Breakfast Table" (a.k.a. Oliver Wendell Holmes Sr.) regarding euthanasia and commenting: "Perhaps logically it is difficult to justify a passive more than an active attempt at euthanasia; but certainly it is much less abhorrent to our feelings. To surrender to superior forces is not the same thing as to lead an attack of the enemy upon one's own friends."[19]

While anesthesia, the germ theory of disease, better diagnostic tests, and effective surgical operations were helping allopathic physicians of the 1880s to consolidate their intellectual authority as well as their control over licensing and medical school training requirements, their authority was far from secure.[20] They faced the old challenges from Sectarians—homeopaths and Eclectics—as well as new ones from Christian Science and osteopathy. In this precarious position, allopathic physicians perceived Williams's ideas on euthanasia as another effort to undermine them. In a characteristic editorial, *JAMA* attacked euthanasia as a "euphemistic term for what may be called *professional murder*" (emphasis in the original), and went on to call Williams's proposal a "ghastly idea" that would make the "physician don the robes of an executioner."

By the 1890s the euthanasia debate expanded beyond the medi-

cal profession to include lawyers and social scientists. The antago-
nism between physicians and lawyers was present even then, with
lawyers attacking physician authority and calling for greater patients' rights. During the early 1890s Albert Bach, a New York
lawyer and Vice President of the Medico-Legal Society of New
York, spoke at numerous conferences advocating euthanasia and
physician-assisted suicide. At the 1895 Medico-Legal Congress,
for instance, he endorsed euthanasia because patients should
have a right to end their lives: "There are also cases in which the
ending of human life by physicians is not only morally right, but
an act of humanity. I refer to cases of absolutely incurable, fatal
and agonizing disease or condition, where death is certain and
necessarily attended by excruciating pain, when it is the wish of
the victim that a deadly drug should be administered to end his
life and terminate his irremediable suffering."[21]

One of the more controversial speeches on euthanasia at the
end of the nineteenth century was made by Simeon Baldwin in his
1899 Presidential Address to the American Social Science Association. Baldwin delivered a blistering attack on the medical profession, claiming that terminally ill patients are "kept panting for
breath so, and screaming with pain, by medical skill." The problem, according to Baldwin, is that the modern physician "has the
power to hold us back from the grave, in a state of long-drawn
agony, for a few days, a few weeks, a few years, to which the
physician of antiquity was a stranger," and he uses this power
despite the irreversibility of the disease and the suffering created
by the treatment. Baldwin concluded his denunciation by stating,
"I do say that it is not right that [a terminal and painful] life
should be prolonged in hopeless misery, by medical art, against
the sufferer's will, when nature has plainly called him away."

While from our perspective Baldwin's remarks seem mostly an
effort to exhort physicians to withdraw their life-sustaining and
death-prolonging interventions from terminally ill patients, he
was interpreted by his contemporaries as endorsing euthanasia.
But Baldwin went even further than advocating euthanasia for
competent adults to advocating it for children. Baldwin claimed
that just as the elderly should have the right to die, so too should
"the unfortunate babe, that is born into the world with physical

defects." Physicians vigorously contested these positions, claiming, among other things, that they would "bring the profession into discredit."[22]

Twentieth-Century Perspectives

At the turn of the century, euthanasia debates continued on the editorial pages of medical journals and in formal presentations at meetings of learned societies. But more importantly, they moved into the lay press and political forums. Probably the most notable event occurred in 1905–06. Professor Charles Eliot Norton, a renowned classicist at Harvard and member of Harvard's Board of Overseers, delivered a speech advocating euthanasia. His position inspired a wealthy woman, Anna Hill, whose mother was suffering from cancer, to campaign for the legalization of euthanasia in Ohio. Representative Hunt introduced a bill entitled "An Act Concerning Administration of Drugs Etc. to Mortally Injured and Diseased Persons" into the Ohio legislature to legalize euthanasia.

Hunt's bill prompted significant interest in the medical and lay press. *The New York Times* reported on the bill, wrote editorials against it, especially condemning Norton's role, and published charged letters for and against euthanasia:

> Careful and accurate observation would reveal, we think, that the periodic raising of this equally absurd and outrageous question [of euthanasia] is due, not to an exceptionally tender regard for the victims of accident and disease, but to a morbid sensitiveness at the sight of what is or seems to be uselessly prolonged suffering. A too suspicious critic of the euthanasiasts might charge them, or some of them, with a selfish disinclination for taking the trouble and enduring the annoyances which the sight and care of a certain class of patients imposes on friends and relatives.[23]

The normally judicious and moderate *British Medical Journal* denounced the notion of legalizing euthanasia in a highly impassioned editorial, which among other things asserted that "America is a land of hysterical legislation" in which "every now and again [the legalization of euthanasia] is put forward by literary *dilettanti* who discuss it as an academic subtlety or by neurotic 'intellectuals' whose high-strung temperament cannot bear the thought of pain. The medical profession has always sternly set its face against a measure that would inevitably pave the way to the grossest abuse and would degrade them to the position of executioners." And the editors of *JAMA* attacked the advocates of euthanasia for their utilitarianism: "On a purely utilitarian basis, old people past their productive period could be easily disposed of, but this is not the tendency of modern civilization. Any civilization that adopted such a course would be taking a long step backward toward savagery." Hunt's bill was rejected by the Ohio legislature, 79 to 23.[24]

After 1906 the intensity of the British and American interest in euthanasia dwindled, although, as one editorial stated, the issue was "like a recurring decimal" with periodic reappearances on both sides of the Atlantic.[25] In 1906, for instance, Dr. Russell Wells addressed the Medico-Legal Society in London on the question "Is euthanasia ever justifiable?" In 1912 Abraham Jacobi, President of the American Medical Association, wrote an editorial denouncing euthanasia because it would "make true what Plato said of the practice of medicine 'It was no respectable calling.'" In 1913 the *Medical Review of Reviews* solicited the opinions of major Americans, ranging from Eugene Debs and the historian Charles Beard to Drs. William Welch and Roswell Park, and printed them as a "symposium on euthanasia." But at no time was there sustained interest in the topic either within the medical profession or in the larger American and British polities.

The public had begun turning against unfettered competition, survival of the fittest, and economic gains as the only measure of success. These philosophies were being replaced by Progressivism in America, and there was election of Liberals in Britain. The new views advocated that government should promote general welfare and viewed harmony through cooperation as more desirable than the gains of raw competition. The idea that professional expertise could solve problems better than the market was also sanctioned. This corresponded to a time in which the profession had consolidated its authority over medical education and practice.[26]

But just as interest in euthanasia and physician-assisted suicide was subsiding in Britain and the United States, it was increasing and developing academic credibility in Germany. Interest in euthanasia in Germany began in the mid-1890s, coinciding with the rediscovery of Mendel's laws of genetics and the rise of scientific racism and eugenics. Among the first important German publications on euthanasia or "mercy killing" was *The Right to Death* by Adolf Jost in 1895. Over the next few decades there was examination of issues surrounding suicide and consensual murder among German legal scholars, culminating in *The Right to Destroy Life Unworthy of Life* published in 1920. Karl Binding, a Professor of Law at Leipzig, and Alfred Hoche, a Professor of Psychiatry at Freiburg, "turned out to be the prophets of direct medical killing" in this work.[27]

Binding and Hoche claimed that euthanasia should be possible for individuals with "terminal cancer, untreatable tuberculosis, and mortal wounds . . . who, fully understanding their situation, possess and have somehow expressed their urgent wish for release." Of greater prominence in both space and rhetorical stress, however, were their arguments favoring euthanasia based on the need to preserve the *Volk* and reduce social costs. Binding and Hoche favorably quoted and echoed Jost's claim that certain individuals have a duty to be euthanized for the good of the state. Binding also argued that "incurable idiots . . . [who] are a fearfully heavy burden both for their families and for society" could be killed. Hoche, the psychiatrist, went even further, arguing that individuals with brain damage and "the incurably insane [are] . . . mentally dead having value neither for society nor for the individual." They place "economic and moral burdens upon the environment, the institution, and the state . . . It is easy to estimate what *incredible capital* is withdrawn from the nation's wealth for food, clothing, and heating." Hoche then calculates the annual cost of each mentally dead person—1300 marks in 1920—and concludes: "In the prosperous times of the past, the question of whether one could justify making all necessary provision for such dead weight existences was not pressing. But now [after World War I] things have changed, and we must take it up seriously . . . There is no room for half-strength, quarter-strength, or eighth strength members." Thus, the German advocacy of "mercy killing" based on "compassion and relief of suffering of the incurably ill" was over-shadowed by very strong claims that euthanasia would relieve the *Volk* of economically burdensome individuals.

In 1931 the debate about euthanasia in Britain exploded back into medicine.[28] Dr. C. Killick Millard, a prescient advocate of compulsory vaccination and the use of birth control and a well-respected public health official in England, became the President of the Society of Medical Officers of Health in Britain in 1931. In his presidential address, Millard presented a scholarly review of the history of euthanasia and suicide, ending with a forceful recommendation to legalize voluntary euthanasia in Britain. Millard even delineated a model bill.[29]

Millard's view and the interest it generated prompted the creation of the Voluntary Euthanasia Legislation Society. The Euthanasia Society proposed legislation to legalize euthanasia which required the patient to "sign an official application form; his signature duly attested by two witnesses, one of them of a specified status. He must also obtain two independent medical certificates that he was suffering from incurable disease likely to involve severe pain. These would be sent to an official whose duty it would be to ensure that the case was a proper one to come under the Act, and if satisfied he would grant the necessary permit, not to be acted upon until after an interval of seven days. The practitioner who was to administer euthanasia [who may not be the patient's usual physician] would be named in the permit, and would hold a [euthanasia] license from the Minister of Health."[30]

The leaders of this society were all prominent physicians. The President was a famous surgeon and former President of the Royal College of Surgeons, Lord Moynihan; the medical Vice-President was a former President of the Royal College of Physicians, Sir Humphry Rolleston; Millard was the secretary; and the chairman of the executive committee was D. J. Bond, a consulting surgeon to the Leicester Royal Infirmary. To pre-empt objections based on religion, the inaugural meeting included endorsements by a number of prominent religious leaders, such as the past and current Deans of St. Paul's. The first meeting of the Voluntary Euthanasia Society was held in the British Medical Association (BMA) House in Tavistock Square, London.[31]

During this period, the idea of legalizing euthanasia was vigorously debated at many public forums and in the British medical journals. Many argued the ethics of the matter and others objected to the elaborate safeguards, permitting extensive intrusion of bureaucrats into the physician-patient relationship. In late 1935 the public's interest in the subject was fanned by the London *Daily Mail*, which published an interview with an unnamed "elderly country physician" who confessed that he had committed euthanasia on five suffering patients over his career. This story created a public stir both in Britain and in the United States; newspapers and magazines rivaled one another in printing lurid requests for euthanasia from patients, sensational testimonials on past incidents of euthanasia from physicians, and denunciations of the requests and stories by physicians and medical organizations. *Time* ran three articles on euthanasia, including one that portrayed a suffering patient who desired euthanasia.[32]

In Britain a formal bill to legalize euthanasia was submitted to the House of Lords. On its second reading, it was debated on December 1, 1936. Lord Moynihan, President of the Voluntary Euthanasia Society, had died before the debate. The two physician peers, Lord Dawson and Lord Horder, argued against the bill, strongly contributing to its defeat, 35 to 14. The bill, therefore, was never sent to the House of Commons.[33]

Quickly after the defeat of the Voluntary Euthanasia Society's efforts came World War II and the discovery of the Nazi death camps and elucidation of the relationship between genocide and German physicians. These factors combined to mute interest in euthanasia. Beginning in the late 1950s, however, Ganville Williams and Yale Kamisar revived the debate over the ethics of euthanasia in the British and American legal literature. In 1969 the first bill to legalize euthanasia since 1936 was introduced into the British Parliament. During the 1970s and early 1980s euthanasia became a subject of more extensive academic debate in many countries and a point of public contention mainly in the Netherlands. But it was not until the late 1980s that euthanasia and physician-assisted suicide began to attract substantial medical and public interest in the United States and Britain.[34]

The Arguments Then and Now

While the mere occurrence of these debates about the ethics and legality of euthanasia is extremely interesting, of even greater interest is the fact that the arguments and justifications advanced both for and against euthanasia have not changed over a century. British and American authors of the past use the language of contemporary bioethics, such as right, autonomy, beneficence, justice, much more sparingly; nevertheless the moral grounds of their arguments are just the same as those advanced today. Indeed, aside from some elements of style and phrasing, the articles of 1885 or 1890 could be dated 1985 or 1990.

Those arguing for the legalization of euthanasia and physician-assisted suicide typically began by making two preliminary observations that set the context for their claims. First, they claim that physicians have been excessively aggressive in prolonging the lives of terminally ill patients. "In civilized nations and particularly of late years, it has become the pride of many in the medical profession to prolong [the lives of the terminally ill] at any cost of discomfort or pain to the sufferer, or of suspense and exhaustion to his family" (Baldwin, 1899). Second, that it is only humane to put terminally ill animals suffering pain out of their misery. "In the case of an animal suffering from some incurable and painful disease, or which has been hopelessly mutilated by some accident, common humanity demands that we should 'put the poor creature out of its pain.' This is not only regarded as an act of mercy but as a positive duty, the neglect of which amounts to actual cruelty" (Millard, 1931).

After these background observations, the argument for euthanasia typically begins with the claim that patients have a right to control the manner of their death and, more particularly, that terminally ill patients should have the right to a quick and painless death by euthanasia or physician-assisted suicide. As Eugene Debs and Dr. Millard, respectively, put it: "Human life is sacred, but only to the extent that it contributes to the joy and happiness of the one possessing it, and to those about him, and it ought to be the privilege of every human being to cross the River Styx in the boat of his own choosing, when further human agony cannot be justified by the hope of future health and happiness" (1913). "The proposition merely is that individuals, who have attained to years of discretion, and who are suffering from an incurable and fatal disease which usually entails a slow and painful death, should be allowed by law—*if they so desire* and if they have complied with the requisite conditions—to substitute for the slow and painful death a quick and painless one. This, I submit, should be regarded not merely as an act of mercy, but *as a matter of elementary human right"* (emphasis in the original, 1931). Furthermore, it is argued that euthanasia promotes the well-being of patients racked by pain. "There can, however, be no doubt that if such a system [legalizing euthanasia] could be introduced with sufficient safeguards, it would put an end to a great quantity of human suffering" (Williams, 1872).

Next, those advocating the legalization of euthanasia argue that there is no substantive ethical distinction between withdrawing life-sustaining treatments or administering narcotics for pain relief and actively administering medications to curtail a patient's life.

The very medical attendant who would revolt from the bare idea of putting a hopelessly suffering patient to death outright, though the patient implored him to do so, would feel no scruple in giving temporary relief by opiates, or other anaesthetics, even though he were absolutely sure that he was shortening the patient's life by their use. Suppose, for instance, that a given patient were certain to drag on through a whole month of hideous suffering, if left to himself and Nature, but that the intensity of his sufferings could be allayed by drugs, which nevertheless would hasten the known inevitable end by a week;—there are few, if any, medical men who would hesitate to give the drugs . . . Is it not clear that if you once break in upon life's sacredness, if you curtail its duration by never so little, the same reasoning that justifies a minute's shortening of it, will justify an hour's, a day's a week's, a month's, a year's; and that all subsequent appeal to the inviolability of life is vain? (ibid.)

In addition, it is argued that permitting euthanasia would not only relieve pain of the terminally ill but have the added benefit of reassuring people in general that death would not be painful.

"If this remedy [of euthanasia] were of recognized and general use, the greatest evil man has to submit to would be so far modified as to lose its chiefest dread; death might then be faced calmly by the timid as well as the brave; its sufferings might be met without quailing by the weak as well as by the strong" (ibid.).

Finally, it is claimed that the legalization of voluntary euthanasia and physician-assisted suicide for the terminally ill is not a "slippery slope" that would ultimately permit involuntary euthanasia; there is a clear ethical distinction between granting euthanasia to a patient who requests it and committing involuntary euthanasia on the incompetent. Only the former, it is argued, is deemed ethical. According to an editorial in the *St. Louis Medical Review* (1906):

> As regards any application of this principle to the elimination of the unfit or the degenerate, the imbecile, etc. as such, we find no such suggestion . . . It would be entirely out of keeping with the consistently expressed individualism . . . The fact that [euthanasia] may be justifiable, perhaps even a duty of humanity, under certain circumstances, exceptional circumstances, if you like—to yield to the pleas of the sufferer himself for "the end of pain," in no sense supports the idea that any person or persons may properly decide to eliminate the degenerate or the imbecile against or in the absence of his express consent and desire.

It is important to note that the arguments for euthanasia and physician-assisted suicide in the United States and Britain differ from those offered by Binding and Hoche in Germany. As in Germany, there was a vigorous eugenics movement in the United States. The passage of the first involuntary sterilization bill for eugenics occurred in 1907 in Indiana, and the Eugenics Record Office was founded at Cold Spring Harbor in 1910. And there were vigorous debates on eugenics in the 1920s among British and American physicians.[35] The arguments used to advocate for eugenics, however, were disconnected from the advocacy of euthanasia and physician-assisted suicide in Britain and the United States.

True, some British and American writers advocated euthanasia as a means to rid society of unproductive and burdensome dependents. For instance, at the 1906 meeting of the London Medico-Legal Society a participant claimed that he would "raise no protest against a law ordaining the use of the lethal chamber for absolute idiots, incurably demented persons, and convicted murderers." But the more common view was one expressed by a British physician opposed to euthanasia who favored eugenics of the "socially burdensome." The justification for euthanasia and physician-assisted suicide that resonated with the American and British public stressed patients' rights to self-determination and the relief of pain and suffering. Arguments for euthanasia based on economics and purifying society of the "feeble-minded" were made with less frequency, less sharply, by less prominent individuals, and garnered less public support.

Those American and British physicians and writers who opposed euthanasia and physician-assisted suicide made arguments related to the medical practice at the time of death, to the ethics of euthanasia itself, and to the adverse consequences of its legalization. Most critics of euthanasia and physician-assisted suicide noted that the cases requiring euthanasia and physician-assisted suicide are much fewer than its proponents suggest and that in fact death and the approach of death are usually not accompanied by pain. "Contrary to popular belief, the process of dying, or the act of death itself, is *rarely* and exceptionally attended with pain or severe bodily suffering. Physicians who have had ample opportunities of observation from their connection with hospitals or in their private practice, clergymen, and intelligent nurses will all bear witness to the truth of the statement" (Williams, 1894).

Next it is argued that in the past physicians may have been overly aggressive in prolonging life, but now physicians are more sensitive and willing to treat pain aggressively, even if it might shorten life, and to withdraw futile interventions. Indeed, an exchange in the correspondence section of *The Lancet* (1899) illustrates the willingness to use narcotics. A physician asks about a patient who had invasive uterine cancer with severe pain. Because of the pain, her "death struggle was an awful and most pitiable experience." He then asks of his *"confreres"* "would it be justifiable to use morphia hypodermically? or to what extent would the inhalation of chloroform be admissible in mitigation of so great agony and distress?" A correspondent writes back claiming not only is the physician justified but he is duty-bound to use hypodermic morphine.[36]

Similarly the editors of *The Lancet* reply that "it would have been perfectly justifiable for him to have used morphia hypodermically and patients are frequently kept under chloroform cautiously administered for hours to mitigate the sufferings . . . We consider that a practitioner is perfectly justified in pushing such treatment to an extreme degree, if that is the only way of affording freedom from acute suffering . . . If the risks be explained to the friends we are of opinion that even should death result the medical man has done the best he can for his patient."

The sentiment that physicians are ethically and professionally justified in using high-dose morphine to relieve terminal pain even if it shortens life seems to have been widely shared. It was noted, however, that this use of morphine for pain relief is ethically distinct from intentionally using medications to kill a patient. As many physicians and editorials in medical journals argued, there is a distinction between deliberately killing a patient and allowing the patient to die by withholding interventions or acting to relieve pain. Here are two typical presentations of the argument:

> Perhaps logically it is difficult to justify a passive more than an active attempt at euthanasia; but certainly it is much less abhorrent to our feelings. To surrender to superior forces is not the same thing as to lead an attack of the enemy upon one's own friends. (*Boston Medical and Surgical Journal*, 1884)

> I should not hesitate to use morphia, or even chloroform, freely, with the intent to relieve pain; but surely it should not be beyond the power of a capable physician to so grade the dosage as to keep the patient free from pain but short of killing him. And should he accidentally or unintentionally in such a case as this administer an overdose, this is a very different thing from willingly and knowingly poisoning the patient. (*St. Louis Medical Review*, 1906)

Having made these arguments about the ethics of caring for dying patients, opponents of euthanasia and physician-assisted suicide typically examined four deleterious practical consequences of legalizing euthanasia and physician-assisted suicide. First is the claim that legalizing euthanasia and physician-assisted suicide is likely to lead to abuse. Euthanasia and physician-assisted suicide, it is argued, "would put into the hands of unscrupulous parties a certain and easy method of being rid of an objectionable relative" (*JAMA*, 1885) and "physicians might, under the pretense of doing a merciful act, really commit a deed of felony" (*JAMA*, 1901).

Second, the legalization of euthanasia and physician-assisted suicide would place tremendous pressure on patients to request it to relieve their families' distress. "The patient knows that he is being a burden to his loved ones, who are certainly sharing his agony. If the agonized patient know that he alone can cut short their mental suffering by consenting to, or perhaps suggesting euthanasia, he will find himself faced with a hideous dilemma: he must either be so selfish as to discard euthanasia and let his dear ones suffer, or, by being generous, he must bid farewell to those last sweetest, still hopeful, moments of life" (1936).[37]

Third, and more importantly, legalizing euthanasia and physician-assisted suicide would undermine the trust at the heart of the physician-patient relationship and thereby destroy the profession. "Once an alteration was made in that conception of a physician's duty [by legalizing euthanasia] the whole public confidence in the medical profession would go" (*JAMA*, 1919). Indeed, legalizing euthanasia would "degrade [physicians] to the position of executioners."

The doctor is eagerly awaited with the hope, not that he will put the man out of pain, but that he will put the pain out of the man. . This new society aims at putting the man out of existence. Let us make no mistake about this; the change is so fundamental that it will reach much further than even we contemplate, and the whole status of the profession will be altered in the minds of the people . . . Every doctor knows that there are already enough shadows in the sick-room without adding that of the lethal chamber. (*British Medical Journal*, 1936)

Finally, opponents of euthanasia and physician-assisted suicide argue that legalizing voluntary euthanasia for terminally ill patients is "only the thin end of a very big wedge" (ibid.). Initially, the terminally ill with uncontrolled pain could voluntarily request euthanasia and physician-assisted suicide, then the elderly, and then involuntary euthanasia for "absolute idiots, incurably demented persons, and convicted murderers" would become socially tolerated and justified.

What Can We Make of This History?

It is always difficult to interpret historical events and draw definitive conclusions about their causes and effects. Nevertheless, if we are to draw on history to help guide our current action, we must venture some interpretations, no matter how tentative. At least three important conclusions can be drawn from this historical record: (1) There is no consistent or causal link between advances in life-sustaining medical technology and interest in euthanasia and physician-assisted suicide. (2) Interest in euthanasia and physician-assisted suicide is associated with the dominance of philosophies that celebrate individualism and personal initiative. And (3) interest in euthanasia and physician-assisted suicide is associated with challenges to the authority of physicians.

While the current advocates of euthanasia claim that advances in life-sustaining technology create interest in euthanasia, the historical record suggests that there is no inherent or causal link between actual advances in biomedical technology and interest in euthanasia.[38] Physicians' capability to utilize life-sustaining interventions and to prolong the death of patients postdates, by many decades, the debates in ancient Greece as well as interest in euthanasia expressed by More and Bacon.

More importantly, these late-nineteenth and early-twentieth-century Anglo-American campaigns for the legalization of euthanasia occurred before medicine had life-sustaining interventions. Medicine in the late nineteenth century was becoming scientific with the recognition of the importance of the biological sciences, the identification of the role of microorganisms in disease etiology, the implementation of the first diagnostic laboratory tests, and the like. Yet the therapeutic interventions available to physicians were quite meager and ineffective. It was not until the turn of the twentieth century that anesthesia and aseptic techniques combined to enable surgery to be a safe, curative intervention.[39]

Life-sustaining medical interventions lagged even further. It was 1927 when Drinker and Shaw developed the first respirator ("the iron lung"); 1928 when penicillin was discovered, and 1941 when it became widely available; and 1932 when sulfonamides were introduced.[40] The speeches by Williams, Bach, and Baldwin and the legislation in Ohio all pre-date the development of effective life-sustaining medical technology. When effective life-sustaining medical technology did become widely available after World War II, there was no immediate resurgence of interest in euthanasia and physician-assisted suicide. During the 1950s and 1960s medicine could sustain the lives of brain-damaged patients. As Pope Pius XII's comments on this issue make clear, there was concern about keeping patients alive but no popular interest in euthanasia and physician-assisted suicide.

This is not to say that advances in medical technology have had no impact on the debate regarding euthanasia and physician-assisted suicide. It is true that advances in the use of morphine and the discovery of ether and chloroform anesthesia did precede the nineteenth century's debates about euthanasia. And these advances in medical technology are cited by the advocates of euthanasia and did seem to influence their arguments. But what a paradox and irony! Advances in the technology of *pain relief*—just when physicians had the capabilities to effectively alleviate pain and when interest was growing within the medical profession in understanding and teaching about how to ease the dying process—seem to be associated with an upsurge of interest in euthanasia. This historical survey suggests that it is not technological advances in sustaining life but technological advances in easing the dying process that stimulates interest in euthanasia.

While fear of being kept alive by medical technology may be a necessary factor motivating interest in euthanasia, clearly it is not sufficient. Indeed, almost all the arguments made today to justify euthanasia were made before modern medical technology existed and could prolong life. Nevertheless, it is part of "conventional wisdom" that the development of modern life-sustaining technologies is the cause of the contemporary rise in interest on euthanasia and physician-assisted suicide. Typical of this view is the long discussion on the interaction of life-sustaining technology and the desire for euthanasia that occurs in the 1996 ruling of the Ninth Circuit Court recognizing a constitutional right to assisted suicide. (See chapter 9 for a further exploration of this legal ruling.) Unfortunately, it does not comport with the historical facts. Life-sustaining technology is not the cause of interest in euthanasia.

In contrast to the technology explanation, I want to suggest that social values drive interest in euthanasia and physician-assisted suicide—in particular the dominance of individualism, which creates a hospitable environment for interest in these practices. This suggestion postulates that societies may be more receptive to appeals for permitting and legalizing euthanasia during periods when economic recession is extended, when a survival-of-the-fittest mentality is more accepted, when *laissez faire* economic policies predominate, and when the rights of the individual are strongly affirmed over social harmony.

In America and Britain, the worst economic recessions or depressions over the last 120 years occurred in the mid-1870s, mid-1890s, the 1930s, and the 1980s.[41] These have also been periods of unsentimental economic individualism—celebrating self-assertion and accumulation of wealth rather than democratic individualism. It accepts the circumstances of the less fortunate as being of their own making rather than a failure of the social order, and it restricts governmental actions to the promotion of economic competition rather than social welfare. In these periods, the language of social Darwinism, such as "survival of the fittest," becomes the idiom of public discourse. And when recessions strain government budgets, it legitimates resentment of those who cannot compete and are dependent—the poor, old, and disabled—and justifies cuts in safety-net programs.

This public philosophy also changes the individual's own perceptions. It legitimates the adoption of the utilitarian logic of business—contract, calculations of costs and benefits, success and profit—as the proper guide for individual action. Individuals forsake traditional bonds and respect for authority. And with self-sufficiency viewed as the highest virtue, dependence seen as a vice, acceptance of governmental aid considered a drain, and rationalist calculations of the value of life as proper, the old and sick become identified with the "unfit." More importantly, the old and sick come to see *themselves* as "unfit" and as burdens on others. With a shrinking safety net, individuals come to fear sickness, especially chronic and terminal illness, as a threat to their family's well-being and their own self-esteem and social standing. Thus, social policies reinforce self-understandings; as social supports disappear, the sick and aged do as a matter of fact become economic burdens on their family, and their self-perception as burdens is reaffirmed by the way the world is.

Often advocates of euthanasia appealed directly to social Darwinian ideas for legitimation. Williams's speech was suffused with references to Darwin and the "universal struggle . . . of the strong over the weak." Similarly, Baldwin in 1899 invoked the "one great all-dominating lesson which the nineteenth century has taught, the law of evolution" in support of a calm passage to death through euthanasia. Advocates frequently attacked the belief in the "sacredness of life [as] still tinctured with ancient superstition and with metaphysical haziness. Life is sacred when it is pleasant . . . But a life of pain, agony, and anguish is not sacred." They also mocked "the greater sensibility and the greater power of sympathy which [the euthanasia opponent] implies are worth preserving, even at the cost of the poor old parent who is forcibly maintained in a world which has become a torment to him."[42]

Conversely, the nineteenth-century opponents of euthanasia frequently attacked social Darwinian ideas to undermine support for euthanasia. For instance, they attacked the "purely utilitarian [calculations in which] old people past their productive periods could be easily disposed of [by euthanasia] as a long step backward toward savagery." A 1905 editorial claimed advocates misused Darwinism and rejected the notion that medicine's opposition to euthanasia was "preserving the unfit."[43]

The 1980s were reminiscent of the 1880s. Deep recessions occurred just when the economic and social policies of Reagan in the United States and Thatcher in Britain revived the celebration of raw individualism, unfettered capitalistic competition for sur-

vival, antiunion sentiments, wholesale governmental deregula-
tion, and curtailment of social safety-net programs for the poor,
old, and sick. As the historian Eric Foner and others have suggested, there has been a "resurrection in the 1980s of . . . the
social Darwinism mentality, if not the name itself."

Today it is not respectable to appeal openly to social Darwinism
to justify euthanasia or any other social policy. Nevertheless,
contemporary opponents and advocates of euthanasia do appeal
to individualism and individual rights in justifying euthanasia.
They also explicitly worry that discrimination against vulnerable
groups and cost containment focused on the elderly and terminally ill do influence support for euthanasia. Similarly, it is during
these years that there has developed interest in age-based rationing of health care resources. Consistent with this public philosophy, Americans are worried about their future and have indicated
that the single most important reason for endorsing euthanasia is
to avoid being a burden on their family.[44]

Some may detect a superficial similarity between these periods
of social Darwinism in Anglo-American tradition and the German praise of euthanasia because it reduced the social cost of
"economically burdensome" patients. But there are fundamental
differences. Germans viewed the benefits from the perspective of
the state or the *Volk;* as Hoche put it, euthanasia of the mentally
dead is important for the health of the "civil organism."[45] The
Anglo-American appeal to social Darwinism is individualistic;
the state should be as insignificant as possible, following *laissez
faire* policies, not reformist ones. The social Darwinism that might
make Americans receptive to euthanasia rejects the German attachment to a community as antirationalist sentimentality.

In addition to these general social and economic factors that
might inspire interest in euthanasia are factors that impinge more
directly on medical practice itself. There is a continuous social,
cultural, and legal process of delineating the extent of physician
authority. It appears that the periods of powerful and prominent
challenge to physician authority are precisely the periods of interest in euthanasia. The last third of both the nineteenth and
twentieth centuries were such periods.

In the late nineteenth century, medicine was being transformed from a suspect and divided profession to one with socially recognized authority. Americans became willing to "surrender [their] private judgments" in matters of health to physicians. Allopathic physicians were confronting and overcoming the challenges posed by Sectarians, Christian Scientists, and others. During this period, advocates of euthanasia frequently couched their appeals in attacks on the "pride of many in the medical profession." Some advocates justified euthanasia by arguing that patients, not physicians, had a right to decide when their life should end. Concomitantly, many in the medical profession viewed euthanasia as another threat to their authority, as a way to undermine the very "foundations of the existence of the profession." As Abraham Jacobi, President of the AMA, put it: If you legalize euthanasia, then "you would make true what Plato said of the practice of medicine: It was no respectable calling."[46]

Again, there is striking similarity between the past and today. In contrast to the situation of the nineteenth century, the authority of the medical profession was widely accepted in the early 1970s. Then began a concerted attack on it in the name of patient autonomy. This challenge is embodied in the progressive enumeration of patient rights, which carves out a sphere where patients' private judgments about the value of medical care reign supreme. Central to the patient rights movement has been the expansion of patients' right to refuse medical care, even life-sustaining care. The motivation has been to remove physicians from decision-making and let individual patients weigh the benefits and burdens of continued life. As one court put it: "The right to refuse medical treatment is basic and fundamental . . . Its exercise requires no one's approval . . . The controlling decision belongs to a competent informed patient . . . It is not a medical decision for her physicians to make."[47]

In the view of many, the general acceptance of the patient's rights to refuse medical care and concomitant restriction of physician authority has set the stage for acceptance of euthanasia; the arguments for patient control over their lives that justify refusal of life-sustaining treatment logically extend to euthanasia. And many have viewed the interest in euthanasia as a public condemnation of physician control over patients' deaths. As leading proponents of Washington State's Proposition 119 argued: "My sense is that people do feel in many aspects of their lives as if they are out of control. I suspect in this one area people are saying 'Dammit, this is the one thing that I ought to be able to control for myself.'"[48] In this way, the current interest in euthanasia may be the culmination of a twenty-year effort to curtail physician authority over end-of-life decision-making and over health care more generally. Technology, and physicians' control over technological interventions, may actually be a more easily characterized, but less accurate, surrogate for this struggle to constrict the bounds of physician authority.

One use of history is to show us similarities and differences between the past and present that help us better understand our current era and social practices. This historical review of previous euthanasia debates, especially those in the last third of the nineteenth century, provides three important insights about the sources and causes of the current debate on euthanasia. First, it is very difficult to argue that advances in medical and surgical technologies cause or create public interest in legalization of euthanasia. Long before any medical technologies could prolong life, the legalization of euthanasia was vigorously debated. Ironically, if any association between technological advances and interest in euthanasia exists, it seems to be with advances in the management of pain. Immediately preceding the nineteenth-century debates, new pain relief techniques, including hypodermic morphine and ether and chloroform anesthesia, were developed and used. Similarly, the 1970s and 1980s witnessed renewed attention on improving care of the dying through better pain management, use of palliative and hospice care, and the withdrawal of life-sustaining technologies.

Second, this historical review suggests an association between interest in legalizing euthanasia and moments when social Darwinism and raw individualism, free markets and wealth accumulation, and limited government are celebrated. Finally, public support for euthanasia seems to be correlated with periods of intense struggle over professional dominance and the authority of the physician over death and dying.

9

The Bell Tolls for a Right to Suicide

GEORGE J. ANNAS

The sometimes deafening and always distracting national debate on the constitutional "right" to physician-assisted suicide ended abruptly when a unanimous U.S. Supreme Court declared a winner on June 26, 1997. On that date the Court issued two 9–0 decisions that reversed the opinions of two U.S. Circuit Courts of Appeal that had each found a constitutionally protected right to physician-assisted suicide in the Fourteenth Amendment. Because this outcome must have been foreseen even by the proponents, the opinions can be seen as a form of "judicial-assisted suicide" for the movement to establish a constitutional right to physician-assisted suicide. In this chapter I describe these two cases, explain why the U.S. Supreme Court reversed them, and discuss some of the implications of the Court's decisions for patients and their physicians.[1]

The Circuit Courts

In the spring of 1996, within a month of each other, U.S. Circuit Courts of Appeals on both coasts ruled state prohibitions of assisted suicide unconstitutional when applied to physicians who prescribe overdoses of medication for terminally ill, competent adults who wish to end their lives. The Ninth Circuit includes Alaska, Arizona, California, Hawaii, Idaho, Montana, Nevada,

Oregon, and Washington, and the Second Circuit includes New York, Connecticut, and Vermont. Both courts reached the same conclusion, but for different legal reasons.

In the Ninth Circuit *(Compassion in Dying v. Washington)*, four physicians and three patients (one dying of AIDS, one of cancer, and one of emphysema) challenged a Washington law that prohibits aiding another person to commit suicide. In the Second Circuit *(Quill v. Vacco)*, three physicians and three patients (two dying of AIDS and one of cancer) challenged New York laws that prohibit aiding another person in committing or attempting suicide. None of these patients was currently suicidal, but all wanted prescription drugs that they could take to end their lives if their suffering became unbearable. Taking an overdose of prescription drugs is the suicide method that has long been advocated by Derek Humphrey and his Hemlock Society. All the physicians said that they felt unable to comply with the requests because of state laws against assisting suicide (there are no laws against committing suicide).[2] Two primary stories by the physicians were used to illustrate their concerns about legal liability.

Dr. Harold Glucksberg, for whom the Ninth Circuit case was named after it went to the U.S. Supreme Court, recounted the story of a 34-year-old AIDS patient of his in his affidavit. Glucksberg had been treating the patient during the last year of his life, and through four months of "excruciating pain." Having wasted away, and in danger of becoming blind, the patient asked him "to prescribe drugs that he could take to hasten his inevitable death," instead of entering a hospital and "lingering in a drug-induced stupor." The patient was competent, and Glucksberg believed he "should" accommodate this request. However, he writes, "because of the statute [prohibiting assisted suicide] I was unable to assist him in this way." The patient later committed suicide by "jumping from the West Seattle bridge," and, the doctor continues, because of his weakened physical condition "it is my belief that he was aided by close family members."

The second story, by Dr. Timothy Quill, after whom the Second Circuit case was named, is much more famous because Quill wrote about his patient, Diane, in the *New England Journal of Medicine*.[3] Diane was suffering from cancer which, if treated, has a 25

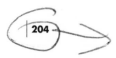

percent chance of remission. She refused the cancer treatment but was very concerned that she would die in terrible pain. She asked Quill for a prescription for drugs she could take to end her life if her suffering became unbearable. Unlike Glucksberg, Quill did write a prescription, instructing Diane to keep in touch. He also put her in touch with the Hemlock Society. A few months later Diane took the drugs and died. After Quill published an article about this case, a district attorney brought him before a grand jury, but it failed to indict him. The New York medical licensing board also investigated the case but concluded that Quill followed good medical practice.

Each of the circuit court cases presented the same two issues: Is there a constitutional right to the assistance of a physician in committing suicide? And if so, does the state nonetheless have a sufficient interest to prohibit the exercise of this right? Lurking in the background throughout was Jack Kevorkian, a former Michigan pathologist who uses carbon monoxide gas to assist in the suicides of his clients, who may or may not be terminally ill.

The Ninth Circuit Court adopted the term "physician-assisted suicide" to describe "the prescription of life-ending drugs for use by terminally ill, competent adult patients who wish to hasten their deaths," but the court was not happy with it, saying, "We have serious doubts that the terms 'suicide' and 'assisted suicide' are appropriate legal descriptions of the specific conduct at issue here." Instead of simply ruling that the assisted-suicide laws do not apply to such drug prescriptions, the court's ambitious 8 to 3 opinion, written by Judge Stephen Reinhardt, relied on a substantive due process approach (based on the Due Process Clause of the Fourteenth Amendment) to create a new constitutional right: the right to determine "the time and manner of one's own death."

This new right was broadly worded, but the court nonetheless ruled that only a narrow category of patients may lawfully exercise it: competent, terminally ill adults who have "lived nearly a full measure" of life and who want to die with dignity. For such patients, "wracked by pain and deprived of all pleasure, a state-enforced prohibition on hastening their deaths condemns them to unrelieved misery or torture." Surely, the court concluded, choosing "whether to endure or avoid such an existence" is a liberty every bit as vital as that involved in deciding whether or not to proceed with a pregnancy. In the court's words, "Like the decision of whether or not to have an abortion, the decision how and when to die is one of 'the most intimate and personal choices a person may make in a lifetime,' a choice 'central to personal dignity and autonomy.'" The court cited as "highly instructive" and "almost presumptive" Justice Kennedy's poetic language in *Casey*, the Court's most recent abortion decision: "At the heart of liberty is the right to define one's own concept of existence, of meaning, of the universe, and of the mystery of human life. Beliefs about these matters [personal decisions relating to marriage, procreation, contraception, family relationships, child rearing, and education] could not define the attributes of personhood were they formed under compulsion of the state."[4]

The other analogy the Ninth Circuit relied on was the removal of feeding tubes. A majority of the U.S. Supreme Court had assumed that there was a constitutionally protected liberty interest in "refusing unwanted medical treatment" in the case of Nancy Cruzan, a young woman in a persistent vegetative state whose family sought to have a feeding tube discontinued on her behalf. Because Nancy Cruzan would die without a feeding tube, the Ninth Circuit Court characterized the decision in *Cruzan* as having "necessarily recognize[d] a liberty interest in hastening one's own death," thus permitting "suicide by starvation."

The court thought that "as part of the tradition of administering comfort care, doctors have been supplying the causal agent of patients' deaths for decades," and understood that physicians have justified this prescribing pattern on the basis of the "double effect—reduce the patient's pain and hasten [his or her] death." But the court rejected the double-effect rationale, saying, "We see little, if any, difference for constitutional or ethical purposes between providing medication with a double effect and providing medication with a single effect . . . [or] between a doctor's pulling the plug on a respirator and . . . prescribing drugs which will permit a terminally ill patient to end [his or her] own life."[5]

After this new constitutional right was defined, the only remaining question was whether the state has a sufficient interest to prohibit its exercise. The court concluded that it did not:

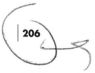

"When patients are no longer able to pursue liberty or happiness and do not wish to pursue life, the state's interest in forcing them to remain alive is clearly less [than] compelling." The court did, however, call on states to regulate the practice, suggesting procedural safeguards—such as witnesses, waiting periods, second medical opinions, psychological examinations, and reporting procedures—to help avoid "abuse."

One month later, in April 1996, the Second Circuit summarily rejected the Ninth Circuit's entire substantive due process analysis, concluding simply, "The right to assisted suicide finds no cognizable basis in the Constitution's language or design, even in the very limited cases of those competent persons who, in the final stages of terminal illness, seek the right to hasten death." But the Second Circuit nonetheless found a new constitutional right to a doctor's lethal prescription, based on the Equal Protection Clause of the Fourteenth Amendment.

The Equal Protection Clause requires states to treat people who are similarly situated in a similar manner. Although this is superficially a different constitutional approach from that of the Ninth Circuit, the Second Circuit also had to implicitly discover a new right (the right to hasten death) before it could conclude that the right was being protected unequally by the state because all persons in New York had the right to refuse treatment, and no one had the right to assistance in suicide.

The Second Circuit did this by making two related assertions: the right to refuse treatment is the same as the right to "hasten death," and there is no distinction between a person who is dependent on life-support equipment and one who is not. Neither assertion is persuasive. As to the first, the court argued that New York treats similarly situated people unequally because its law permits people "in the final stages of terminal illness who are on life support systems . . . to hasten their deaths by directing the removal of such systems," but those not receiving life support cannot hasten their deaths "by self-administering prescription drugs." The primary cases cited for this proposition are *Cruzan* and *Eichner*, even though neither of the two patients involved, who were both in persistent vegetative states, was terminally ill and neither had expressed any desire to commit suicide.

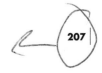

207

The patient in the *Eichner* case, Brother Joseph Fox, was an elderly Catholic brother of the Society of Mary who had said to his friend, Father Phillip Eichner, before hernia surgery, words to the effect, "If I wind up like Karen Quinlan, pull the plug."[6] Since suicide is a mortal sin in the Catholic Church, it is likely that Brother Fox would have been horrified at the notion that his refusal of a ventilator constituted suicide. As both *Eichner* and *Cruzan* make clear, both the courts and the real people involved in these cases believe the right at stake is the right to refuse treatment (even if refusal results in death), not the right to commit suicide. Moreover, there is no legal requirement that a person be terminally ill, suffering, or in pain to exercise the right to refuse treatments. Americans have never been obligated to accept any or all manner of medical treatment available to prolong life; the essence of the legal right at stake is the right to be free from unwanted bodily invasions.

Even more striking is the court's second assertion, which is based on its acceptance of Justice Antonin Scalia's strange concurring opinion in the *Cruzan* case (an opinion no other Justice on the Court joined). Scalia had argued that refusals of treatment which result in death are all suicides, and any notion that the patient dies a "natural" death from the underlying disease is nonsense. The Second Circuit adopted Justice Scalia's position, concluding that death after the removal of a ventilator is "not natural in any sense"; rather, it brings about "death through asphyxiation." Likewise, the Second Circuit stated that the removal of artificially delivered fluids and nutrition causes "death by starvation . . . or dehydration." In the court's words, "The ending of life by these means is nothing more nor less than assisted suicide."

Because it considered both refusing treatment and taking an overdose of drugs as equally constituting suicide, the Second Circuit concluded that giving citizens equal protection under the law means that the state must treat both acts in the same manner. The court argued that because doctors are permitted to "assist" patients being sustained by various life-support mechanisms to commit suicide by removing them, patients who do not need these medical interventions to continue to live should also be entitled to the assistance of a physician in committing suicide.

As to the state's possible interests in distinguishing between these acts, the court concluded that the state has no interest "in requiring the prolongation of a life that is all but ended." The court continued, "What business is it of the state to require the continuation of agony when the result is imminent and inevitable?" The court did not believe it was giving physicians a new license to kill, since, it believed, "physicians do not fulfill the role of 'killer' by prescribing drug [overdoses] to hasten death any more than they do by disconnecting life support systems." The court did, however, specifically reject euthanasia, distinguishing it from assisted suicide: "In euthanasia one causes the death of another by direct and intentional acts . . . Euthanasia falls within the definition of murder in New York."

Because avoiding the slippery slope to euthanasia is probably the primary state interest in prohibiting physician-assisted suicide, the ability to distinguish objectively between good and bad suicides is critical. The opinion of the Ninth Circuit overruled a 1995 decision in the same circuit in which Judge John Noonan, writing for a 2-to-1 panel, had concluded that any attempt to define the category of constitutionally protected assisted suicides is "inherently unstable," such that any right to assisted suicide would ultimately have to be available to all adults.[7] In contrast, the 1996 Ninth Circuit decision, issued by an *en banc* panel of 11 judges on that court, concluded that doctors can accurately distinguish worthy suicides from unworthy and irrational suicides. In the court's words: "One of the heartaches of suicide is the senseless loss of a life ended prematurely. In the case of a terminally ill adult who ends his life in the final stages of an incurable and painful degenerative disease, in order to avoid debilitating pain and a humiliating death, the decision to commit suicide is not senseless, and death does not come too early. Unlike the depressed twenty-one-year-old, the romantically devastated twenty-eight-year-old, the alcoholic forty-year-old . . . a terminally ill competent adult cannot be cured . . . [but] can only be maintained in a debilitated and deteriorating state, unable to enjoy the presence of family or friends."

The court found that frustrating the wishes of such terminally ill patients is "cruel indeed," and quoted Kent's lines from *King*

Lear, spoken immediately after Lear dies, to buttress its argument: "Vex not his ghost: O! let him pass; he hates him / That would upon the rack of this tough world / Stretch him out longer." Courts almost never resort to quoting literature, and when they do it, it is usually because they have no legal argument to support their conclusion. I believe that is true here, and the court's misreading of *King Lear* only serves to emphasize how difficult it is to draw lines or make objective assessments in this area. Thus, the seemingly marginal use of a quotation turns out to be central to understanding the entire opinion.

Lear did not die because he was terminally ill or in severe pain. Rather, Lear is much more like the person who dies because of a personal emotional tragedy: in Lear's case he had just learned that his one faithful and loving daughter, Cordelia, had been murdered, and has just uttered his famous line over her dead body: "Why should a dog, a horse, a rat, have life, / and thou no breath at all?" Earlier that same day, Lear was prepared to spend many years in prison with Cordelia. But after her murder, Lear dies of a broken heart. There is no suicide and no assistance; instead, to the contemporary reader, Kent acts as Lear's health care agent and exercises Lear's right to refuse treatment by ordering that resuscitation not be attempted. No legal changes are needed to protect the right of someone in Lear's position to refuse treatment.

Taking a line out of context from *King Lear* parallels the way the Ninth Circuit also took a line out of context from *Casey* to use as the basis for the new constitutional right it enunciated. There are some striking similarities between abortion and assisted suicide. Perhaps the most notable is the tendency of proponents and opponents to use overblown language that obscures rather than clarifies. Thus in the abortion debate, opponents use words like "killing babies" and "murder" and "right to life"; and similar language is used by opponents of physician-assisted suicide. Proponents also adopt "prochoice" rhetoric to support assisted suicide, using words like "personal choice," "liberty," and "control" to express their view. Contrary to such political slogans, notions of control and choice are either illusory or incredibly limited at both ends of life. The other striking image is the use of suffering.

The antiabortion camp tends to concentrate on the suffering of the fetus, such as in the film *Silent Scream* and descriptions of "partial birth" abortions; whereas the proponents of physician-assisted suicide focus on the suffering of the terminally ill person. Religion and religious beliefs also play a major role in both debates. The challenge is to get beyond the sloganeering to try to understand the real differences and their relevance to the constitutional analysis.

The most important difference is defining the constitutional right involved. In abortion, it is the right to decide whether or not to continue a pregnancy. In contrast, although suicide has been decriminalized, there is no constitutional right to commit suicide, and it would be difficult to know what such a right would look like. Perhaps this is why neither the Ninth nor the Second Circuit discussed directly a "right to suicide." Instead, both courts used phrases like "a right to hasten death" and "a right to determine the time and manner of death." This is important because, as *Casey* teaches, the right of a physician to perform an abortion is entirely derivative from the right of the pregnant woman to have one. If there is no constitutional right to commit suicide, there can be no constitutional right to have a physician's assistance in committing suicide.

A second distinction involves the basis for the constitutional right at issue. To the extent that both are asserted to be liberty rights found in the Due Process Clause of the Fourteenth Amendment, the parallel holds. However, no such parallel exists in an equal protection analysis. Abortion applies only to women, and pregnancy itself is sui generis. In this aspect, abortion cannot be seen as parallel to suicide, since there is no issue of gender equality involved in suicide. In this same regard, the right to terminate a pregnancy is limited to a narrow and very easily defined class of people: pregnant women. There is no bright line that can limit the category of people to whom a right to commit suicide (or assistance in suicide) would apply.[8]

A third distinction involves the role of the physician. Abortion is a medical procedure. Because abortion endangers the life and health of women if performed by the woman herself or by unlicensed or "back alley" practitioners, the state has a sufficiently compelling interest in protecting women's health to require that only licensed physicians be permitted to perform abortions. No such rationale exists regarding suicide. Almost all competent adults are capable of successfully committing suicide, and tens of thousands do so every year. Suicide is not a medical procedure, and there is no health or safety reason why physicians must be involved in an individual's suicide. Jack Kevorkian's use of carbon monoxide poisoning illustrates this point.

A fourth major distinction is what is being killed. The heart of what makes abortion a political, religious, and social-policy issue is the belief many people hold that protectable human life begins at conception, and that to purposely kill an embryo or a nonviable fetus is "murder." The U.S. Supreme Court (with no Justice ever disagreeing on this), however, has consistently ruled that a fetus does not become a person under the Constitution until birth (although it is so similar to a person at viability that the state has a compelling interest in protecting its life at this point). This is what makes "near birth" feticide so problematic. What is killed in pregnancy termination is human and alive, but it is not a person. On the other hand, the entity being killed (or killing him or herself) in physician-assisted suicide is always a person under the Constitution. And the state has a compelling interest in protecting the lives of all persons, including those who are suffering and near the end of life.

Reliance on *Cruzan* is as problematic as relying on *Casey*. *Cruzan* involved the clearly definable right to refuse treatment, not the indefinable right to "hasten death." Nor did anyone involved, including Nancy Cruzan's parents, the state of Missouri, the Missouri Supreme Court, and the U.S. Supreme Court, see a refusal of artificial fluids and nutrition by Nancy Cruzan, or her parents on their daughter's behalf, as a possible violation of Missouri's law against assisted suicide. Suicide and assisted suicide were simply not at issue in *Cruzan* because refusing treatment, even when the refusal will certainly end in death, has never been equated with suicide by courts, legislatures, or patients and their families.

The patients whose cases were presented to these two courts are all sympathetic, and it is not surprising that the circuit courts

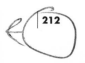

wanted to help them. Cancer and AIDS often lead to "hard deaths," and patients dying of these two diseases make up the vast majority of patients in hospices, as well as of those who seek the assistance of physicians in committing suicide, probably because the final stages of these illnesses are relatively predictable. What is surprising is that these courts failed to acknowledge explicitly that it has never been illegal to prescribe pain medication that competent, terminally ill patients *might* use to commit suicide, as long as the physician's *intent* is to foster their patients' well-being by giving them more control over their lives, and as long as the drugs have an independent legitimate medical use. Such a prescription can legitimately be intended as suicide prevention rather than suicide assistance. Neither court could point to even one case of a physician ever being criminally prosecuted for the conduct they approve of, and both courts would have been on much stronger ground if they had simply acknowledged that intent matters in criminal law and that prescriptions written under these very limited circumstances do not legally constitute assisted suicide, by definition.[9]

In this regard, it should be noted that the Ninth Circuit's restatement of the principle of the double effect, which treats pain relief and death as equally intended, is false: the principle is that treating the patient's pain is acceptable even if the treatment hastens death (which it will, of course, not always do). Providing medication to control pain has always been a legitimate and lawful medical act, even if death or suicide is risked; just as performing surgery is a legitimate and lawful medical act even if death is risked. There is a difference between an intended result and an unintended but foreseen and accepted consequence.

Thus, no physician should have concluded on the basis of the Ninth Circuit that providing pain medication that increases the risk of death is either assistance in suicide or homicide. As one of the dissenting judges in the Ninth Circuit's opinion, Judge Andrew Kleinfeld, properly noted, when General Dwight D. Eisenhower ordered American troops to the beaches in Normandy, he knew he was sending many to certain death, but his intent was to liberate Europe from the Nazis. Judge Kleinfeld continued, "The majority's theory of ethics would imply that this purpose was legally and ethically indistinguishable from a purpose of killing American soldiers." Intent really does matter.

Neither court's logic about the cause of death after refusal of treatment is persuasive. If one accepts that Nancy Cruzan "died of starvation" and not from the vegetative condition that made continued artificial feeding necessary for her survival, one would also have to accept the conclusion that when physicians stop attempted cardiopulmonary resuscitation on a patient in cardiac arrest, what kills the patient is not the cardiac arrest but rather the act of the physician who intentionally stops compressing the heart. Since failure to perform cardiopulmonary resuscitation always "hastens death," under each court's logic, patients who instruct their doctors not to resuscitate them in the event of a heart attack would always be committing suicide, and doctors who write do-not-resuscitate orders would always be assisting this suicide. The failure to distinguish real causes of death from various medical tools and techniques that may temporarily substitute for particular bodily functions is fatal to the logic of both these opinions.

This logical failure also helps explain why neither court could define the right they had discovered nor persuasively limit its exercise to prescriptions written by physicians for competent, terminally ill patients, limitations that have no basis in constitutional law.[10] The *Cruzan* and *Eichner* cases, after all, support the proposition that the right to refuse treatment is not lost by incompetence but can be exercised in advance by means of a living will or the designation of a health care proxy, and also that an adult need not be terminally ill to refuse treatment. Of course, no one can commit suicide by proxy. On the other hand, nothing in the logic of these opinions would have prohibited physicians from actually injecting lethal doses into patients who met their other criteria and who were unable to commit suicide themselves, although the Second Circuit explicitly prohibited this.

The Ninth Circuit (but not the Second) also explicitly protected family and friends working under direction of a physician, but never explained why either a physician or a prescription drug is constitutionally required. For example, neither court suggested any reason why a physician could not recommend suicide by gun and instruct a patient or family member about where to aim it before the patient pulled the trigger. Since both courts admitted that there is no constitutional definition of terminal illness, the group of covered patients may encompass many with years to live (like Lear) whose lives no longer bring them joy or happiness, and certainly seems to include early HIV infection, Alzheimer's disease, or cancer. To the extent that states have an interest in protecting these persons from physicians who might encourage suicide for reasons other than unrelievable pain or suffering at the end of life, these opinions cannot prevent a slide down the slippery slope.

Recognizing the dangerousness of the right they were espousing, both courts called on states to regulate physician-assisted suicide. The Ninth Circuit also seemed to approve of Oregon Ballot Measure 16, which provides legal immunity to physicians who follow certain procedures when prescribing lethal drugs to terminally ill patients with the intent that they use them to commit suicide. Under the Second Circuit's equal protection analysis, the state is permitted to adopt the same or substantially similar regulations for refusals of treatment that "hasten death" as for physician-assisted suicide. If states adopt such regulations, the hard-won rights that the great majority of patients can and do now exercise to refuse medical treatments are put at risk, since mandatory procedural safeguards can actually frustrate rather than foster the self-determination of patients.[11]

The opinions could also be read as undercutting all laws relating to Schedule I drugs (drugs which have a high potential for abuse and have no accepted medical use), as well as regulation of medical experimentation, at least with regard to patients near the end of life. If laws against assisted suicide are unconstitutional because they deprive terminally ill patients of relief from suffering, how can laws that restrict their access to heroin or LSD be constitutional? Contrary to the actions of these courts, the Supreme Court has previously and unanimously endorsed the view of the Food and Drug Administration that drug laws that require demonstrated safety and efficacy forbid everyone, including the terminally ill, to obtain unapproved drugs.[12]

By ignoring the past two decades of jurisprudence concerning the right to refuse treatment (including the rulings by state supreme courts that explicitly hold that refusals of treatment are neither suicide nor homicide), and by failing to make such basic distinctions as those between the right to refuse treatment and the "right to die," between suicide and assisted suicide, between law and ethics, and between ends and means, these courts virtually guaranteed that their decisions would not be the last word on the subject.

The U.S. Supreme Court

The U.S. Supreme Court agreed to review both of these decisions in September 1996 and heard oral arguments on January 8, 1997. At the oral argument, which was widely anticipated and covered by the press as potentially the most important case of the term before the Court, the advocates on behalf of physician-assisted suicide dramatically shifted their arguments. Harvard law professor Laurence Tribe, who argued for upholding *Quill,* centered his argument on an alleged medical practice that had not even been mentioned in either lower court: "terminal sedation." Professor Tribe described terminal sedation as drugging a patient into a coma and then starving the patient to death by withholding fluids and nutrition. He argued that this practice was the same as assisting suicide (homicide?), since death is the intended end. Because this practice is legally permitted, Professor Tribe argued that the state must also permit the patient to be sedated, the alternative of taking an overdose and dying at once. According to Tribe, assisted suicide would avoid forcing the patient to be subjected to this degrading procedure, which might undermine the patient's firmly held values and drain the meaning from his death.

New York Attorney General Dennis Vacco argued that terminal sedation (which he termed "sedation in the imminently dying") is only legally permitted as a last resort, in extreme cases, after carefully titrating medication until it effectively eliminates pain or the other symptoms it is designed to treat. It is thus consistent with an intent to treat the patient, not an intent to kill, and is justified by the principle of the double effect.

Attorney Katherine Tucker, who represented the organization Compassion in Dying, argued that physician-assisted suicide should be heavily regulated and limited only to those very near death. Asked specifically by Justice Ruth Bader Ginsburg if a suffering, terminally ill patient who met all of her qualifications but who could not physically take the drug overdose herself could be given an injection of lethal drugs by a physician, she replied "no," saying that the drugs must be self-administered to ensure that the decision is "authentic and voluntary." Justice Ginsburg also asked the U.S. Solicitor General, Walter Dellinger, what he knew about the alleged practice of doctors to defy the law by using "winks and nods." Dellinger replied that he knew of no evidence to support this characterization of current practice.

The fundamental constitutional right proposed was exceptionally narrow, much narrower than that discovered by the two circuit courts. In the words of the *Quill* brief, authored primarily by Professor Tribe, it was the "right of a terminally ill, mentally competent adult who is in the process of dying to end her own intolerable suffering, pain and physical disintegration by obtaining, within the context of the doctor-patient relationship, a prescription for medication that will allow her to end her own life." The Justices were skeptical that such a right existed, and wondered, if it did and was so important, why it shouldn't apply to more people. They also indicated that they believed there was a real difference between suicide and refusing treatment, and that too little was known about the entire area of end-of-life care for the Court to take the issue away from the states and rule definitively on it for all U.S. citizens.

Virtually all who observed the oral arguments agreed that it was likely that the Supreme Court would reverse both cases, and by a wide margin. Nonetheless, the overwhelming 9-to-0 opinions were stunning. Both opinions were written for the Court by Chief Justice William Rehnquist. Five Justices also wrote concurring opinions.

In the case of *Washington v. Glucksberg,* the Chief Justice stated the question before the Court in straightforward terms: "The question before us is whether the 'liberty' specially protected by the Due Process Clause [of the Fourteenth Amendment] includes a right to commit suicide which itself includes a right to assistance in doing so."[13]

Justice Rehnquist described the Court's "established method of substantive due process analysis" as having two features: (1) The fundamental right or liberty must be "deeply rooted in this nation's history and tradition . . . or so fundamental to ordered liberty . . . that neither liberty nor justice would exit if [it] were sacrificed." (2) The asserted fundamental right or liberty interest must have a "careful description." As to the first, the Court concluded there is no historic tradition of treating suicide as a fundamental right, noting that to find such a right the Court would instead "have to reverse centuries of legal doctrine and practice, and strike down the considered policy choice of almost every state."

In a review of the history of laws against suicide and assisted suicide, the Court noted that the decriminalization of suicide was not done because the states approved of suicide or wanted to encourage it. Rather, "this change reflected the growing consensus that it was unfair to punish the suicide's family for his wrongdoing." It is, of course, impossible to punish the person who commits suicide. Thus, for deterrence, public health prevention rather than criminal sanction makes more sense. Suicide, though not punishable by law, "remained a grievous, though nonfelonious, wrong . . . confirmed by the fact that colonial and early state legislatures and courts did not retreat from prohibiting assisting suicide." Nor was there ever any exception for those who were "near to death."

In this context the Court reviewed the Ninth Circuit's reliance on *Cruzan* and *Casey*. The Court characterized *Cruzan* as a case which involved the constitutional right to refuse unwanted medical treatment, a right supported in common law battery and informed consent doctrine, and by "the long legal tradition protecting the decision to refuse unwanted medical treatment." And in footnote 17 the Court abandoned the language it used in *Cruzan* to "assume" a constitutional right to refuse treatment, and said simply that in *Cruzan* "we concluded that the right to refuse unwanted medical treatment was so rooted in our history, tradition, and practice as to require special protection under the Fourteenth Amendment." The Court then concluded that suicide "has never enjoyed similar legal protection" and that the "two acts are widely and reasonably regarded as quite distinct." The Court noted finally that it recognized in *Cruzan* itself that most states outlawed assisted suicide, and in *Cruzan* "we certainly gave no intimation" that the right to refuse treatment could be "somehow transmuted into a right to assistance in committing suicide."

The Court dealt even more summarily, if less persuasively, with *Casey* and the poetic language of Justice Kennedy. The Court noted simply that such generalities as "the mystery of life," are used to describe the types of "personal activities and decisions" that the Court has previously identified as deeply rooted in our history or fundamental to ordered liberty that they are protected by the Fourteenth Amendment—not as support for "the sweeping conclusion that any and all important, intimate, and personal decisions are so protected."

Because the Court concluded that no fundamental constitutional right could be found in either our nation's history or in "the concept of constitutionally ordered liberty," all the state of Washington had to demonstrate was that their assisted suicide ban was "rationally related to legitimate government interests." The Court concluded that "this requirement is unquestionably met here." The Court went on to list the following legitimate governmental interests: (1) the preservation of human life, noting that states may put all of their citizens, including their dying ones, "under the full protection of the law"; (2) preventing suicide, which the Court notes is a "serious public-health problem"; (3) protecting the integrity and ethics of the medical profession; (4) protecting vulnerable groups from abuse, neglect, and mistakes; (5) preventing a start "down the path to voluntary and perhaps even involuntary euthanasia." Noting that the Ninth Circuit seemed to permit surrogate decision-making, and "in some instances" lethal injection by a physician or family member, the Court concluded, "it turns out that what is couched as a limited right to 'physician-assisted suicide' is likely, in effect, a much broader license, which could prove extremely difficult to police and contain. Washington's ban on assisting suicide prevents such erosion."

The Court also cited the experience in the Netherlands as support for Washington's concern about preventing euthanasia, noting the 1991 study that disclosed "more than 1,000 cases of euthanasia without an explicit request," and another "4,941 cases where physicians administered lethal morphine overdoses without the patients' explicit consent." The Court did not compare the more recent Netherlands study to this one to try to determine whether or not things were getting worse in the Netherlands. The Court's point was more limited and precise: "This study suggests that, despite the existence of various reporting procedures, euthanasia in the Netherlands has not been limited to competent, terminally ill adults who are enduring physical suffering, and that regulation of the practice may not have prevented abuses in cases involving vulnerable persons, including severely disabled neonates and elderly persons suffering from dementia."

The opinion concluded with the holding, a footnote to the holding, and a final paragraph. The holding is simply that Washington's assisted suicide law "does not violate the Fourteenth Amendment, either on its face or as applied to competent, terminally ill adults who wish to hasten their deaths by obtaining medication prescribed by their doctors." The footnote acknowledges that there is a "possibility" that a specific individual might be able to prevail in a more particularized challenge, noting: "Our opinion does not absolutely foreclose such a claim. However, given our holding that the Due Process Clause of the Fourteenth Amendment does not provide heightened protection to the asserted liberty interest in ending one's life with a physician's assistance, such a claim would have to be quite different from the ones advanced . . . here." The opinion concludes, "Throughout the Nation, Americans are engaged in an earnest and profound debate about the morality, legality, and practicality of physician-assisted suicide. Our holding permits this debate to continue, as it should in a democratic society."

In the case of *Vacco v. Quill,* the Chief Justice, again writing for the Court, stated the question before the Court as whether the state of New York, by making it a crime to aid another to commit or attempt suicide while permitting patients to refuse even life-saving treatment, thereby violates the Equal Protection Clause of the Fourteenth Amendment. The Court held that "it does not."[14]

The Court began its analysis with a statement of what the Equal Protection Clause requires: "It embodies a general rule that States must treat like cases alike but may treat unlike cases accordingly." State statutes will be upheld as long as they bear "a rational relation to some legitimate end" unless the statute "burdens a fundamental right [or] targets a suspect class." As previously summarized in *Washington v. Glucksberg,* the Court had concluded that statutes outlawing assisted suicide "neither infringe fundamental rights nor involve suspect classification," and also that such statutes are reasonably related to legitimate state interests. Thus the only real question in *Vacco v. Quill* was whether there is a rational difference between assisting a patient to commit suicide and withdrawing life-sustaining treatment. The Court answers this question at the outset, stating that on their face New York's laws draw no distinctions between people but treat all New York citizens the same: "Everyone, regardless of physical condition, is entitled, if competent, to refuse unwanted lifesaving medical treatment; no one is permitted to assist a suicide."

The Second Circuit missed this point, probably because it performed its analysis only on the universe of terminally ill people near the end of life and had tried to find a new right by mischaracterizing the right to refuse treatment as suicide in this context. It had concluded that since ending or refusing life-sustaining medical treatment is "nothing more nor less than assisting suicide," the laws prohibiting assisted suicide for those terminally ill people who are not dependent on medical treatment to maintain their lives effectively deny them equal protection of laws. The Supreme Court emphatically disagreed, and specifically upheld as rational the historic legal distinction between refusing treatment and committing suicide: "Unlike the Court of Appeals, we think the distinction between assisting suicide and withdrawing life-sustaining treatment, a distinction widely recognized and endorsed in the medical profession and in our legal traditions, is both important and logical; it is certainly rational."

The Court explained (contrary to abstract philosophy) that causation and intent are the critical distinguishing characteristics in the criminal law. As to causation, the Court agreed with previous legal rulings that "when a patient refuses life-sustaining medical treatment, he dies from an underlying fatal disease or pathology;

but if a patient ingests lethal medication prescribed by a physician he is killed by that medication." But since medications prescribed for legitimate medical purposes can kill as well, the real distinction in close cases is the physician's *intent* in prescribing the medications. The Court explained that when a physician provides aggressive palliative care, "in some cases, pain killing drugs may hasten a patients' death, but the physician's purpose and intent is, or may be, only to ease his patients' pain." On the other hand, a doctor who assists a suicide necessarily intends that the patient dies. Similarly, a patient who commits suicide with a doctor's aid "necessarily has the specific intent to end his or her own life, while a patient who refuses or discontinues treatment might not." The Court noted that the law has historically distinguished between actions done "because of" a given end and actions done "in spite of" their unintended but foreseen consequences, and quoted as authority Judge Kleinfeld's example of General Eisenhower ordering American soldiers to battle to liberate Europe, knowing many American soldiers would certainly die because of his order.

The Court then noted that other courts, including those in New York, have routinely made this distinction, citing thirty-four prior decisions and discussing specifically the first major life-sustaining treatment refusal case, the case of Karen Ann Quinlan, and the more recent Michigan Supreme Court opinion involving the actions of Jack Kevorkian. In short, it is simply a legal error to characterize the refusal of life-sustaining treatment as the equivalent of a suicidal act, just as it is an error to assume that because courts have authorized treatment refusals where death is predictable, courts have thereby also authorized suicide and assisted suicide. The Court similarly noted that legislatures in virtually all states have also adopted this distinction between refusing treatment and committing suicide in their laws, and that New York specifically has repeatedly made this distinction in its laws.

Finally, the Court examined its own opinion in *Cruzan*, noting that *Cruzan* "also recognized, at least implicitly, the distinction between letting a patient die and making that patient die." *Cruzan*, the Court tells us, was not based on the recognition of any "general and abstract 'right to hasten death' but on well-es-

tablished, traditional rights to bodily integrity and freedom from
unwanted touching." The Court therefore (unsurprisingly) concluded: "By permitting everyone to refuse unwanted medical
treatment while prohibiting anyone from assisting a suicide, New
York follows a long-standing and rational distinction."

The example on which the case was fought at oral argument—terminal sedation—was relegated to a footnote. The
Court's discussion of terminal sedation is nonetheless useful,
since the Court applied the reasoning of its opinion to that example. The Court accepted the proposed definition of terminal sedation as "inducing barbiturate coma and then starving the person
to death." Even with this bizarre definition, the Court concluded
that a state can legally countenance this medical practice as a
form of palliative care if it is "based on informed consent and the
double-effect." In the Court's words: "Just as a state may prohibit
assisting suicide while permitting patients to refuse unwanted
life-saving treatment, it may permit palliative care related to that
refusal, which may have the foreseen but unintended 'double effect' of hastening the patients' death."

There were five votes for each of the opinions written by the
Chief Justice (his own and Justices Sandra Day O'Connor, Antonin Scalia, Anthony Kennedy, and Clarence Thomas). All nine
Justices agreed that state laws prohibiting assisted suicide violate
neither the Due Process nor the Equal Protection clauses of the
Fourteenth Amendment to the U.S. Constitution, even as applied
to physicians who prescribe overdoses of medications to competent, terminally ill patients who want to commit suicide. Nonetheless, five Justices wrote concurring opinions to express additional
or different reasons for this conclusion than those so far summarized.

Justice O'Connor, whose concurring opinion in *Cruzan* helped
energize the health care proxy movement, wrote a four-paragraph
concurring opinion, more of a short essay, which suggested she
believes there might be a right to avoid "great" suffering near
death that might be articulated by the Court in a different case.
She made three points: (1) All the parties agree that in Washington and New York states there are no legal barriers to prevent "a
patient who is experiencing great pain" from "obtaining medica-

tion, from qualified physicians, to alleviate that suffering, even to the point of causing unconsciousness and hastening death." (2) Since this is true, the state's interests justify a prohibition against physician-assisted suicide, even if the Court had recognized a right to assistance in suicide. (3) State legislatures are the proper forum for an "extensive and serious evaluation of physician-assisted suicide and other related issues." Justice O'Connor concluded:

> In sum, there is no need to address the question whether suffering patients have a *constitutionally cognizable interest in obtaining relief from the suffering that they may experience in the last days of their lives.* There is no dispute that dying patients in Washington and New York can obtain palliative care, even when doing so would hasten their deaths. The *difficulty of defining terminal illness,* and the risk that a dying patient's request for assistance in ending his or her life might not be *truly voluntary* justifies the prohibition on assisted suicide we uphold here. (emphasis added)

Justice Ruth Bader Ginsburg joined in both judgments of the Court, "substantially for the reasons stated by Justice O'Connor." Justice Stephen Breyer also joined Justice O'Connor's opinion, "except insofar as it joins the majority." It is difficult to discern exactly what Justice Breyer meant, but he is concerned about dying patients who get insufficient pain medication. Breyer opined that our legal tradition, while not supporting a right to suicide, might support something "roughly like 'a right to die with dignity.'" Breyer acknowledged, however, that such a right would likely have to include "the avoidance of severe physical pain (associated with death)," and that this interest is not implicated in these cases (as Justice O'Connor noted). Breyer concludes that if a state did prohibit a physician from providing sufficient palliative care—"including the administration of drugs as needed to avoid pain at the end of life"—the Court would be presented with a different case, "and might have to revisit its conclusions in these cases."

Justices John Paul Stevens and David Souter each wrote much

longer concurring opinions. Like Justice Breyer, neither got any other Justice to join in their concurring opinion. Nonetheless, each opinion merits comment. Justice Stevens was the one Justice that many observers thought might vote to uphold at least one of the two circuit court opinions. He, of course, did not. Justice Stevens fully agreed that there is no constitutional right to commit suicide or to have assistance in committing suicide. Stevens is the only Justice to cite literature to justify this conclusion but is on firmer ground than was the Ninth Circuit when it relied on a line from *Lear*. Stevens chose John Donne's *Meditation* on death, quoting the entire text in a footnote and highlighting perhaps its most famous sentence in the body of his opinion: "No man is an island." It is Donne's concept of community, Stevens believes, that supports the right of states to outlaw suicide and assisted suicide: "The value to others of a person's life is far too precious to allow the individual to claim a constitutional entitlement to complete autonomy in making a decision to end that life." In this case, Stevens could have added, the bell tolls for the constitutional right to physician-assisted suicide that had been recognized by the circuit courts.

Stevens agreed with the Court's distinction between treatment refusals and suicide. Nonetheless, he noted that in at least some cases the terminally ill patient who refuses treatment may in fact intend to die as certainly as the suicidal patient, and the physician's intent "might also be the same in prescribing lethal medication as it is in terminating life support." Since outsiders cannot always know individual intentions "beyond a reasonable doubt," Justice Rehnquist felt obligated to respond to this point of Justice Stevens in footnote 12 of *Vacco*. There he notes that the Court does "not insist" that in all cases there is in fact a significant difference of intent in the two circumstances. The point is a much more precise one: "In the absence of omniscience . . . the state is entitled to act on the reasonableness of the distinction."

Finally, Justice Souter wrote the longest concurring opinion to set forth his alternative suggestion for how the Court should perform substantive due process analysis. He is alone in this. Souter is also the only Justice to find the abortion analogy persuasive, perhaps because he reads *Casey* as recognizing a woman's "right to a physician's counsel and care." Like Breyer, he also saw the right at stake in these cases as broader than suicide, and more akin to a right to die with dignity that would include a physician's medical assistance if a person is in untreatable pain or conscious of unacceptable "dependency and helplessness as they approached death." Ultimately, however, Souter concludes that "the case for the slippery slope is fairly made out here," and too many facts are disputed for the Court to rule: "Legislatures . . . have superior opportunities to obtain the facts necessary for a judgment about the present controversy."

Death Rights

In retrospect it is easy to see how the "right to physician assistance in suicide" failed to gain constitutional recognition in the Supreme Court. To find such a constitutional right, the Court had to find a constitutional right to suicide itself, and there is no historical or legal support for this. Second, the analogies the proponents relied on—abortion and the right to refuse treatment—were easily distinguishable. The Court itself remains deeply divided on abortion, and notwithstanding some expansive, poetic language, *Casey* limited the abortion rights articulated in *Roe v. Wade*; it did not expand them.[15] The right to refuse treatment is deeply rooted in American law, and so are the principles of intent and causation in the criminal law—principles that distinguish suicide from treatment refusal, and assisted suicide from withdrawing or withholding treatment. This distinction is one that virtually every court since *Quinlan* has made, and virtually every legislature that has passed living will and health care proxy legislation.

Third, although the Court only had to find the states' interests in outlawing assisted suicide "rationally-related to a legitimate state interest," it seems reasonable to conclude that a majority of the Court would have permitted the states to continue to outlaw physician-assisted suicide even if the Justices thought it was a fundamental constitutional right, because at least some of these interests, especially avoiding the slippery slope to active euthanasia, are compelling. The Court was not fazed by learning what it did about "terminal sedation," and gave physicians who engage in this practice a ringing endorsement of trust (perhaps too ringing). The Court ruled that terminal sedation was fully justified legally if it accorded with good medical practice, and if the physician's intent was to alleviate suffering with the use of drugs and to follow the patient's competent refusal of treatment by withholding fluids and nutrition after the patient became unconscious. Thus, the Court explicitly endorsed the principle of the double effect, also endorsed by the American Medical Association, as a legally valid doctrine.[16]

The Court did not directly apply the double effect to writing drug prescriptions. Nonetheless, the logic of the opinion supports the conclusion that a physician can write a prescription for medically necessary drugs even if the physician knows that the patient might use the drugs to commit suicide, as long as the physician's intent is that the patient live longer or better. A physician who writes a drug prescription under these circumstances is *not* engaged in physician-assisted suicide, by legal definition.[17]

The Court implicitly sanctions what Dr. Timothy Quill did with his famous patient Diane as consistent with good medical practice. As Quill has written, he never intended Diane to commit suicide, and prescribed the drugs she ultimately used primarily so that she could stop worrying about her final days and better live her final months.[18] Specifically, it is legal for a doctor to prescribe drugs that could be used to commit suicide (and to risk such a suicide) if the drugs have an independent legitimate medical purpose, including the prevention of suicide; but states can outlaw the prescription of the same drugs if the physician's intent is to assist a suicide.

Suicide advocates tried to "spin doctor" this case by arguing that the Court did not completely "close the door" to future constitutional litigation, and that the Court's opinions gave a "green light" to states to adopt laws approving of and regulating physician-assisted suicide. The first argument is tenable but irrelevant. Courts never absolutely foreclose any argument; but no Justice suggested any specific case they might have in mind, nor have any of the litigants suggested another case they think will be a winner here. If patients dying of cancer and AIDS and in the last weeks of their lives are not persuasive, what case would be?

The type of case the Justices may be talking about is a patient at the very end of life who is suffering intolerably, whose physician wants to provide adequate pain medication but where the local district attorney intervenes and threatens the physician with prosecution if he or she prescribes or administers the pain medication. There has never been a case like this in the history of the United States (and none of the litigants could find one even close), and there is unlikely ever to be one. It is a statement of the misplaced emphasis on physician immunity in this litigation that such a wildly hypothetical possible future case is held out as the potential basis for more litigation over a constitutional "right to die."

The "green light" argument is simply another way of saying that the entire series of lawsuits on the constitutionality of assisted suicide laws was a waste of time and energy. States always had (and retain) the right to modify or abolish their assisted-suicide laws, as they have already all abolished their suicide laws. These Court decisions made no change at all in this area of the law. To the extent that some suicide advocates continue to see the law as an obstacle to their agendas, we may see more legislative activity at the state level—but whatever statutes are enacted, they are unlikely to improve the medical care of any patients in the real world.

The Oregon law, Ballot Measure 16, for example, is so cumbersome and confusing that in practice it will be less flexible than current law based on intent and the double effect. It requires that a physician actually intend that the patient commit suicide by using an overdose of drugs, prescribed for that purpose (thereby requiring that the doctor violate both medical ethics and the drug laws) to obtain legal immunity. It also requires that the patient endure a minimum 17-day waiting period, make a written, witnessed request for an overdose prescription, and be examined by a second physician. Legislation like this confuses law with medical ethics, makes the practice of medicine more bureaucratic and burdensome, and less private and accountable, and encourages the abandonment of patients at the end of life.

Granting physicians legal immunity for prescribing drug overdoses to a few suicidal terminally ill patients who cannot now get them from their physicians is an insufficient reason to put disadvantaged Oregonians, who are already relegated to the country's only formally rationed medical service delivery system, at even higher risk of underservice, alienation, and abandonment. The New York Task Force on Life and the Law, whose report on suicide and euthanasia was often cited as authority by the Court in *Washington v. Glucksberg* and *Vacco v. Quill,* unanimously concluded that "ideal" cases, like that described by Quill, are an insufficient basis for changing public policy in a country where medicine continues to be practiced in the context of bias and social inequality, and where hospice care is not generally available. The Task Force rightly concluded that in the real world, legalizing assisted suicide would "pose the greatest risks to those who are poor, elderly, members of a minority group, or without access to good medical care."[19]

No sympathy can be found in either of these opinions for the idea that physicians should be granted prospective legal immunity from criminal prosecution for writing drug prescriptions. The Court did not specifically deal with the affidavit of Harold Glucksberg in this regard, but perhaps by ignoring it the Court has made its comment. Unlike Quill, Glucksberg abandoned his dying AIDS patient, who he says then threw himself off a Seattle bridge to his death with the help of his family. This is a shocking story, but not because it illustrates problems with the assisted suicide laws. Rather the shocking part is that Dr. Glucksberg sees himself as the victim in this case, rather than his former patient or the patient's family. This, even though no physician in the history of the United States has ever been indicted (let alone tried or convicted) or had his or her medical license suspended or revoked for complying with such a request.

It would have been more comforting for physicians had the Court more explicitly ruled that what the physicians wanted to do in these cases was not assisted suicide by definition, and thus the constitutionality of the statutes as applied to them did not even have to be adjudicated.[20] The avoidance of this central question, and the hand-wringing of the five Justices who wrote or joined in

concurring opinions about hypothetical cases of suffering terminally ill patients that were not before the Court, indicate that the
Justices—like all Americans—have a very difficult time coming to
grips with the dying process. The abstract nature of all the opinions can also be explained by the fact that there was no trial in
either case, and thus there are only physician affidavits of fear of
the law and the stories of already dead patients before the Court.

Only physicians who really believe they are intentionally killing their patients with overdoses of drugs, and who would feel the
same if they shot their patients with a gun—or provided their
patients with a loaded gun with the intent that they use the gun
to kill themselves—should change their behavior to comply with
the laws against homicide and assisting suicide after this opinion.
Doctors who provide palliative care with the primary intent of
relieving pain and suffering, and with the patient's consent, are
strongly encouraged to continue to do so by the Court. Indeed, at
least five members of the Court seem to think there is something
akin to a "right not to suffer," at least near death, and that states
have no constitutional authority to prohibit or inhibit physicians
from doing all in their medical power to prevent such suffering.

Changing American Medicine

There are real problems with the way Americans die; but the
solution to these problems is not to be found in the U.S. Constitution, or in making it even easier for patients to kill themselves.
Thus, unless these cases help us to focus our efforts on taking care
of real people instead of constructing grand constitutional theory, they will have been a waste of time and a missed opportunity.
Americans consistently say they want to die at home, with friends
and family, quickly and without pain. Instead, most Americans die
in hospitals, surrounded by strangers, and in varying degrees of
pain. There are many reasons for this, but I think the most important one is that patients' rights are not taken seriously during a
person's life, and therefore they are not likely to be taken seriously just before death.

Problems in dying exist in the extreme in the contemporary
teaching hospital, in which patient care is often a distant third

goal after teaching and research. In this high-tech, high-pressure environment, there is little room for thoughtfulness, for the intrusion of human values, or for conversation with the patient or family. The primary values are action-and technology-oriented; the imperative is to use all available medical technologies possible for the patient or for practice.

As hospitals become more and more like large ICUs, this impersonal, technological emphasis has increased. Add the cost pressures of managed care to treat patients more quickly, and care of the dying in hospitals is getting worse, not better. Hospice care remains marginalized, and death is still seen as failure. Medical students and residents are taught that talking is a waste of time, distracting from the time available to do real medicine. And when doing "real medicine" cannot help the dying patient, students and residents quickly learn that the attendings are uninterested in having discussions with patients or families about death or pain.

These attitudes are such a pervasive part of contemporary medical culture that the only realistic way to improve the care of dying patients in the short run is to get them out of hospitals and to keep them from going to hospitals at the end of their life. A recent study, for example, showed that an astonishing "41 percent experienced moderate or extremely severe pain most of the time" during their last three days of life in a hospital intensive care unit.[21] There is no excuse for this indifference to human suffering, which amounts to systematic patient abuse; and observing such callous "care" is at least one reason why physician-assisted suicide has been seen by the public as a reasonable option.

Medical sociologists teach that there are three basic ways to change professional behavior: convince the profession that it is in their best interests to change; change the norms of the profession; and change the incentives. The first strategy hardly ever works, since professionals generally think they know their own best interests better than any outsider. The second works, but takes a very long time. Perhaps we are now in a cultural lag period in medicine, but if so we are at the very beginning. The third produces much more rapid change, and is why changing the payment rules for hospital services has already drastically changed the role and nature of the hospital in medical care in the United

States, and will ultimately transform hospitals into institutions that actually take patient-centered care seriously if they want to survive. Our payment rules should also encourage hospice care and home care, both of which place the patient in the center of the enterprise.

If we really want to enable patients in hospitals to have their pain properly treated and to exercise their right to refuse treatment near the end of life, we must have much stronger prevention methods and establish much more effective patient-centered interventions. Changing the treatment incentives, rather than trying to develop a grand constitutional theory of suicide, is probably the most effective way to proceed. What is needed is not immunity for discretionary acts but incentives to actually care for patients and follow effective pain-relief regimes. Medical licensing boards must make it clear to licensees that painful deaths are presumptively ones that are incompetently managed, and should result in license suspension or revocation in the absence of a satisfactory explanation.

A more effective way to use law than constitutional adjudication would be to establish a system of not-for-profit public interest health care law firms whose sole mission is to promote patient rights by educating the public and the medical community about their rights, and by bringing lawsuits on behalf of patients whose rights are not honored in the hospital setting. Patients would learn of the availability of the law firm to help them through advertising, the Internet, a hotline, and paralegals who would act as patient advocates on request. The firms would take cases on a contingency fee basis, and all of the contingency fee would go to help fund the firm (whose lawyers would all be on salary). The firms would continue in existence until there were insufficient cases of patient abuse to support them, at which point one might be able to conclude that the culture of hospital-based medicine had changed sufficiently to honor patient refusals and keep patients pain-free as a routine matter.[22]

This plan would require a national network of public interest firms, but a pilot program could be started in three or four major cities and expanded from this base if it proved a successful model for enhancing patient rights in a health care system much more dedicated to its own interests and survival. Alternatively, established law firms could offer their services pro bono in this area. They could also work with the state attorneys general separately, or in concert in a manner analogous to the legal strategy the attorneys general adopted against the tobacco companies to fund Medicaid that recently led to a possible settlement. The problem of pain and suffering near death is pervasive in America, and only a very powerful challenge to existing medical practice is likely to change it. Lawyers are likely to get the ear of physicians, hospitals, and health plans that have been deaf to the pleas of patients, families, and nurses.

Resort to the courts means that the system has broken down, and lawyers should be primarily engaged in prevention. In addition to education and development of a system of patient advocates, it will also be helpful for patients if "report cards" are developed on both hospitals and physicians that include their attitudes and actions on informed consent and other patient rights, and their actual track records in areas such as availability for discussions with the patient and family, adherence to advance directives, providing adequate pain management, writing do-not-resuscitate orders upon request, and keeping dying people out of the ICU.

The bell has tolled for constitutional adjudication. Nonetheless, to the extent that law continues to dominate medical ethics in the United States, changes in the ethical behavior of physicians will continue to require legal action. Litigation to protect dying patients from pain, and legislation to promote universal hospice care, seem reasonable places to begin.

10

A Question of Balance

LINDA L. EMANUEL

Physician-assisted suicide and euthanasia have been debated since before Hippocrates. And yet the questions must be rendered anew for society's current context. To begin, the major arguments must be clearly understood and balanced. The major arguments represented in this volume divide roughly along two lines: those that address the interests of individuals versus those that address the interests of society on the one hand; and on the other, those opposing versus favoring physician-assisted suicide (see table). In this concluding chapter I will attempt to line up these arguments for a series of point/counter-point analyses, and offer for each one a balanced summary (printed in italic type, for convenience).

But the job of evaluation does not stop there. Deliberative wisdom is distinguishable from practical wisdom, if only by the latter's origins in confrontations with reality. Considerations that seem minor within the contexts of reading or reflection may be major in the real world, and vice versa. Therefore, the juxtaposing and balancing in the first part of this chapter is followed by a series of practical points for consideration by those who must make difficult decisions in individual cases, and by those who must make policy. This section is not drawn extensively from the authors' contributions, and indeed there is a general paucity of practical writing on preparing for death. Its pressing importance and absence in the literature propelled inclusion here.

Arguments in Favor of Physician-Assisted Suicide and Euthanasia	Arguments against Physician-Assisted Suicide and Euthanasia	
1. Mercy dictates these practices.	1. Pain is not the main motivator; palliative care is sufficient.	Individual considerations
2. Some killing is justified.	2. Killing human life is an intrinsic evil.	
3. Dignity lies in exercising control, avoiding being a burden.	3. Dignity lies in suffering, humility.	
4. Decisions to act or remain passive are morally equivalent.	4. Actions are not morally equivalent to omissions.	
5. Self-determination, voluntariness support these practices.	5. Autonomy is lost; voluntariness is impossible.	
6. Private matters should be free of interference.	6. Implications are a public matter.	Collective considerations
7. Professions are at society's command.	7. Professions have independent values.	
8. Legal trends support assisted suicide.	8. U.S. Constitution does not support assisted suicide.	
9. Legalization permits restraints.	9. Slippery slope would be worse with legalization.	
10. Holland's policy works all right.	10. Holland's policy is not safely reproducible in U.S. culture.	

But the job still does not stop there. A number of state rulings on the matter have come up, two of them reaching the United States Supreme Court, variously to declare illegal or declare a right to physician-assisted suicide or euthanasia. Society, professionals, and individuals are in need of a policy position, not perhaps for all time but for our patients in this society in this time. Therefore this volume ends with a personal position on the question of policy regarding physician-assisted suicide and euthanasia.

Major Arguments Regarding Physician-Assisted Death

Individual Case Considerations

WHAT DOES MERCY DICTATE? That mercy can require actively, intentionally ending life is a possibility that has pulled at the hearts of more than a few physicians and family members of the seriously ill. Many physicians deeply desire to help those who suffer, including by physician-assisted suicide or euthanasia, as Angell points out. Mercy, according to Battin, is one of the premier medical values, and Loewy would have society, at least as a tentative trial, extend the option of merciful death through euthanasia to those who are unable to but would commit suicide.

On the other hand, Wolf points out that physician-assisted suicide and euthanasia are all too likely to be born of a misguided, ambivalent, or nonauthentic request, and both Wolf and Childress note that many believe euthanasia to be a generally misguided interpretation of mercy. People in states of disability value their life quality higher than nondisabled people would and fault the unsupportive environment for much of their suffering. Consistent with this, Pellegrino argues that ideal palliative care can manage almost all suffering adequately. Others assert even more strongly that in cases of unmanageable suffering, anesthetic coma can be induced until death comes, so that all suffering is potentially manageable without resort to physician-assisted suicide and euthanasia. Importantly, van der Maas indicates that pain alone is a rare (3 percent) motivator for euthanasia requests. For 46 percent of requests, pain is one of several motivations; and for the remaining 51 percent of requests, pain is not a cited factor at all.

The epidemiology of unbearable terminal suffering is also relevant to the mercy argument. Van der Maas and I note a World Health Organization estimate that up to 10 percent of all dying people might experience intolerable suffering even in the presence of palliative care. (This estimate presumably omits the possible use of anesthetic coma for otherwise untreatable suffering.) Not all of these suffering patients would both want and be eligible for physician-assisted suicide or euthanasia (criteria would presumably include—in addition to terminality—mental competence, absence of clinical depression, and full information on all alternatives and risks). The final proportion of dying patients who might for mercy's sake receive physician-assisted suicide or euthanasia is probably a fraction of 1 percent.

A balance of deliberation suggests that the traditional pro-euthanasia mercy argument, if accepted as valid in principle, applies in a very small proportion of deaths.

IS MERCY A JUSTIFICATION FOR KILLING? For this small population where the suffering of dying provokes requests for mercy, is killing justified? The view that killing is an intrinsic evil and can never be justified fails to acknowledge widely accepted situations of justifiable killing, such as in the line of war duty or in self-defense. Childress notes that major monotheistic religions support justifiable killing. If killing is a bad and generally proscribed act (as both sides of the debate accept), the question has to come down to whether or not physician-assisted suicide and euthanasia can be counted among the rare justifiable killings.

The view that human beings are made in the divine image and therefore that their lives must not be taken except to avert some greater desecration is persuasive to some (including myself). The main religious arguments that oppose euthanasia on this ground, which Childress describes, are countered in positions such as those of Angell, Loewy, and Battin. To euthanasia proponents it is a desecration to needlessly let a dying human being suffer. Both groups agree that human life is precious, but their inferences are divergent. The difference appears to hinge on what is needlessness in suffering and what is the greater desecration.

The related argument that our lives are only lent to us and are therefore not our own to end as we choose is one that has great sway over many people (again, including myself). Nonetheless, the reverse logic, namely that stewardship requires that human life be cared for in ways that include physician-assisted suicide and euthanasia, is also possible. A good steward could as logically be required to hasten immanent dying for avoidance of suffering as to assume a passive position.

These questions are apparently answered differently depending on a larger interpretation of meaning in life. Only if the argument is supported with other arguments—for instance, about the legitimate actions of human beings or interpretations of the meaning of holiness and desecration—can the desecration or the stewardship determinations be complete. That is, spiritual arguments require a nexus of associated interpretations and beliefs. If these religious arguments carry weight only as part of a larger committed understanding, then they will not carry intrinsic weight for adherents of a different framework.

Another type of response to the question of whether or not mercy can be a justification for killing is not religious but logical. As Wolf notes, ending suffering should not be achieved by ending the life that suffers. This is a powerful argument, especially if all suffering can be and is controlled, if only with anesthetic coma. Battin provides a counterargument by noting that some people do not want to die in a coma but rather want to be conscious up to the last moment, surrounded by, and aware of, those they love. The degree of suffering entailed by ending life in a coma rather than by physician-assisted suicide and euthanasia is, however, not compelling if the former involves no moral concern and the latter does.

The balance of deliberation suggests that killing is sometimes justified even in major monotheistic traditions, but the question of whether mercy killing is ever justified is not resolved by the logic of these religious arguments alone. In circumstances where palliative care can eliminate physical suffering, the patient's misery is reduced to the inability to choose physician-assisted suicide or euthanasia over medication-induced coma. This degree of suffering does not, in my view, justify mercy killing.

ARE ACTS AND OMISSIONS MORALLY DIFFERENT? To justify physician-assisted suicide and euthanasia, several philosophers (as Battin, Angell, and Loewy describe) and some legal decisions have taken the view that there is no moral difference between withholding or withdrawing life-sustaining treatment and actively causing death. The justification is that the intent (avoidance of suffering) and outcome (death) are the same whether the means is an omission or an act. Commentators tend to describe paired cases where the intent and outcome are indistinguishable and only the active and passive means distinguishes the cases.

If the nondistinction is accepted, it neutralizes an objection to certain narrowly defined cases of physician-assisted suicide. Further, cases abound where act and omission both require responsibility for choosing death and argue persuasively against making simplistic distinctions in which all omissions are permissible and all acts are not.

However, this argument does not thereby justify physician-assisted suicide and euthanasia more generally, since not all acts and omissions that share intent and outcome are automatically equivalent. It is not a persuasive argument for the general absence of a moral distinction. Further, if the distinction is erasable, it argues for caution with both types of decision; it does not follow that both are automatically acceptable. Childress describes how religious argumentation relies on the distinction, for instance, to provide a definition of natural death, while still requiring responsibility for both acts and omissions. Nonreligious arguments can use similar logic and aspirations for natural death.

Van der Maas indicates that empirical data show a tangible difference in the descriptions Dutch physicians have of their intent and the outcome depending on whether life-ending decisions use active or passive means. Physicians who withhold or withdraw life-sustaining interventions intend to cease prolonging the dying process, while those who assist in death intend death itself. The patients of the former group die over a longer period, usually days, while patients of the latter group die more immediately.

A balance of deliberation suggests that the act/omission distinction in some specific and rather theoretical circumstances may not matter, but that in most cases the distinction is morally relevant.

IS PHYSICIAN-ASSISTED DEATH MORE DIGNIFIED THAN NATURAL DEATH? Different people have different conceptions of dignity. A personal experience illustrates the point. I was privileged to watch Ute Pippig win among women at the Boston Marathon in 1996. That it was her third win was not the most remarkable thing; nor was it the last dash that brought her from a lagging second place into first place. The inspiring thing was that she was suffering from uncontrolled diarrhea and menstrual bleeding during the race. She chose to run on despite not only the physical pain but the indignity of running in public covered with her own blood and stool. When she arrived at the finish line, spectators were stunned by her beauty, humility, and courage—complete with what might be considered extraordinary indignity. She reached through to a greater dignity. Something similar can happen for those who are dying, as was illustrated by Cardinal Bernadine when, dying of pancreatic cancer in 1997, he allowed an unusually public witnessing of the process. In the bodily disintegrations of the dying process there is an opportunity to respond with a greater vision of glory.

But what of people who do not wish to face the challenge, or who have a different conception of dignity that does not include a romantic or spiritual vision to overcome the many miseries of natural dying? Battin provides a real story (personal communication) that puts this counterpoint into perspective. An elderly hospitalized woman, whose illness reminded her painfully of the suffering she sustained during World War II, repeatedly requested physician-assisted suicide or euthanasia. Her request was denied, but when a nurse brought the woman her usual sedative, the patient erroneously thought it was her lethal drug. She sat up, smiling, took the pills and settled peacefully into her pillows, saying "Thank you, thank you," and went to sleep. On awaking, she realized the error, and wept. Angell's description, data from Van der Maas's chapter, and other publications also indicate that a nontrivial number of people see indignity in natural death, quite often when there are associations with prior experiences of suffering.

There seems little objective ground (only subjective perceptions of correctness) to trump one vision with another. To demand that a person espouse a vision that does not ring true or seems unrealistic for them risks coercion.

A balance of deliberation suggests that, unless bolstered with arguments that make either natural or controlled dying better for independent reasons, the dignity argument seems to lend itself to either direction.

WHEN MIGHT PHYSICIAN-ASSISTED SUICIDE AND EUTHANASIA HONOR OR VIOLATE AUTONOMY? Self-determination is the strongest argument for physician-assisted suicide and euthanasia, and Angell, Battin, and Loewy all use or presume it. Dying stages provide the last and in some ways the most enduring personal legacies, so people's legitimate interest in how they die is strong. Its recurrent emergence in history, as E. J. Emanuel describes, points to a connection between physician-assisted suicide and euthanasia issues and strong human claims.

The self-determination argument, however, cannot be a simple and unrestricted application of rights for three reasons. First, the principal—the dying person—who exerts the autonomy is destroyed thereby, as Wolf points out. Autonomous choices for self-destruction tend to fall outside the usual justifications for self-determination. For instance, few permit the "right" to sell oneself into slavery or prostitution. Thus, autonomy may not require that a request—even an apparently free request—for physician-assisted suicide and euthanasia be followed.

Second, all autonomy rights are limited by the rights of others not to be interfered with or injured. Since there are many ways in which physician-assisted suicide and euthanasia may affect not only the patient but the physician (as van der Maas reports), family, friends and society, a range of other restrictions to this form of self-determination may also apply. Battin considers some limits to the restrictions, but there is general consensus that restrictions apply.

Third, and importantly, the basic right in autonomy is to be free of unwanted intervention. While this supports the right to have medical intervention withheld or withdrawn, it does not logically extend to physician-assisted suicide and euthanasia where there is no unwanted intervention. It is possible that self-determination arguments more akin to surviving interest exist, but these have not been well articulated.

Does self-determination in matters of physician-assisted suicide and euthanasia lend itself intrinsically to losing autonomy in the process, as Pellegrino suggests? Given the profound connectedness of people to one another, and the different agendas connected people have, it would be startling if free will were easily defined. It must be hard for a patient to avoid internalizing the projected burden of exhausted caregivers or an unwelcoming society, for example. Further, some have argued that proper informed consent to self-destruction is so difficult to conceive that it may be unattainable or at least unassurable. But is such lost autonomy in assisted suicide a tendency or an inevitability? Wolf and Pellegrino have argued persuasively that it is a strong tendency and, in the aggregate, an inevitability. E. J. Emanuel's argument that pro-mercy-killing movements emerge in times of social depression and belief in competition as a quality necessary for survival seems consistent with this view. On the other hand, van der Maas presents data confirming that many prior wishes are honored in both assisted and natural death and many false requests by the vulnerable or misguided are appropriately denied.

A balance of deliberation suggests that existing strong autonomy arguments may not apply well to physician-assisted suicide and euthanasia. However, subjection to others' control is not inevitable either. While assisted suicide could often be enactments of pretenses or complex subjugations rather than real autonomy, such misuses are not inevitable.

SUMMARY A balance of deliberation for individual cases suggests the follow conclusions: The strength of the pro-physician-assisted suicide and euthanasia arguments is that they do not (or should not) claim to apply in any but a few well-defined situations. At extremes of suffering for some who are actively dying, mercy might justify requested killing. Opposing arguments show strength in establishing that physician-assisted suicide and euthanasia justifications pertain in very few situations, that the act/omission distinction is often morally relevant, that killing is usually evil, and that dignity is possible even in the face of great suffering and dependence. However, proof that physician-assisted suicide and euthanasia are always categorically wrong is unestablished.

Collective Considerations

ARE DECISIONS FOR PHYSICIAN-SECURED DEATH A PURELY PRIVATE MATTER? Dying is a profoundly personal experience. Personal, however, is distinct from private. Dying is often about as private as childbirth, when many people are in immediate or proximate attendance and responses to the event include the larger community. The reason is only partly that dying and childbirth often require assistance for those immediately involved. Connections among people make the fact and circumstances of almost anyone's dying meaningful and of legitimate concern to others, as Pellegrino notes. Opposers of physician-assisted suicide and euthanasia are not alone in arguing this position. The rather common reason for requesting physician-assisted suicide and euthanasia, namely to avoid being a burden, also underscores the interdependence of people. Indeed, depending on the views and feelings of relatives, concern for survivor's feelings often sways requesters either toward or away from physician-assisted suicide and euthanasia. The influence of individual cases on the larger society is not contested. The public importance of this matter, its private nature notwithstanding, seems to be a point of consensus.

A balance of deliberation suggests that the profoundly personal nature of dying does not command unmitigated privacy for decisions about physician-assisted suicide and euthanasia.

SHOULD THE MEDICAL PROFESSIONAL EVER SECURE DEATH? The argument that doctors *qua* doctors should never intentionally kill, even in extreme situations, stands most pivotally on one assumption, namely that physician-assisted suicide and euthanasia are contrary to the values of medicine. Although I agree that physicians should not kill, a position indicated by Pellegrino and Wolf, it is also clear that agreement depends on an interpretation of the values of medicine. The Hippocratic tradition may be one of the more admirable traditions but it is only one interpretation of medical values, and non-Hippocratic medical traditions have either remained silent on the matter or openly endorsed physician-assisted suicide and euthanasia, as Battin and Loewy point out. Agreement on the medical profession's mandate to minimize harm to patients and advocate for their health needs does not entail obvious agreement on where to draw the line in assisting individual patients who face inevitable death.

The profession should advocate for the overall best interests of patients and the health of society and take a stand against activities that are to the detriment of either. But the application of this duty to support or resist physician-assisted suicide and euthanasia depends on an assessment of how it serves or does disservice to the collective best interests of patients and the health of society. As the chapter by van der Maas demonstrates, much empirical assessment of the relevant practices and context is necessary for this assessment.

A balance of deliberation suggests that the values of medicine can be defined and applied to support or oppose physician-assisted suicide and euthanasia. An appropriate professional position may be determined by assessment of overall benefit to patients and society.

SHOULD PHYSICIAN-ASSISTED SUICIDE AND EUTHANASIA BE PROTECTED EVEN IF MANY FIND THEM ABHORRENT? This question has been examined in several chapters, mostly under the rubric of legal theory. Pellegrino argues that the U.S. Constitution does not and should not be argued to support physician-assisted suicide and euthanasia, and Annas explicates the support for this position by the U.S. Supreme Court, while Angell builds an argument that case law and the Fourteenth Amendment to the Constitution do support it.

The fashion in which the Constitution applies to health care generally is tenuous. Consideration of physician-assisted suicide and euthanasia as a liberty interest is uncomfortable since achievement of the objective kills the individual who had the interest, as Wolf points out, and liberty provides a right to be free of intervention, not to demand assisted self-destruction. The right to be free of interference in accomplishing rational suicide might be easier to defend, but physician-assisted suicide and euthanasia are not accomplished by mere noninterference. However, as Oregon recently demonstrated, state protection remains possible by democratically established legislation.

A balance of deliberation suggests that U.S. Constitutional Law does not lend itself well to protection of physician-assisted suicide and euthanasia. State protections may, however, be established by popular will.

WHAT IS THE BEST WAY TO GUARD AGAINST THE SLIPPERY SLOPE? There is little disagreement over the presence of a "slippery slope," that is, a situation whereby physician-assisted suicide and euthanasia could play a part in a deteriorating trend to kill unjustifiably. Both sides of the debate concur that a potential slippery slope exists—Angell, Loewy, Pellegrino, and Wolf all make this point—and also on the need for procedures or limits to resist the decline.

The disagreement is over where and how to draw the line. Opponents of physician-assisted suicide and euthanasia claim that the act/omission and intent distinctions provide a very good place to draw the line. Under this arrangement procedural assurances could fall within the realm of existing medical, civil, and criminal monitoring. While it is potentially cruel to those who genuinely want physician-assisted suicide and euthanasia if their suffering must be endured for the sake of society, it is fair and important that relief of their suffering should not be at the price of greater suffering and wrong to others.

Data noted in van der Maas's and my chapter confirm that physician-assisted suicide and euthanasia practices in the United States occur despite their illegal status. Proponents of legalization argue that since physician-assisted suicide and euthanasia already occur, they should be done in the open where monitoring can be improved. Physicians who assist in suicide or perform euthanasia in the United States, for instance, often fail to involve colleagues in the process, possibly because of the illegal standing of these practices. Angell, Loewy, and Battin note that several groups have proposed legislation with safeguards intended to resist misuse and the slippery slope. Others assert that continued illegal status is necessary to keep the incidence low. They claim that regulation is impossible, at least in the United States. Data from van der Maas's and my chapter note that open regulation in the Netherlands results in neither slippery slopes nor in reduced misuse rates. Whether or not retaining the illegal status of physician-assisted suicide and euthanasia would improve due process and safeguards in the United States is unproven. Optimized implementation of acknowledged claims to nonintervention and to comfort care is widely assumed to be capable of reducing needless calls for and misuse of physician-assisted suicide and euthanasia.

A balance of deliberation indicates that concern over a slippery slope is universal, but there are no empirical studies that would allow us to assess whether legalizing physician-assisted suicide and euthanasia in the United States would reduce or increase misuse. Better end-of-life care could reduce misguided calls for and use of these practices.

WHAT DO DIFFERENT CULTURAL PRACTICES REVEAL? Different cultures and historical periods vary markedly in their approaches to physician-assisted suicide and euthanasia. The United States is a dominantly Western and monotheistic culture, so analogies to non-Western and nonmonotheistic cultures are of limited applicability. Among more analogous cultures, one that started endorsing physician-assisted suicide and euthanasia was disastrous (Nazi Germany), and one has remained tolerant and civilized (Holland). Has the United States sufficient similarity to or difference from either that inferences are possible?

Differences between the culture of Nazi Germany and that of present-day United States are obvious and stark. But repulsion at the analogue should not prevent recognition that the United States is vulnerable to social undercurrents that could lead to misuse of assisted dying, as Wolf notes.

In Holland, the contrasts with the United States are in a different category. Holland has universal health coverage, more availability of hospice care, and a legal system that distinguishes between illegal and punishable. The distinction allows the society to declare that physician-assisted suicide and euthanasia are bad but that prosecuting physicians for these practices is not always in the public interest. Holland also differs from the United States in having a tradition of pragmatism mixed with Calvinism, as well as a more ethnically and culturally homogeneous population. In the United States, by contrast, citizens do not have universal access to health care; palliative care is not widely available; legal initiatives currently hinge on rights rather than obligation or pragmatism; and much of the legal system is state-based. U.S. culture is idealistic and has well-documented tendencies to testing limits, to self-centeredness, and to violence. Current U.S. culture has little place for dying or preparation for it. Death is rarely discussed even by family members; and physicians, pastors, and other professionals are not trained to recognize patients' readiness to prepare for dying or to assist them in thinking through and discussing their preparations.

Studies of other cultures' practices are few and are rarely made relevant. In the end, the question about how assisted suicide is best regulated requires a fuller social science perspective. Of all the arguments in the physician-assisted suicide and euthanasia debate, this is the least studied, most difficult, and perhaps the most determinative. Recent legalization of physician-assisted suicide provides something of a social laboratory in the United States. Careful study and interpretation will be critical.

A balance of deliberation is hard to attain from cross-cultural studies, since social science research is sparse on the topic. Assisted suicide can probably be sustained in a stable civilized society, but one of the most genocidal societies included physician-assisted suicide and euthanasia in its early and probably seminal activities. A policy involving legal physician-assisted suicide or euthanasia that works for the United States may be hard to attain, at least for the current time, although results from Oregon's experience may be helpful.

SUMMARY A balance of deliberation for collective considerations suggests the following conclusions: The obligations of the profession and the best legal approach to physician-assisted suicide and euthanasia cannot be established until further empirical, theoretical, and social science scholarship is available. Concerns about misuse and policy problems suggest that before widely legalizing physician-assisted suicide and euthanasia in the United States, our society should first move to provide quality palliative care, advance planning, and widespread access to general health care, as well as to improve the debate and provide more suitable legislative possibilities.

A Practical Approach

If preparing for one's own death or the death of a loved one or patient, there are practical things to think about and arrangements to make. Because this area is rarely talked about in present-day U.S. society, there is little practical wisdom to be had. This is unfortunate since practical-minded wrestling is critical to making the best possible judgment.

The real world and the realities of our human condition sometimes bring about more common ground between positions than debate and deliberation ever could. In the realities of my own clinical care there has been rather little difference between the way patients who did or did not want assisted suicide or euthanasia needed assistance. Even acknowledging that I bring my own approach to the issues that might influence my patients—those patients who started out being interested in physician-assisted suicide and euthanasia ended, as I had hoped, by wanting well-planned and aggressive palliative care instead—it is still remarkable that polarized positions do not necessarily result in opposing actions, and that practical wisdom can create common ground between otherwise incompatible groups. What follows is an approximation to the practical approach I have come to offer, constituted from the thought of many, rendered through seeing patients and editing this book, and offered in the second person as prescriptive advice.

Considerations in Preparing for Your Own Death

TAKE A PURPOSEFUL APPROACH Consider that terminal stages prepare for one last job in life, or the last chapter of your personal story, and consider what the right job or best chapter might be. If you think in this way, you ▸ prepare for the legacy you want to leave behind, and ▸ avoid acting on impulse, even if time is short.

DO SOME ADVANCE PLANNING Consider a range of dying circumstances and figure out what your goals for medical care would be for each, checking your goals against your larger beliefs and against some specific medical interventions. Worksheets are now available that help people to think through the issues, some of which have been researched to ensure that they cover the main medical dilemmas and that they generally facilitate articulation of preferences that are internally consistent and durable. Use these worksheets to help structure decisions with those who are likely to care about your dying, including your doctor.

Just going through worksheets within your mind and with relevant people will accomplish a number of things: ▸ People who care about your dying will begin to be able to talk about issues that are hard to talk about. You will learn how different types of dying would leave people you care for either proud or pained, burdened by sacrifice or by shame, able to go on with comfortable memories or unable to do so. ▸ People who care for you will not be left with the burden of regrettable undiscussed acts (such as suicide or prolonged periods of medical intervention) or of proxy decision-making that could not be guided by direct knowledge of your own hopes. ▸ You and your loved ones will see in a tangible way what your medical options are. ▸ You will find out something about from where and from whom your support may come. ▸ You will be reminded of or hear stories of others' dying and how they, their caregivers, and survivors handled things. ▸ You will have an opportunity to understand and articulate what dying scenarios are most fearsome to you. ▸ You will be able to ask your doctor and talk through with your loved ones how likely dying is to occur, and what can be done to avoid or mitigate it. Ask, for example, about patients' last few days, which are often the most difficult, and plan some ways to cope. ▸ For all concerned, expectations of abandonment, indignity, and meaningless suffering may seem different.

MAKE PRACTICAL INQUIRIES AND ARRANGEMENTS Comprehensive palliative care is more and more available. Find out what may be available to you. Comprehensive home hospice or nursing care is more widespread than before, as are institutional or assisted living arrangements. Social service departments of health care facilities, associations, and government organizations have information. Think about and discuss with your friends and family how care for life-threatening illness might affect you all. Try to end up with arrangements that respect the diverse needs and aspirations of family groups. You will thereby have helped ▸ minimize your physical suffering; ▸ minimize your indignity; ▸ minimize the practical burden your illness may cause others; and ▸ minimize personal and financial or other losses to your survivors.

REFLECT AGAIN; ADJUST YOUR PLANS IF NEED BE People have deep but little expressed reasons for wanting assistance during dying. People who want care during natural death may have similar motivations to those who want physician-assisted suicide and euthanasia. Fear, altruism, love, humility, piety, control are all common motivations behind the diverse plans we create for ourselves. Appraise candidly the reasons for your plans. Be fair to yourself, but put aside reasons you would not be proud to be remembered by, and put aside plans that might likely be mistaken for unworthy goals. Be sure that your plans are not coercing anyone and that you are not being coerced, and that the plan has instead been persuasive to all or to as many as possible. Remember that many others have died before, and not a few have managed to make something fulfilling of this overwhelmingly sad transition. Aim to ▸ feel peaceful; and ▸ help those who care about you feel peaceful.

Considerations in Preparing for the Death of a Family Member or Friend

TAKE A PURPOSEFUL APPROACH Caring for a dying person can be one of the most punishing and demeaning or one of the most privileged and uplifting experiences in your life. Often it is a mixture. You do not have complete control or responsibility over how things go, but you do have a lot. Try to think of the burden as a difficult but privileged job.

DO SOME ADVANCE PLANNING Know the job of preparing that the dying person faces. To support the person, facilitate dialogue, especially advance care planning as described above, help find out about and secure practical resources, help with adjustments if plans change, and get to know your role (health care proxy, home care person, companion, and so on). When you participate in going through a worksheet and making practical arrangements you will ▸ benefit from the same kind of insights the preparing person benefits from, but for yourself; ▸ be privileged to witness how someone you care for reconciles himself or herself to mortality, and prepares for it; ▸ have the honor of helping a person in one of the most difficult and important acts in life.

MAKE PRACTICAL INQUIRIES AND ARRANGEMENTS FOR YOUR-SELF Set up your own supports, practical and emotional. Burdens are great, and bereavement grief starts long before and continues long after death. Find out about practical resources and sources for caregiver support. No one can give of themselves indefinitely without being given to in return. By preparing your own supports you will help yourself: ▸ care well for the person who is dying, without exhausting yourself; ▸ grow through the experience into a wiser person.

REFLECT ON YOUR GOALS AND MOTIVES; ADJUST THEM IF NEED BE Caring for the dying is a big job and a challenge. Caregivers need to be comfortable with the reasons why they are doing this extraordinary work. Caregivers have deep and conflicting emotions. Examine your hopes, resentments, fears, emotional gains. Resolve and replace ones that will make you feel bad when all is said and done. Look for possible false hopes, for instance to avoid unavoidable losses (remember that life-sustaining intervention cannot prevent all death and that some who are saved are very diminished until they do eventually die) or to avoid burdens without paying the price (some hope to avoid burdens through physician-assisted suicide and euthanasia and forget that it may involve personal turmoil and leave survivors with enduring burdens of guilt, failure, and ruined legacy). Think things through and be realistic. By engaging in these reflections, ▸ regrets you may have will be minimized; ▸ gratifications you may have will be maximized.

Considerations in Preparing for the Death of a Patient

BE SURE YOU ARE COMPETENT Most physicians are not trained to know, recognize, or handle the needs of patients who are preparing, or should be preparing, to die. Even physicians who rarely attend the dying need to have training in the area as much as they need training in, say, the physical examination of the heart; if there is a need, any physician must be able to detect it and either respond or refer the patient to the appropriate colleague. Physicians who do attend the dying must have complex interdisciplinary skills that were not part of most physicians' training. Physicians must take the responsibility of seeking out continuing medical education to acquire the skills. To avoid the uncomfortable feeling that your dying patient has exhausted your ability to help—that day should not come until *after* their death when you have helped the surviving family through the early steps of bereavement—you need training in two areas: comprehensive advance care planning and comprehensive palliative care.

If you are trained in the deliberative skills of comprehensive integrated advance care planning, and routinely provide it for your patients, and are willing to return to the discussion whenever it becomes relevant; and if you are trained in the interdisciplinary approaches and philosophy of palliative care and provide it to appropriate patients, ▸ you will be released from the fears of impotence and incompetence aroused in many physicians by the prospect of caring for the dying, freeing yourself to continue regular unabbreviated visits and thereby avoid abandoning your patient; ▸ you will be able to understand patients' goals for care, which differ greatly, and tailor your interventions to deliberated and agreed upon goals; ▸ you will be able to offer your patients their full range of interventionist and supportive care options, whether they are terminal or not (physicians palliate symptoms of many chronic conditions, not just terminal conditions, and palliative care skills apply in many situations). The fundamental obligation of physicians, to care for patients from cradle to grave, curing where possible and caring when cure cannot be had, cannot be fulfilled without these skills. Once you have them, ▸ you will also be able to experience care of the dying as one of the most fulfilling and gratifying care experiences available to physicians.

HAVE A MENTAL CHECKLIST WHEN ASSISTING IN DECISIONMAK- ING Know your own reflected moral positions, and discuss the relevant congruence or disagreement you have with your patient. As you assess your patient's frame of mind, be sure you have addressed possible confounding reasons for patient requests, whether they are for life-sustaining intervention when the grounds for hope are slim or for physician-assisted suicide and euthanasia. Have in mind: ▸ fear of abandonment, by you or someone else; ▸ false hopes of avoiding burden; ▸ false fears of terminal suffering; ▸ treatable depression; ▸ other contributing psychological or psychiatric conditions; ▸ masked personal agendas (suicide as a means to get back at someone, life-sustaining intervention as an avoidance of existential reality); and ▸ reversible social or personal situations (isolation, unsatisfactory care, and so on).

CONSULT MULTIPLE COLLEAGUES Talk with other professionals about ▸ your patient's pathophysiological issues; ▸ your patient's psychosocial and spiritual issues; ▸ ethical and legal issues; ▸ your own personal needs—avoid "burnout." As always, but especially when a decision has questionable moral standing, be sure all alternatives have been exhaustively pursued. Be sure you know its legal standing, and possible consequences to you. Be sure that anything you do you would be prepared to justify in public.

Looking at these considerations all together, some may wonder how helpful they can be in such a charged situation. This is an empirically testable question, but data are not yet available. Anecdotal evidence suggests they are very helpful. Also the practically wise know well that the quiet, sane, and practical approach is often the best solution to charged situations. If your patient wants you to do something morally challenging (whether to provide physician-assisted suicide and euthanasia or medical intervention with no limits) these practical and noncontroversial steps are as likely as anything we know to dissolve the challenging request, leaving you on therapeutic common ground.

Collective Considerations

Whether or not physician-assisted suicide and euthanasia are accepted as justifiable in rare circumstances, several major steps are necessary before legalization could be as measured in the United States as it appears to be in the Netherlands. They include:

WIDESPREAD MEDICAL EDUCATION IN END-OF-LIFE CARE
Training in palliative care, advance care planning, and euthanasia-request assessment skills is essential for all physicians.

WIDESPREAD COMPREHENSIVE PALLIATIVE CARE SERVICES
Physician skills must be supported by the infrastructure in health care delivery organizations so that centers of expertise and continued training and progress can be achieved.

COMPREHENSIVE STUDIES Good empirical studies are needed to assess the needs, cultural context, and practice trends under various systems and safeguards. These have been hampered by taboos around death-related topics. To rush to legalization before permitting open-minded and impartial study seems foolish.

ACCESS TO BASIC HEALTH CARE FOR ALL CITIZENS Currently death and abortion are argued to be constitutional rights when no other medical service is a constitutional or even a social right. Access to basic health care for all is probably a precondition for safe physician-assisted suicide and euthanasia.

A WELL-DEVELOPED LEGAL APPROACH What is needed is an approach that can balance the rightful protections of patients who wish to die with the rightful protections of those who may be vulnerable to misuses of physician-assisted suicide and euthanasia. As it currently stands, Michigan was recently unable to call unconstitutional the physician-assisted suicide and euthanasia of two nonterminal patients by Kevorkian. With this kind of legal precedent there is ground for skepticism that it is possible to regulate physician-assisted suicide and euthanasia well. Oregon's experiment may bring a helpful perspective.

A MODERATED, CARING CULTURE Equally important, but more challenging, is to foster and achieve a culture that does not tend so severely to aggression and extremes. The United States has a long history—proud in some cases—of testing the limits of freedom. The limits of freedom may well lie shy of legalized physician-assisted suicide and euthanasia in a society where people routinely push their rights so hard. Paradoxically perhaps, a society less obsessed with rights might be able to give more freedom in this matter without risking so much safety for others.

The first set of requirements, to improve medical care at the end of life, is so obviously worthwhile on its own merit that there seems little reason to push ahead with legalization of physician-assisted suicide and euthanasia until these requirements have been accomplished. Given the vicissitudes of public opinion in history, the moral ambiguity of physician-assisted suicide and euthanasia, and the possibility that improved palliative care and access to health care would satisfy much of the drive toward physician-assisted suicide and euthanasia, it is quite likely that after taking these morally noncontentious steps, physician-assisted suicide and euthanasia will no longer be in demand.

Taking a Position

Thus far, this overview has dwelled on an impartial balancing of arguments and then on common existential themes and practical general advice. What of the decisions about policy and practice that must be made? When balancing is said and done and practical advice has been heard, even followed, can physician-assisted suicide and euthanasia occasionally be justified for today's patients, and what is the right policy decision for today's society? Of all the pertinent arguments and facts that came forward in creating this book, some stand out.

First, there is no *right* to physician-assisted suicide and euthanasia. There is an ethical and legal right to be free of unwanted intervention, of unwanted presence within one's own body. This underlies the existing right to withdraw or withhold life-sustaining intervention and is strongly justified by autonomy arguments, among others. It does not, however, extend to an act which transgresses an individual's body boundaries, even if it is desired, for the purposes of that individual's destruction. Such an extension is illogical and an error in categories of reasoning. These argument were noted above and are taken up in Wolf's chapter.

By contrast there is a *professional obligation* to provide comfort to the suffering. This is a value, not a right, but it is a basic part of all major codes and declarations in medicine. The physician's accepted duty is to attempt cure when possible and to seek comfort when cure is impossible. Suffering does justify concerted attempts to use fully and well the existing patient rights to withdrawal or withholding of unwanted intervention, and it justifies concerted attempts to use full professional ability to provide aggressive comfort care to all who need it. But this justification does not apply by logical extension to physician-assisted suicide and euthanasia.

Second, although alleviation of suffering is far from adequate in the United States at present, in the history of medicine there has probably never been an era or a culture with less physical suffering than ours, or with better potential to relieve it. So, if physical suffering were ever to justify physician-assisted suicide and euthanasia, here and now would not be the time. So it seems that the strongest justification for physician-assisted suicide and euthanasia is minimally operative in the U.S. debate. The justification proffered in favor of physician-assisted suicide and euthanasia are much more effective in justifying continued pursuit of quality end-of-life care under existing regulations as they have been established in the last decades for withdrawing and withholding intervention and aggressive comfort care.

Third, arguments against physician-assisted suicide and euthanasia based on professional standards alone are also persuasive, even for rare individual cases. These include: the difficulty of ever establishing reliably that a request for assisted death is a reflection of the patient's unmitigated wish; the difficulty of making such a request freely, without undesirable social and contextual influence; the availability of alternative treatments for pathophysiological suffering, including terminal coma for pain relief with accepted-although-not-sought death; and the moral weightiness and irreversibility of suicide.

Fourth, there is an additional professional obligation which must be balanced against the need to seek comfort for suffering patients, and that is the obligation to consider public health and the welfare of other patients. It is too often forgotten that the policies of the United States are emulated by many other countries, not least and perhaps especially in matters of medicine. Imagine what would happen if legal and professional endorsement of physician-assisted suicide and euthanasia was carried to other countries where the favorable circumstances that the United States enjoys do not pertain. Imagine a physician in war-torn Rwanda, the Vietnam of the 1960s, or present-day Russia, where half of hospitals have no running water and procurement of opiods for symptom relief is similarly impeded, or rural areas of Africa where systems of medical care may not penetrate at all. In such places the pathophysiological suffering that might justify physician-assisted suicide and euthanasia is presumably far greater than in the United States today. What would a physician do who felt free, or even obligated, to use physician-assisted suicide and euthanasia as a treatment for such widespread, unrelievable suffering? Many of the strongest proponents of physician-assisted suicide and euthanasia shudder at the thought of such a physician "shooting the wounded." So the circumstances when this strong justification of suffering pertains most fully are the same circumstances which present the greatest risk of professional abandonment or betrayal by acting to end patients' lives.

Fifth, the above points combine to guide our thinking about a slippery slope of misuse, a concern shared by all sides of the debate. The question is: Where should the line on physician-assisted suicide and euthanasia be drawn? There is clear ethical, legal, and intuitive distinction between intent to comfort and intent to kill even as a means to comfort. In fact, physicians' medical actions and patients' outcomes differ depending on whether the intent is comfort and acceptance of death or physician-assisted suicide and euthanasia. This confirms that practitioners' moral intuitions also make a distinction between these types of action, even in the absence of judging one good and the other not. This is apparently a good place to draw the line. Given the weakness of the mercy arguments for these practices in today's United States, and professional obligations to set responsible precedents, the most justifiable and workable line to halt any slippery slope seems to be where it has been brought to in the last decades and currently is: that is, endorsing the right of patients to be free of unwanted intervention and emphasizing physicians' obligation to secure comfort for the dying, but stopping short of physician-assisted suicide and euthanasia. When medical culture has fully accommodated the progress of the last decades, a stable professional and societal boundary should be achieved and should provide maximum comfort and a minimum of misuse for all concerned.

Sixth, and perhaps most important of all, physician-assisted suicide and euthanasia are apparently not the real issues being raised by suffering patients and policymakers, nor the best answer to their concerns. It is essential to have a solid grip on the root motivations for calls for assisted death, whether made by individuals or the larger society, and to respond to the root cause before the overt call is evaluated on face value. Treatment of the root cause is far more reliable, safe, and effective than treatment of the presenting complaint alone. This is a matter of sound clinical and social policy practice. Strong data all point to the predominance of psychosocial, contextual suffering or fear of suffering as motivators, rather than current, unbearable, unrelievable, pathophysiological suffering. Most requesters are motivated not by pain but by fear: fear of future suffering, fear of indignity, fear of burdensomeness, fear of abandonment, and fear of lost control.

The severity of psychosocial suffering need not be understated to stand by this argument. Rather, the point is that psychosocial suffering should be treated by ameliorating its sources, not by eliminating the victim. Unfortunately, the widely acknowledged difficulty of assessing and lessening psychosocial suffering is a factor that could make physicians more prone to misuse of physician-assisted suicide and euthanasia if it were legalized.

So this is the position to which the reflective process of editing this volume has led me: In a very real sense, the current physician-assisted suicide and euthanasia debate in the United States is a false debate. If society takes the call for legally endorsed physician-assisted suicide and euthanasia on face value alone, and if the medical profession as a whole or physicians in particular take patients' calls for physician-assisted suicide and euthanasia on face value alone, society, the profession, and physicians will have made a grave error. Without better understanding of the fears that drive these requests, policies will be enacted and acts taken that not only miss the point but risk abuse. Some of history's great mistakes have been founded on misconceptions no greater than this failure to examine root causes. Positions on whether or not physician-assisted suicide and euthanasia are ever justifiable need not hinder us from reaching a consensus on the need to pursue this investigation. A responsible society and a responsible profession would not wish to pursue contentious policy, and a professional would not wish to act for reasons that turn out to have been beside the point and risky.

This is not the place to examine in depth the root causes of requests for assisted suicide; I am neither a psychologist nor a sociologist, and no spiritual authority either. Nonetheless, it is relevant to note that society in general, and medical culture too, have been in a death-denying era, perhaps since the scientific revolution, or at least since biomedical technology became so powerful in this century. Society sequesters and sanitizes our dying in hospitals, it pursues youth, control, and potency, and it avoids talk of normal dying. We do not have a healthy place in society for the dying and for rituals surrounding death. Cultural health and personal maturity require a balanced place for the realities of normal dying. Perhaps the physician-assisted suicide and euthanasia debate is evidence that society is beginning to climb out of its death-denying phase. Or perhaps it is evidence of imbalance and irrational denial; the call for physician-assisted suicide and euthanasia could be an attempt to be rid of normal dying. Or perhaps death denial is only part of the problem. Perhaps societal selfishness and pride of potency have caused failing members of society to be and feel unwelcome, burdensome, abandoned, undignified, and ashamed to be the frail humans that we all are.

Beginnings can be made to understand and address the root problems, whatever they are. Physicians and others can learn how to discuss and plan for and manage dying, not only with patients but with their proxies and family, thereby simultaneously helping to bring dying back into a healthy balance with living, and to build a care unit for patients who lack one. The larger society can return to emphasizing care networks for the dying, whether provided by family, community, professionals, religious groups, volunteers, or others, or by government safety nets and legislative action. Purveyors of culture—mass media, publishers, artists, religious institutions, educational organizations—can include the theme of normal dying in their programs. Indeed, in recent years, more attention has been paid to this issue in the popular culture, which is encouraging to those of us who specialize in this field.

If this reintegration of mortality into life occurs, and if care of the suffering and dying is done better, the physician-assisted suicide and euthanasia debate will likely become moot. If this prediction is wrong or if future turns of society raise the issue anew, the arguments for and against it will still be available for revisitation in this book.

NOTES
ACKNOWLEDGMENTS
INDEX

1. Helping Desperately Ill People to Die

1. *In re Quinlan,* 70 N.J. 10, 355 A. 2d 647 (1976).

2. President's Commission for the Study of Ethical Problems in Medicine and Biomedical and Behvioral Research, *Deciding to Forgo Life-Sustaining Treatment: A Report on the Ethical, Medical, and Legal Issues in Treatment Decisions* (Washington, D.C.: Government Printing Office, 1983).

3. M. Angell, "The legacy of Karen Ann Quinlan," *Trends in Health Care Law and Ethics* 8, no. 1 (1993): 17–19.

4. *Lane v. Candura,* 376 N.E. 2d 1232 (Mass. App. Ct. 1978).

5. *Cruzan v. Harmon,* 760 S.W. 2d 408 (Mo. 1988), *aff'd sub nom. Cruzan v. Director,* 497 U.S. 261 (1990).

6. *Brophy v. New England Sinai Hospital, Inc.,* 497 N.E. 2d 626 (Mass. 1986).

7. The Multi-Society Task Force on PVS, "Medical aspects of the persistent vegetative state," *New England Journal of Medicine* 330 (994): 1499–1508.

8. *Quill v. Vacco,* 80 F.3d 716 (2d Cir. 1996).

9. "It's over, Debbie," *JAMA* 259 (1988): 272.

10. T. E. Quill, "Death and dignity: a case of individualized decision making," *New England Journal of Medicine* 324 (1991): 691–694.

11. Central Committee of the Royal Dutch Medical Association, "Vision on euthanasia," *Medical Contact* 39 (1984): 990–998.

12. P. J. van der Maas, J. J. M. van Delden, L. Pijnenborg, and C. W. W. Looman, "Euthanasia and other medical decisions concerning the end of life," *Lancet* 338 (1991): 669–674.

13. G. J. Annas, "Death by prescription: the Oregon initative," *New England Journal of Medicine* 331 (1994): 1240–1243.

14. M. A. Lee, H. D. Nelson, R. P. Tilden, L. Ganzini, T. A. Schmidt, and S. W. Tolle, "Legalizing assisted suicide: views of physicians in Orgeon," *New England Journal of Medicine* 334 (1996): 310–315. C. J. Ryan and M.

Kaye, "Euthanasia in Australia: the Northern Territory Rights of the Terminally Ill Act," *New England Journal of Medicine* 334 (1996): 326–328.

15. R. A. Knox, "Poll: Americans favor mercy killing," *Boston Globe,* November 3, 1991, p. 1.

16. Ibid.

17. *Compassion in Dying v. Washington,* 79 F.3d 790 (9th Cir. 1996). *Quill v. Vacco,* 80 F.3d 716 (2d Cir. 1996).

18. "Courts cross the Styx," *Wall Street Journal,* April 8, 1996, p. A18.

19. A. Solomon, "A death of one's own," *New Yorker,* May 22, 1995, pp. 54–69.

2. Is a Physician Ever Obligated to Help a Patient Die?

1. The Boston Working Group's model statue provides: "No individual who is conscientiously opposed to providing a patient with medical means of suicide may be required to do so or to assist a responsible physician in doing so." Charles H. Baron, Clyde Bergstresser, Dan W. Brock, Garrick F. Cole, Nancy S. Dorfman, Judith A. Johnson, Lowell E. Schnipper, James Vorenberg, Sidney H. Wanzer, "A model state act to authorize and regulate physician-assisted suicide," *Harvard Journal on Legislation* 33, no. 1 (1996): 1–34.

2. Oregon Death with Dignity Act, Section 4.04. The Act does require, however, that if a health care provider is unable or unwilling to carry out a patient's request under the Act, and the patient transfers his or her care to a new health care provider, that the prior health care provider shall transfer, upon request, a copy of the patient's relevant medical records to the new health care provider (Section 4.04). To be sure, a health care provider would be legally obligated to transfer the patient's records at the patient's request in any case.

3. Many of these arguments can also be made for and against physician performance of active euthanasia, though since that is no longer the focus of most legislative proposals in the U.S., I won't discuss it further here.

4. For example, Dan Brock uses the term mercy in his *Life and Death* (Cambridge: Cambridge University Press, 1993). I've discussed at some length the relationship between the principles of nonmaleficence and beneficence, now canonical in the bioethics literature, and what I like to call the principle of mercy. The former are comparatively narrow principles, requiring not doing harm and doing good, respectively. The latter, the principle of mercy, is a broader principle that amalgamates both in

the context of suffering. Thus the principle of mercy requires not just refraining from causing pain or suffering, which the principle of non-maleficence would require, but also acting to relieve pain or suffering, as the principle of beneficence would require.

To call this principle the principle of mercy, then, is to use shorthand for much more cumbersome terms, but it is also to invoke traditional conceptions of the physician's role in the matter of pain and suffering. See my account "Euthanasia: the fundamental issues," originally appearing in *Health Care Ethics,* ed. D. Van DeVeer and T. Regan (Philadelphia: Temple University Press, 1987), reprinted in Margaret P. Battin, *The Least Worst Death* (New York: Oxford University Press, 1994).

5. The SUPPORT Principal Investigators, "A controlled trial to improve care for seriously ill hospitalized patients," *JAMA* 274, no. 20 (1995): 1591–1598. Objections to the methodology of this study include the fact that these reports were taken from family members or other survivors, not the patients themselves.

6. When the practices of euthanasia and physician-assisted suicide first came to light in the Netherlands, it became clear that some physicians did not know the appropriate drugs or dosages to use; some attempted to use wholly inappropriate drugs, such as insulin or morphine. In response, anesthesiologist Dr. Pieter Admiraal published the appropriate information in a booklet sent to all Dutch physicians; this information has been revised and updated repeatedly. See Gerrit K. Kimsma, "Euthanasia and euthanising drugs in the Netherlands," *Journal of Pharmaceutical Care in Pain and Symptom Control* 3, nos. 3/4 (1995) and 4, nos. 1/2 (1996), also published as *Drug Use in Assisted Suicide and Euthanasia,* ed. Margaret P. Battin and Arthur G. Lipman (Binghamton, NY: Haworth Press, 1996).

For information on methods of physician assistance in suicide used by Compassion in Dying, Seattle, see Thomas A. Preston and Ralph Mero, "Observations concerning terminally ill patients who choose suicide," in the same volume. Derek Humphrey's *Final Exit: The Practicalities of Self-Deliverance and Assisted Suicide for the Dying* (Eugene, OR: The Hemlock Society, 1991), has also provided drug information to the general public.

7. Some authors argue for the legitimacy of directly caused death on grounds of mercy in the absence of patient request when the patient is no longer competent and cannot make a request or express any wishes but is suffering severely. No contemporary writer with whom I'm familiar argues for directly caused death where that is contrary to the patient's wishes.

8. The term "patient-directed" is from Totie Oberman, personal communication, American Association of Suicidology, May 1995. The term "self-enacted" is from Stephen Jamison.

9. Actual cost savings from physician-assisted suicide may be far smaller than generally believed. See E. J. Emanuel and M. P. Battin, "The economics of euthanasia: what are the potential cost savings from legalizing physician-assisted suicide?" (*New England Journal of Medicine*, forthcoming), where we estimate that the cost savings from patients who would choose physician-assisted suicide or euthanasia, were these legal, would be less than 1 percent of the total U.S. healthcare budget. For a more detailed discussion of safeguards against abuse, see Battin, "Voluntary euthanasia and the risks of abuse," in Battin, *Least Worst Death*, pp. 163–181.

10. Ludwig Edelstein, "The Hippocratic Oath: text, translation, and interpretation," in *Supplements to the Bulletin of the History of Medicine* no. 1 (1943), and in *Ancient Medicine: Selected Papers of Ludwig Edelstein,* ed. Owsei Temkin and C. Lillian Temkin (Baltimore: Johns Hopkins University Press, 1967). Also see Danielle Gourevitch, "Suicide among the sick in classical antiquity," *Bulletin of the History of Medicine* 43 (1969): 501–518; Darrel W. Amundsen, "The physician's obligation to prolong life: a medical duty without classical roots," *Hastings Center Report* 8, no. 4 (1978): 23–30; Margaret Pabst Battin, *Ethical Issues in Suicide* (Englewood Cliffs, NJ: Prentice-Hall, 1995); and Ezekiel Emanuel, "The history of euthanasia debates in the United States and Britain," *Annals of Internal Medicine* 121, no. 10 (1994): 793–802.

11. Paul J. van der Maas, Johannes J. M. van Delden, Loes Pijnenborg, and Caspar W. N. Looman, "Euthanasia and other medical decisions concerning the end of life," *The Lancet* 338 (1991): 609–674. The first Remmelink report is available in full in English as a special issue of *Health Policy* 22, nos. 1 and 2 (1992); the follow-up report is available in condensed form in Paul J. van der Maas et al., "Euthanasia, physician-assisted suicide, and other medical practices involving the end of life in the Netherlands, 1990–1995," *New England Journal of Medicine* 335 (1996): 1699–1705.

12. See Loes Pijnenborg, Paul J. van der Maas, Johannes J. M. van Delden, and Caspar W. N. Looman, "Life-terminating acts without explicit request of patient," *The Lancet* 341 (1993): 1196–1199. This more detailed examination of the approximately 1,000 cases of euthanasia without explicit request uncovered in the original Remmelink Commission report shows that in about 59 percent of them the physician did have some information about the patient's wish, though short of a full, current request; in nearly all of the other 41 percent of cases, the patient had

become no longer capable of discussion, was suffering unbearably, there was no chance of improvement, and palliative possibilities were exhausted. While the Dutch do not seek to defend every case that occurs, it is clearly not the case, as outside observers often insinuate, that in the Netherlands patients are routinely killed against their will.

13. Kevin W. Wildes, S.J., "Conscience, referral, and physician assisted suicide," in *Journal of Medicine and Philosophy* 18, no. 3 (1993): 323–328, a special issue entitled "Legal Euthanasia: Ethical Issues in an Era of Legalized Aid in Dying," ed. Margaret P. Battin and Thomas J. Bole, III.

14. Thomas A. Preston and Ralph Mero, "Observations concerning terminally ill patients who choose suicide," *Journal of Pharmaceutical Care in Pain and Symptom Control* 3 (1995): 3–4; also in *Drug Use in Assisted Suicide and Euthanasia,* ed. Battin and Lipman.

15. See Margaret Battin, "The eclipse of altruism: the moral costs of deciding for others," in Battin, *The Least Worst Death,* pp. 40–57.

3. Harming, Healing, and Euthanasia

1. I. Kant, *Foundations of the Metaphysics of Morals,* trans. Lewis White Beck (Indianapolis, IN: Macmillan Publishing, 1986), p. 47.

2. The point that patients in hospitals today rarely die when nothing to prolong their life can be done is evident to all who have worked as nurses, physicians, or ethics consultants in a hospital. See E. H. Loewy, "Futility and its wider implications," *Archives of Internal Medicine* 153 (1993): 429–431, and "Futility and the goals of medicine," *European Philosophy of Medicine and Health Care* 1, no. 2 (1993): 15–27.

3. P. Carrick, *Medical Ethics in Antiquity* (Boston: D. Reidel, 1985).

4. In the first century, early Christianity forbade all killing, whether as capital punishment, in war, or even in self-defense. This posed a great problem for the Roman empire: on the one hand, they could not ignore an ever-growing segment of their population; on the other hand, they could not give citizenship to persons who refused to serve in the army or to condone capital punishment. The first church–state accord resulted: the Church permitted killing those who were fighting an unjust war and those who had broken a just law. The definition of what was "just" and what "unjust" was left up to the State. Curiously enough, killing in self-defense remained proscribed until about the time of St. Augustine. An excellent description of this "doctrine of innocence" can be found in J. Rachels, *The End of Life* (New York: Oxford University Press, 1986), pp. 11–13.

5. See Sir Thomas More, *Utopia,* trans. Robert M. Adams (New York: Norton, 1975). One of the best and earliest discussions of this book can be

found in K. Kautsky, *Thomas More and His Utopia,* trans. Russel Ames (New York: Russell & Russell, 1959). Another excellent source is G. M. Logan, *The Meaning of More's Utopia* (Princeton: Princeton University Press, 1983).

6. Euthanasia as conceived by the Nazis was neither a "good death" nor a death brought about so as to benefit (or to prevent harm to) the person killed. While this program was carried on in semisecrecy, the propaganda made for abandoning persons termed "nutzlose Fresser" ("useless eaters") was clearly visible to all. The extermination of the Jews was not termed "euthanasia": the euphemism "euthanasia" was too evidently a euphemism to allow its use even at that late date. It is frightening to realize that the tentative lists of persons believed to be "genetically unfit" and proper subjects at least for sterilization was later used in the Nazi "euthanasia" program (that is, "the feeble-minded, the pauper class, the criminal class, the epileptics, the insane, the constitutionally weak, or the asthenic class, those predisposed to specific diseases or the diathetic class, the deformed, those having defective sense organs, as the blind and the deaf"). This list was first suggested by an American, Bleeker Van Wagenen, at a conference in at the University of London in 1912 (Preliminary report of the Committee of the Eugenics Section of the American Breeders' Association to study and to report on the best practical means for cutting off the defective germ plasm in the human population. In *Problems in Eugenics* (Adelphi, WC: The Eugenics Education Society, 1912). The most definitive work on this subject is E. Klee, *Euthanasie im NS-Staat* (Frankfurt a/M). As background, the following also can be recommended: L. Alexander, "Medical science under dictatorship," *New England Journal of Medicine* 241 (1949): 39–47; R. J. Lifton, *The Nazi Doctors* (New York: Basic Books, 1986), and K. Moe, "Should the Nazi research data be cited?" *Hastings Center Report* 14, no. 6 (1984): 5–7.

7. E. H. Loewy, "Drunks, livers and values: should social value judgments enter into transplant decisions?" *Journal of Clinical Gastroentrololgy* 9 (1987): 436–441.

8. L. R. Churchill, "Bioethical reductionism and our sense of the human," *Man & Medicine* 5 (1980): 229–247.

9. As Thomasina Kushner has pointed out in "Having a life versus being alive," *Journal of Medical Ethics* 1 (1984): 5–8, we must distinguish between the two senses in which the same word "life" is used.

10. Rachels, *The End of Life.*

11. The general views against physician participation are well expressed in W. J. Curran and W. Cascells, "The ethics of medical partici-

pation in capital punishment by intravenous drug injection," *New England Journal of Medicine* 302, no. 4 (1980): 226–230, and in W. Cascells and W. J. Curran. "Doctors, the death penalty and lethal injection," *New England Journal of Medicine* 307 (1982): 1532–1533.

12. E. H. Loewy, "Healing or killing: health-professionals and execution," in E. H. Loewy, *Ethical Dilemmas in Modern Medicine: A Physician's Viewpoint* (Lewiston, NY: Edwin Mellen Press, 1986).

13. Of course, one can and with some justification argue that the "free consent" of persons whose livelihood depends on such a risky activity is rather less than free. In a capitalist society and given the economic conditions of the times, many will doubt the actual freedom of workers in such industries.

14. W. Gaylin, L. R. Kass, E. D. Pellegrino, and M. Siegler, "Doctors must not kill," *JAMA* 259 (1988): 2139–2140.

15. D. W. Amundsen, "The physician's obligation to prolong life: a medical duty without classical roots," *Hastings Center Report* 8, no. 4 (1978): 23–31.

16. E. D. Pellegrino, "Toward a reconstruction of medical morality: the primacy of the act of profession and the fact of illness," *Journal of Medicine & Philosophy* 4, no. 1 (1979): 32–56.

17. Churchill, "Bioethical reductionism and our sense of the human."

18. H. Krall, *Shielding the Flame: An Intimate Conversation with Dr. Marek Edelman, the Last Surviving Leader of the Warsaw Ghetto Uprising*, trans. Joanna Stasinska and Lawrence Wechsler (New York: Henry Holt, 1986).

4. The False Promise of Beneficent Killing

1. D. Dworkin, T. Nagel, R. Nozick, J. Rawls, T. Scanlon, and J. J. Thomson, "Assisted suicide: the philosopher's brief," *New York Review,* May 27, 1997, pp. 41–47. See, for example, R. Brandt, "A moral principle about killing," in *Beneficent Euthanasia,* ed. M. Kohl (Buffalo, NY: Prometheus Books, 1975); M. Kohl, *The Morality of Killing* (New York: Humanities Press, 1974); J. Wrable, "Euthanasia would be a humane way to end suffering," *American Medical News,* January 20, 1983, pp. 31–33; N. Abrams, "Active and passive euthanasia," *Philosophy* 53, no. 204 (1980): 257–263. D. Maguire, "Death and the moral domain," *St. Luke's Journal of Theology* 20, no. 3 (1977): 197–216; J. Fletcher, *Morals and Medicine* (New Jersey: Princeton University Press, 1979). *Quill v. Vacco,* 80 F.3d 716 (2nd Cir. 1996), and *Compassion in Dying v. State of Washington,* F.3d, 1996 WL 294445 (9th Cir. 1996).

2. J. Rachels, "Active and passive euthanasia," *New England Journal of Medicine* 292 (1975): 78–80; J. Rachels, *The End of Life: Euthanasia and Morality* (New York: Oxford University Press, 1986); and T. L. Beauchamp, "Introduction" to *Intending Death,* ed. T. L. Beauchamp (New Jersey: Prentice Hall, 1996), pp. 1–22.

3. Beauchamp, "Introduction."

4. Rachels, *End of Life,* pp. 6, 64–67, 178–180.

5. For a detailed and telling discussion of the metaethical justification for the distinction between killing and letting die, see D. P. Sulmasy, "Killing and allowing to die," diss. (Washington, DC: Georgetown University, 1995).

6. F. G. Miller and H. Brody, "Professional integrity and physician-assisted death," *Hastings Center Report* 25 (1995): 5.

7. K. Binding and A. Hoche, "Permitting the destruction of unworthy life," trans. W. E. Uright, P. G. Derr, and R. Salomn, *Issues in Law and Medicine* 8 (1992): 231–265.

8. E. Cassell, "The nature of suffering and the goals of medicine," *New England Journal of Medicine* 306, no. 11 (1982): 639–645.

9. K. M. Foley, "The treatment of cancer pain," *New England Journal of Medicine* 313 (1985): 84–95; New York State Task Force on Life and the Law, *When Death Is Sought: Assisted Suicide and Euthanasia in Medical Contexts* (New York, 1994); S. Saxon, *Pain Management Techniques for Older Adults* (Springfield, IL: Charles E. Thomas, 1991); United States Department of Health and Human Services, Agency for Health Care Policy and Research, *Clinical Practice Guidelines: Acute Pain Management: Operative or Medical Procedures and Trauma* (Washington, D.C.: U.S. Government Printing Office, 1992). See also citations to a variety of recent pharmacological, surgical, and anesthesiological advances in pain management in R. D. Truog and C. B. Berde, "Pain, euthanasia, and anesthesiologists," *Anesthesiology* 78, no. 2 (1993): 353–360.

10. Cassell, "The nature of suffering."

11. E. D. Pellegrino, "The clinical ethics of pain management in the terminally ill," *Hospital Formulary,* November 1982, pp. 1493–1496. F. Brescia, "Killing the known dying: notes of a death watched," *Journal of Pain Management* 6, no. 5 (1991): 336–339; J. Lynn, "The health care professional's role when active euthanasia is sought," *Journal of Palliative Care* 4 (1988): 100–102; C. Saunders, ed., *Hospice and Palliative Care: An Interdisciplinary Approach* (London: Edward Arnold, 1990); D. Cundiff, *Euthanasia Is Not the Answer: A Hospice Physician's View of the Death with Dignity Debate* (Totowa: Humana Press, 1992).

12. N. I. Cherny, N. Coyle, and K. M. Foley, "The treatment of suffering

when patients request elective death," *Journal of Palliative Care* 10, no. 2 (1994): 71–79.

13. Saunders, *Hospice and Palliative Care*. N. H. Cassem, "Treatment decisions in irreversible illness," *Massachusetts General Hospital Handbook of General Psychiatry*, ed. N. H. Cassem (St. Louis: Mosby Year Book, 1991), pp. 618–639.

14. 101st United States Congress, 1st Session, *Senate Bill 1766: Patient Self-Determination Act of 1989* (Washington, DC: United States Congress, 1989).

15. The SUPPORT Principal Investigators, "A controlled trial to improve care of seriously ill, hospitalized patients: the Study to Understand Prognosis and Preferences to Outcomes and Risks of Treatment (SUPPORT)," *Journal of the American Medical Association* 274, no. 20 (1995): 1591–1598.

16. L. A. O'Brien, J. A. Grisso, G. Maislin, K. LaPann, et al., "Nursing home residents' preferences for life-sustaining treatments," *JAMA* 274, no. 22 (1995): 1775–1779.

17. B. Lo, "Improving health care near the end of life: why is it so hard?" *JAMA* 274, no. 20 (1995): 1634–1636.

18. *Compassion in Dying v. Washington*, 850 F. Supp. 1454 (W.D. Wash. 1994). *Quill v. Koppel*, 870 F Supp. 78 (S.D. N.Y. 1994). *Ninth Circuit Court of Appeals* 49 F.3d, 586 (9th Cir. 1995). *People v. Kevorkian*, 527 N.W. 2d 714 (Mich 1994) Cert. Denied 115 S. Ct. 1795 (1995). See also D. Orentlicher, "Physician-assisted dying: conflict with fundamental principles of American law," in *Medicine Unbound: The Human Body and the Limitations of Medical Interventions*, ed. R. Blank and A. Donnicksen (New York: Columbia University Press, 1994), pp. 256–228. *Furman v. Georgia*, 408, U.S.238, 286 (1972).

19. *Compassion in Dying v. Washington*, 1995 WL 94679 at 4. *Cruzan v. Director*, Missouri Dept. of Health, 497 U.S. 261 (1990). *Planned Parenthood v. Casey*, 1125 Ct. See, for example, *Matter of Quinlan*, 70 N.J. 10, 355 A.2d 647, 665 (1976); *Superintendent of Belchertown vs. Saikewicz*, 370 N.E.2d 417, 426 n.11 (Mass. 1977); *Matter of Storar*, 52 N.Y.2d 363, 420 N.E.2d 64, 71 n.6 (N.Y. App. 1981); *Matter of Conroy*, 98 N.J. 321, 486 A.2d 1209, 1224 (1985); *Bouvia v. Superior Court*, 225 Cal. Rptr. 297, 306 (1986).

20. *Compassion in Dying v. State of Washington* F.3d, 1996 WL 294445 (9th Cir. 1996). *Quill v. Vacco*, 80 F.3d 716 (2nd Cir. 1996). Verbatim, Oral Arguments in *Washington v. Glucksberg*, Oral Arguments in *Vacco v. Quill*, in *Issues in Law and Medicine* 12 (1997): 393–439. Michael M. Uhlman, "The legal logic of euthanasia," *First Things*, no. 64 (June/July 1996): 39–43.

21. See the conveniently arranged table of court cases in D. C. Thomasma and G. C. Graber, *Euthanasia: Toward an Ethical Social Policy* (New York: Continuum, 1990), pp. 296–298. See also E. D. Pellegrino, "Patient and physician autonomy: conflicting rights and obligations in the physician-patient relationship," *Journal of Contemporary Health, Law, and Policy* 10 (1994): 47–68.

22. Y. Kamisar, "Some non-religious views against proposed 'mercy killing' legislation," *Minnesota Law Review* 42 (1958): 969, 990.

23. S. H. Miles, "Physicians and their patients' suicides," *JAMA* 271, no. 22 (1994): 1786–1788.

24. C. Caine, ed., "Rational suicide and the right to die: reality and myth," *New England Journal of Medicine* 325 (1991): 1101–1102. New York State Task Force on Life and Law, *When Death Is Sought*, p. 126.

25. R. F. Uhlmann, R. A. Pearlman, K. C. Kain, "Physician's and spouse's predictions of elderly patient's resuscitation preferences," *Journal of Gerontology* 43 (1988): M115–M121. Miles, "Physicians and their patients' suicides," p. 1787. M. G. Greene, R. D. Adelman, R. Charon, E. Friedman, "Concordance between physicians and their older and younger patients in the primary care encounter," *Gerontologist* 29 (1989): 808–813. J. Modestin, "Counter-transference reactions contributing to completed suicide," *British Journal of Psychiatry* 60 (1987): 379–385.

26. See H. Hendin, "Seeking death and dignity," *Hastings Center Report* 25, no. 3 (1995): 19–23, for detailed descriptions and interpretations of the deaths of Cees Van Wendel documented on Dutch television and of "Louise" as described in *The New York Times Magazine,* November 14, 1993.

27. G. I. Benrubi, "Euthanasia: the need for procedural safeguards," *New England Journal of Medicine* 326, no. 3 (1992): 197–198.

28. D. Shewmm, "Active voluntary euthanasia: a needless Pandora's box," *Issues in Law and Medicine,* Winter 1987, pp. 219, 220, 231.

29. Cherny et al., "Treatment of suffering," pp. 76–77. S. C. Klagsbrun, "Patient, family, and staff suffering," *Journal of Palliative Care* 10, no. 2 (1994): 14–17.

30. Stephen L. Darwall, "Two kinds of respect," in *Ethics and Personality: Essays in Moral Psychology,* ed. John Deigh (Chicago: University of Chicago Press, 1992), pp. 65–78.

31. Anatole Broyard, *Intoxicated by My Illness and Other Writings on Life and Death,* comp. and ed. Alexandra Broyard (New York: Clarkson Potter, 1992), pp. 33–58.

32. Hippocrates, "The Oath," *Hippocrates I,* trans. W. H. L. Jones, Loeb Classical Library 147 (Cambridge: Harvard University Press, 1972),

pp. 289–302. J. Kevorkian, *Prescription Medicine: The Goodness of Planned Death* (Buffalo, NY: Prometheus Books, 1991). T. Quill, *Death and Dignity: Making Choices and Taking Charge* (New York: Norton, 1993). S. H. Wanzer, D. D. Federman, S. T. Edelstein, et al., "The physician's responsibility toward hopelessly ill patients: a second look," *New England Journal of Medicine* 320 (1989): 884–889.

33. Miller and Brody, "Professional integrity and physician-assisted death." S. H. Miles, "Physician assisted suicide and the profession's gyrocompass," *Hastings Center Report* 25, no. 5 (1995): 8–17.

34. Benrubi, "Euthanasia."

35. R. M. Veatch, "The Hippocratic ethic is dead," *New Physician*, September 1984, pp. 41–42, 48.

36. E. D. Pellegrino, "The metamorphosis of medical ethics: a 30-year retrospective," *JAMA* 269, no. 9 (1993): 1158–1163. R. D. Orr, N. Pang, E. D. Pellegrino, and M. Siegler, "The use of the Hippocratic Oath: a review of 20th century practice and a content analysis of oaths administered in medical schools in the U.S. and Canada in 1993," in press. E. D. Pellegrino, "Dismembering the Hippocratic Oath: the dangers of moral dissection," *Boston University School of Medicine Alumni Report: Medical Ethics & Managed Care,* Fall 1995, pp. 11–17.

37. H. T. Engelhardt Jr., "Death by free choice: modern variations on an antique theme," in *Suicide and Euthanasia* (vol. 35 of the *Philosophy and Medicine* Series), ed. B. Brody (Dordrecht: Kluwer Academic Publishers, 1989), pp. 251–279.

38. See the responses of the disabled cited in N. Hentoff, "Not dead yet," *Washington Post,* June 8, 1996, p. A15.

39. Netherlands, Remmelink Commission, *Medical Practice with Regard to Euthanasia and Related Medical Decisions in the Netherlands: Results of an Inquiry and the Government's View* (Netherlands: Ministry of Welfare, Health, and Cultural Affairs, 1991).

40. Herbert Hendin, *Seduced by Death: Doctors, Patients, and the Dutch Cure* (New York: Norton, 1997).

41. Royal Dutch Medical Association, *Euthanasia in the Netherlands,* 4th ed. (Utrecht: Royal Dutch Medical Association, 1995). A. D. Ogilvie, S. G. Potts, "Assisted suicide for depression: the slippery slope in action," *British Medical Journal* 309, no. 6953 (1994): 492–493. M. D. Hendin, G. Klerman, "Physician assisted suicide: the dangers of legislation," *American Journal of Psychiatry* 150 (1993): 143–145.

42. T. Kushner, "Interview with Heleen Dupius," *Cambridge Quarterly* 2, no. 3 (1993): 275–280.

43. M. T. Muller, G. Van Der Wal, J. T. M. Eijk, M. W. Ribbe, "Voluntary

active euthanasia and physician assisted suicide: are the requirements for prudent practice properly met?" *Journal of the American Geriatric Society* 42, no. 6 (1994): 624–629.

44. B. Cardozo, *Nature of the Judicial Process* (New Haven: Yale University Press, 1949), p. 51. R. Fenigsen, "A case against Dutch euthanasia," *Hastings Center Report* 19, no. 1 (1989): 522–530. *Oregon Death with Dignity Act,* Oregon Ballot Measure 16, passed November 8, 1994. Associated Press, Salem, OR, "U.S. judge bars assisted suicide law in Oregon," *Washington Post,* December 28, 1994, p. A7.

45. M. O'Keefe, "Dutch researcher warns of lingering deaths," *The Oregonian,* December 4, 1994, p. A1. Thomasine Kushner, "Derek Humphrey discusses death with dignity with Thomasine Kushner," *Cambridge Quarterly of Health Care Ethics* 2 (1993): 57, 59. *Michigan v. Kevorkian,* no. 90–39063-A2 (Mich. Cir. Ct., Feb. 5, 1991), reprinted in *Law and Medicine* 107, no. 111 (1991). Royal Dutch Medical Association, *Euthanasia.*

46. L. R. Kass, "Neither for love nor money: why doctors must not kill," *Public Interest,* Winter 1989, pp. 25–46.

47. D. Grossman, *On Killing: The Psychological Cost of Learning to Kill* (Boston: Little, Brown, and Company, 1995).

48. R. F. Diekstra, "Assisted suicide and euthanasia: experience from the Netherlands," *Annals of Medicine* 25 (1993): 5–9.

5. Facing Assisted Suicide and Euthanasia in Children and Adolescents

Thanks to Linda Emanuel, Christine Mitchell, and Robert Truog for originally inviting me to present Grand Rounds on this topic at Children's Hospital in Boston; to Dr. Emanuel as well as to Arthur Caplan, Ellen Clayton, Barry Feld, and Joel Frader for helpful comments on later drafts; to Bridget McKeon and Laurie Nesseth of the University of Minnesota Law School and Thomas G. Horejsi of the University of Minnesota Medical School for research assistance; and to the University of Minnesota Law School and Center for Bioethics for research support.

1. For background, see, e.g., Ezekiel J. Emanuel, "Euthanasia: historical, ethical, and empiric perspectives," *Archives of Internal Medicine* 154 (1994): 1890, 1890, 1892. Note that throughout this chapter I discuss "legitimating" rather than "legalizing" assisted suicide and euthanasia. Outright legalization is only one form of legitimation, as the Dutch have illustrated by opting for legitimation but not full legalization (see note 8 below).

2. Both Supreme Court cases on physician-assisted suicide concerned the constitutionality of state prohibitions as applied only to competent persons. See Compassion in Dying v. Washington, 79 F.3d 790, 793 (9th Cir.) *(en banc)* ("competent adults"), *rev'd sub nom.* Washington v. Glucksberg, 117 S. Ct. 2258 (1997) (same); Quill v. Vacco, 80 F.3d 716, 718 (2d Cir.) ("competent patients"), *rev'd,* 117 S. Ct. 2293 (1997) (same). Note that although the appellate court in *Quill* found the New York statute unconstitutional as applied to "competent, terminally-ill person[s]" (80 F.3d at 731), plaintiffs had sued for a declaration of unconstitutionality "'as applied to . . . competent, terminally ill adults'" (at 719; emphasis added, quoting plaintiffs' complaint). And indeed all plaintiffs in the case who were patients were adults. See Quill v. Vacco, 870 F. Supp. 78, 79 (S.D.N.Y. 1994).

Oregon's statute permitting physician-assisted suicide requires that the patient be an adult, defined as at least 18 years old. Or. Rev. Stat. Ann. § 127.800(1) (Michie Supp. 1996). Bills proposed in other states have imposed comparable requirements. See, e.g., 1995 CA A.B. 1080; 1995 CT S.B. 334, 361; 1995 MA H.B. 3173; 1995 MI H.B. 5015; 1995 N.H. H.B. 339. Other proposals have also required that the patient be at least 18. See, e.g., Charles H. Baron et al., "A model state act to authorize and regulate physician-assisted suicide," *Harvard Journal on Legislation* 33 (1996): 1, 26; Jody B. Gabel, "Release from terminal suffering? The impact of AIDS on medically assisted suicide legislation," *Florida State University Law Review* 22 (1994): 369, 434. An exception is "Model Aid-in-Dying Act," *Iowa Law Review* 75 (1989): 125. Outside the United States, the Northern Territory of Australia's Rights of the Terminally Ill Act 1995, No. 12 of 1995, required that the patient be at least 18 years old before the physician could perform euthanasia or assist suicide. That Act, however, has been struck down by Parliament. See "Euthanasia law struck down in Australia," *New York Times,* March 27, 1997. The Dutch rules are discussed below in text.

3. On abortion and infanticide, see, e.g., Michael Tooley, *Abortion and Infanticide* (1983); John Fletcher, "Abortion, euthanasia, and the care of defective newborns," *New England Journal of Medicine* 292 (1975): 75.

On neonatal termination of treatment and active euthanasia, see, e.g., *Euthanasia and the Newborn: Conflicts Regarding Saving Lives,* ed. Richard C. McMillan et al. (1987); Earl E. Shelp, *Born to Die? Deciding the Fate of Critically Ill Newborns* (1986); Jeff Lyon, *Playing God in the Nursery* (1985); Robert F. Weir, *Selective Nontreatment of Handicapped Newborns: Moral Dilemmas in Neonatal Medicine* (1984); H. Tristram

Engelhardt Jr., "Ethical issues in aiding the death of young children," in *Beneficent Euthanasia,* ed. Marvin Kohl (1975), 180. This literature is confused by inconsistent use of "euthanasia"; it is sometimes limited to active euthanasia but at other times includes termination of life-sustaining treatment.

In addition, there is a literature on the phenomenon of infanticide, apart from any advocacy for physician-assisted suicide and euthanasia. See, e.g., *Infanticide: Comparative and Evolutionary Perspectives,* ed. Glenn Hausfater and Sarah Blaffer Hrdy (1984); Maria W. Piers, *Infanticide* (1978). But terminological confusion surrounds the term "infanticide" too; Shelp, *Born to Die?* p. 155, complains, "Killing by omission is not distinguished from killing by commission."

More rarely do scholars directly debate pediatric euthanasia. See, e.g, John M. Freeman, "If euthanasia were licit, could lives be saved?" in *Euthanasia and the Newborn: Conflicts Regarding Saving Lives,* ed. Richard C. McMillan et al. (1987), 153; Helga Kuhse and Peter Singer, *Should the Baby Live? The Problem of Handicapped Infants* (1985); Joseph Fletcher, *Humanhood: Essays in Biomedical Ethics* (1979), 140–158; *Infanticide and the Value of Life,* ed. Marvin Kohl (1978). Physician-assisted suicide in the pediatric population is even more rarely discussed. Cf. "Model Aid-in-Dying Act," pp. 163–173 (providing for aid-in-dying for terminally ill patients under age 6 and for minors 6 years or older, but not for nonterminal children who are technologically dependent or have an "intolerable dependence"); Harry M. Hoberman, "The impact of sanctioned assisted suicide on adolescents," *Issues in Law & Medicine* 4 (1988): 191 (discussing "assisted suicide").

4. By "assisted suicide" I will consistently mean physician-assisted suicide and will not discuss the problems involved in permitting assistance by family members or other nonphysicians.

5. As noted above, an exception is "Model Aid-in-Dying Act."

6. "Interview with Heleen M. Dupuis, actively ending the life of a severely handicapped newborn: a Dutch ethicist's perspective," *Cambridge Quarterly of Healthcare Ethics* 2 (1993): 275, 279; cf. Robert Burt, "Authorizing death for anomalous newborns," in *Genetics and the Law,* ed. Aubrey Milusky and George J. Annas (1976), 435, 439 ("A generation ago proposals for authorizing voluntary euthanasia for terminally ill adults were met, in part, by assertions that such practices would lead to euthanasia for defective newborns. Proponents of euthanasia rejected this argument, in effect, as implausible and wholly fanciful." (footnote omitted)).

7. Within the United States, see, e.g., "Death at U.C. Med Center," *San Francisco Chronicle,* March 30, 1995 (apparent euthanasia of a 9-year-old

girl who failed to die after termination of life-sustaining treatment); "Doctor faces murder count in premature baby's death," *Orlando Sentinel,* November 13, 1993 (euthanasia of 5 1/2-week-old boy born 13 weeks premature and suffering from kidney failure). Outside the United States, see, e.g., Ben Fenton, "Doctor admits 'mercy killing' of two babies," *Daily Telegraph,* February 15, 1995 (England); Helga Kuhse, "A modern myth: that letting die is not the intentional causation of death: some reflections on the trial and acquittal of Dr. Arthur Leonard," *Journal of Applied Philosophy* 1 (1984): 21, 22 (England). The Dutch situation is discussed below.

There are, in addition, cases in which parents kill their children, claiming it to be a mercy killing. See, e.g., "Mercy killing is murder; Latimer sentence should stand," *Gazette* (Montreal), July 21, 1995 (father convicted in Canada of murdering his 12-year-old daughter with cerebral palsy); Maya Bell, "For the love of Joy: a father's torment over his severely injured daughter drove him over the edge.; Charles Griffin says he killed Joy to end her pain. But is society ready to absolve him?" *Orlando Sentinel Tribune,* August 25, 1991 (father shoots his 3-year-old daughter, who was in a chronic vegetative state; Griffith is convicted, unlike Rudy Linares, who disconnected his 15-month-old son from a respirator, and Michael Hensley, who suffocated his 11-year-old daughter, who had a neuromuscular disorder). See also "Man acquitted in death of infant," *New York Times,* February 4, 1995 (dermatologist acquitted of manslaughter for disconnecting his newborn son from a ventilator).

8. Euthanasia and physician-assisted suicide remain technically illegal in the Netherlands. However, in a series of decisions beginning in 1973 the courts have carved out a domain in which both practices are tolerated. Dutch law has thus demanded voluntary and informed request by the patient, consultation with a second physician, and reporting of euthanasia and assisted suicide by the physician performing the act, among other requirements. See, e.g., Julia Belian, Comment, "Deference to doctors in Dutch euthanasia law," *Emory International Law Review,* 10 (1996): 255, 255–256; John Griffiths, "The regulation of euthanasia and related medical procedures that shorten life in the Netherlands," *Medical Law International* 1 (1994): 137, 138, 143–144; Margaret P. Battin, "Euthanasia: the way we do it, the way they do it," *Journal of Pain and Symptom Management* 6 (1991): 298, 299–300. In 1993 the Dutch parliament enacted legislation on physician reporting but did not legalize the practices outright. See, e.g., John Griffiths, "Recent developments in the Netherlands concerning euthanasia and other medical behavior that shortens life," *Medical Law International* 1 (1995): 347, 347.

9. See, e.g., Tony Sheldon, "Dutch court convicts doctor of murder," *British Medical Journal* 310 (1995): 1028 (gynecologist euthanizes 3-day-old girl with multiple disabilities); "Dutch bring a test case in euthanasia," *New York Times,* December 23, 1994 (another Dutch physician who killed a "gravely ill" newborn); Leonard Doyle, "Dutch doctors pushed on to 'slippery slope' over euthanasia," *Independent,* February 17, 1993 (euthanasia of a newborn with spina bifida and "three other congenital diseases," and noting figure of at least 10 cases per year of active euthanasia of newborns in the Netherlands); Cor Spreeuwenberg, "The story of Laurens," *Cambridge Quarterly of Healthcare Ethics* 2 (1993): 261 (euthanasia of an infant with no cortical activity); Carlos F. Gomez, *Regulating Death: Euthanasia and the Case of the Netherlands* (1991), 83–84 (newborn with Down syndrome and duodenal atresia euthanized). Empirical studies have revealed cases as well. See, e.g., Agnes van der Heide et al, "Medical end-of-life decisions made for neonates and infants in the Netherlands," *Lancet* 350 (1997): 251; P. J. van der Maas et al., "Euthanasia and other medical decisions concerning the end of life," *Health Policy* 22, nos. 1, 2 (1992): 143–145. But see Richard de Leeuw et al., "Foregoing intensive care treatment in newborn infants with extremely poor prognoses: a study of four neonatal intensive care units in the Netherlands," *Journal of Pediatrics* 129 (1996): 661, 663 (finding no "intentional and active termination" in 1993 and only one in 1990). See generally James P. Orlowski et al., "Medical decisions concerning the end of life in children in the Netherlands," *American Journal of Diseases in Children* 147 (1993): 613 (letter); James P. Orlowski et al., "Pediatric euthanasia," *American Journal of Diseases in Children* 146 (1992): 1440; Henk K. A. Visser et al., "Medical decisions concerning the end of life in children in the Netherlands," *American Journal of Diseases in Children* 146 (1992): 1429.

10. See Royal Dutch Medical Association, *Vision on Euthanasia* (1995), 16–17; Committee of the Section on Perinatology, Dutch Pediatric Association, "To do or not to do? Boundaries of medical action in neonatology" (English summary), in *Doen of Laten? Grenzen van het medisch handelen in de neonatologie* (Utrecht: Nederlandse Vereniging voor Kindergeneeskunde, 1992), 11; Royal Dutch Medical Association, Committee on Acceptability of Life-Terminating Actions, "Life-terminating actions with incompetent patients, Part I: severely handicapped newborns: an interim report," *Medisch Contact* 45 (1990): 553, a summary of which is translated in "Report of the Royal Dutch Society of Medicine on life-terminating actions with incompetent patients, Part I: severely handicapped newborns," *Issues in Law & Medicine* 7 (1991): 365. See also

Griffiths, "Recent developments," pp. 354–356; Alex K. Huibers, "Treating and non-treating of critically ill newborns in the Netherlands," *Journal of Legal Medicine* 16 (1995): 227; Zier Versluys and Richard de Leeuw, "A Dutch report on the ethics of neonatal care," *Journal of Medical Ethics* 21 (1995): 14; Henk Jochemsen, "Life-prolonging and life-terminating treatment of severely handicapped newborn babies: a discussion of the report of the Royal Dutch Society of Medicine on 'life-terminating actions with incompetent patients: Part I: severely handicapped newborns,'" *Issues in Law & Medicine* 8 (1992): 167; Royal Dutch Medical Association Committee on Acceptability of Life-Terminating Actions with Incompetent Patients, *Medisch Contact* 43 (1988): 697. Indications of further Dutch approval come from Pieter J. J. Sauer, "Ethical decisions in neonatal intensive care units: the Dutch experience," *Pediatrics* 90 (1992): 729 (1991 report from a committee convened by the Ministers of Justice and Health); Richard Fenigsen, "A case against Dutch euthanasia," *Hastings Center Report,* January–February 1989, S22, S23 (1987 guidelines from the Dutch Health Council).

11. See John C. Moskop, "End-of-life decisions in Dutch neonatal intensive care units," *Journal of Pediatrics* 129 (1996): 627, 628; Sheldon, "Dutch court convicts doctor of murder"; "Dutch doctor free after prosecution proves murder case," *American Medical News,* December 4, 1995, p. 4.

12. See Gary A. Walco et al., "Pain, hurt, and harm: the ethics of pain control in infants and children," *New England Journal of Medicine* 331 (1994): 541; Astrid James, "Perspectives on pain," *Lancet* 342 (1993): 609; C. C. Johnson et al., "A survey of pain in hospitalized patients aged 4–14 years," *Clinical Journal of Pain* 8 (1992): 154; Orlowski et al., "Pediatric euthanasia," p. 1445; Neil L. Schecter et al., "Report of the Consensus Conference on the Management of Pain in Childhood Cancer," *Pediatrics* 86 supp. (1990): 813; Neil L. Schecter, "The undertreatment of pain in children: an overview," *Pediatric Clinics of North America* 36 (1989): 781; Neil L. Schecter et al., "Status of pediatric pain control: a comparison of hospital analgesic usage in children and adults," *Pediatrics* 77 (1986): 11.

13. The percentage of children under 18 living in poverty has long been higher than the percentage of all Americans. From 1980 to 1993 the percentage of children was 17.9 percent to 22 percent, versus 12.8 percent to 15.2 percent. U.S. Bureau of the Census, *Statistical Abstract of the United States: 1995* (115th ed. 1995), 480.

14. See Jane L. Holl, "Profile of uninsured children in the United States," *Archives of Pediatric & Adolescent Medicine* 149 (1995): 398. On recent changes, see note 87 below.

15. The extensive literature on this includes Robert H. Wharton et al.,

"Advance care planning for children with special health care needs: a survey of parental attitudes," *Pediatrics* 97 (1996): 682, 684–685; Anne M. Dellinger and Patricia C. Kuszler, "Infants: public-policy and legal issues," in *Encyclopedia of Bioethics,* vol. 3, ed. Warren T. Reich (rev. ed. 1995), 1214, 1216–1217; Hastings Center Project, "Imperiled newborns," *Hastings Center Report,* December 1987, pp. 5, 17–18; President's Commission for the Study of Ethical Problems in Medicine and Biomedical and Behavioral Research, *Deciding to Forego Life-Sustaining Treatment* (1983), 215–217.

16. See, e.g., N. M. P. King and A. W. Cross, "Children as decision makers: guidelines for pediatricians," *Journal of Pediatrics* 115 (1989): 10; S. L. Leiken, "Minor's assent or dissent to medical treatment," *Journal of Pediatrics* 102 (1983): 169; L. Weithorn and S. Campbell, "The competency of children and adolescents to make informed treatment decisions," *Child Development* 53 (1982): 1589.

17. See, e.g., Compassion in Dying, 79 F.3d 813; Sylvia A. Law, "Physician-assisted death: an essay on constitutional rights and remedies," *Maryland Law Review* 55 (1996): 292; Kathryn L. Tucker and David J. Burman, "Physician aid in dying: a humane option, a constitutionally protected choice," *Seattle University Law Review* 18 (1995): 495. However, the Supreme Court has rejected the assertion that rights to abortion and the termination of treatment ground a federal constitutional right to assisted suicide and euthanasia. See Washington v. Glucksberg, 117 S. Ct. 2258. For commentary doing the same see, e.g., Susan M. Wolf, "Physician-assisted suicide, abortion, and treatment refusal: using gender to analyze the difference," in *Physician-Assisted Suicide,* ed. Robert F. Weir (1997), 167; Seth F. Kreimer, "Does pro-choice mean pro-Kevorkian? An essay on *Roe, Casey,* and the right to die," *American University Law Review* 44 (1995): 803; New York State Task Force on Life and the Law, *When Death Is Sought: Assisted Suicide and Euthanasia in the Medical Context* (1994), 67–75.

18. The literature has become immense. For testimony as to the importance of the debate see, e.g., Ronald Dworkin, *Life's Dominion: An Argument about Abortion, Euthanasia, and Individual Freedom* (1993), 3. In Dworkin's book and elsewhere this debate has become linked to another great American debate, abortion. See, e.g., Kreimer, "Does pro-choice mean pro-Kevorkian?" This linkage became a focal point of discussion as the courts considered whether the U.S. Constitution protects a right to elect physician-assisted suicide or euthanasia. See Washington v. Glucksberg, 117 S. Ct. at 2262, 2269-71, *rev'g* Compassion in Dying, 79 F.3d 790. However, exploring this linkage is not new, especially the linkage

between aborting a fetus and euthanizing a newborn. See, e.g, Fletcher, "Abortion, euthanasia, and the care of defective newborns"; Michael Tooley, "Abortion and infanticide," *Philosophy & Public Affairs* 2 (1972): 37.

19. *Vacco v. Quill* dealt only with the rights of terminally ill, competent patients. See Quill v. Vacco, 80 F.3d 716. Similarly, in *Washington v. Glucksberg* the Ninth Circuit and Supreme Court limited their holdings to adults: "We hold that insofar as the Washington statute prohibits physicians from prescribing life-ending medication for use by terminally ill, competent adults who wish to hasten their own deaths, it violates the Due Process Clause. . . . " 79 F.3d 793–794. See also 117 S. Ct. at 2275. *Lee v. Oregon* has concerned an Oregon statute pertaining only to adults. 891 F. Supp. 1429 (D.Or. 1995), *vacated and remanded,* 107 F.3d 1382 (9th Cir.), *cert. denied sub nom.* Lee v. Harcleroad, 118 S. Ct. 328 (1997). And none of Jack Kevorkian's "patients" thus far has been a minor, so the resultant Michigan litigation has also been about adults. See, e.g., People v. Kevorkian, 527 N.W.2d 714 (Mich. 1994), *cert. denied sub nom.* Hobbins v. Kelley, 115 S. Ct. 1795 (1995). See also Krischer v. McIver, 697 So.2d 97 (Fla. 1997) (competent adult).

There has nonetheless been mention in dicta of minors seeking to end their lives. For example, the Ninth Circuit suggested that a "liberty interest in hastening death is at its low point when . . . [a] person is young and healthy," and that the state might have a strong interest in preventing suicide among the young, as opposed to among terminally ill, competent adults. Compassion in Dying, 79 F.3d at 820–821, 834. The Supreme Court similarly characterized the young as a group vulnerable to suicide and took note, in discussing slippery-slope concerns, that Dutch practice now extends to neonatal euthanasia. Washington v. Glucksberg, 117 S. Ct. at 2272, 2274.

20. See Dworkin, *Life's Dominion.*

21. See Timothy E. Quill, "The ambiguity of clinical intentions," *New England Journal of Medicine* 329 (1993): 1039; Timothy E. Quill, *Death and Dignity, Making Choices and Taking Charge* (1993); Timothy E. Quill et al., "Care of the hopelessly ill: potential clinical criteria for physician-assisted suicide," *New England Journal of Medicine* 327 (1992): 1380; Timothy E. Quill, "Death and dignity: a case of individualized decision making," *New England Journal of Medicine* 324 (1991): 691.

22. See Jack Kevorkian, *Prescription: Medicide* (1991), 195, 200; note 19 above.

23. The American Academy of Pediatrics' reports thus far steer clear of any discussion of assisted suicide and euthanasia. See American

Academy of Pediatrics, Committee on Bioethics, "Guidelines on forgoing life-sustaining medical treatment," *Pediatrics* 93 (1994): 532. See also Committee on Bioethics, "Ethics and the care of critically ill infants and children," *Pediatrics* 98 (1996): 149; Committee on Fetus and Newborn, "The initiation or withdrawal of treatment for high-risk newborns," *Pediatrics* 96 (1995): 362. Yet the proper plea in one of those reports that "physicians and parents should give great weight to clearly expressed views of child patients" raises the obvious question of what weight to give to a child's request for physician-assisted suicide or euthanasia. See American Academy of Pediatrics, "Guidelines," p. 532.

24. See "Death at U.C. Med Center."

25. See "Doctor faces murder count in premature baby's death."

26. Weir, *Selective Nontreatment*, pp. 248–249.

27. Joseph F. Kett, "Science and controversy in the history of infancy in America," in *Which Babies Shall Live? Humanistic Dimensions of the Care of Imperiled Newborns,* ed. Thomas H. Murray and Arthur L. Caplan (1985), 23, 37.

28. Ibid.

29. Cindy Bouillon-Jensen, "Infants: history of infanticide," in *Encyclopedia of Bioethics,* vol. 3, ed. Warren T. Reich (rev. ed. 1995), 1200, 1205.

30. Robert N. Proctor, *Racial Hygiene: Medicine under the Nazis* (1988), 180.

31. Ibid., pp. 179–180.

32. See Robert F. Weir, "Infants: ethical issues," in *Encyclopedia of Bioethics,* vol. 3, ed. Warren T. Reich (rev. ed. 1995), 1206, 1212. For debate over forgoing treatment in neonates see, e.g., Tom L. Beauchamp and James F. Childress, *Principles of Biomedical Ethics* (4th ed. 1994), 217–219; Renee R. Anspach, *Deciding Who Lives: Fateful Choices in the Intensive Care Nursery* (1993); *Compelled Compassion: Government Intervention in the Treatment of Critically Ill Newborns,* ed. Arthur L. Caplan et al. (1992); Hastings Center Project, "Imperiled newborns"; *Which Babies Shall Live?; Ethics of Newborn Intensive Care,* ed. Albert R. Jonsen and Michael J. Garland (1976); Raymond S. Duff and A. G. M. Campbell, "Moral and ethical dilemmas in the special-care nursery," *New England Journal of Medicine* 289 (1973): 890. Analyzing this literature's coverage of active euthanasia is complicated by the fact that some authors use "euthanasia" to refer to forgoing life-sustaining treatment. See, e.g., John A. Robertson, "Involuntary euthanasia of defective newborns: a legal analysis," *Stanford Law Review* 27 (1975): 213.

33. For examples advocating active euthanasia of newborns see Freeman, "If euthanasia were licit, could lives be saved?" p. 153; Shelp, *Born*

to Die?; Kuhse and Singer, *Should the Baby Live?;* Weir, *Selective Non-treatment;* Engelhardt, *Ethical Issues in Aiding the Death of Young Children* (advocating under some circumstances). For an argument challenging this advocacy see Stephen G. Post, "History, infanticide, and imperiled newborns," *Hastings Center Report,* August 1988, p. 14.

34. See, e.g., Shelp, *Born to Die?* pp. 166–172, 175.

35. See, e.g., Tooley, *Abortion and Infanticide,* pp. 332–425; Weir, *Selective Nontreatment,* pp. 152–159 (presenting positions of Tooley, Mary Anne Warren, and Peter Singer that neonates are not yet persons). See also Shelp, *Born to Die?* p. 175.

36. See Tooley, *Abortion and Infanticide.*

37. See, e.g., Johan Legemaate, "Legal aspects of euthanasia and assisted suicide in the Netherlands, 1973–1994," *Cambridge Quarterly of Healthcare Ethics* 4 (1995): 112, 118 ("the crucial role of . . . self-determination"). Indeed, the Dutch definition of "euthanasia" presumes the patient's request. See Griffiths, "Recent developments," pp. 347, 350.

38. Oregon legalized physician-assisted suicide in 1994, but the statute was in litigation for several years after. See Lee v. Oregon 891 F. Supp. 1429 (D.Or. 1996), *vacated and remanded,* 107 F.3d 1382 (9th Cir.), *cert. denied sub nom.* Lee v. Harcleroad, 118 S. Ct. 328 (1997). It then survived a popular re-vote required by the legislature. See "Oregon keeps suicide law; voters reject repeal of doctor-assisted death," *Internationl Herald Tribune,* November 6, 1997. The Northern Territory of Australia legalized voluntary euthanasia in 1995. See Northern Territory of Australia, Rights of the Terminally Ill Act 1995 (No. 12 of 1995); Christopher James Ryan and Miranda Kaye, "Euthanasia in Australia—The Northern Territory Rights of the Terminally Ill Act," *New England Journal of Medicine* 334 (1996): 326. However, the federal parliament struck down that law in 1997. See "Euthanasia law struck down in Australia."

39. For discussion of the legal evolution, see note 8 above.

40. See, e.g., Legemaate, "Legal aspects of euthanasia," p. 114 (five requirements for Dutch euthanasia, including a "voluntary, competent and durable request" by the patient); Griffiths, "The regulation of euthanasia," pp. 143–144 (requirements include that "the doctor must ensure that . . . [the patient's request] is voluntary and informed"); Battin, "Euthanasia," pp. 299–300 (five guidelines, including "that the patient's request be voluntary," which is the central criterion); Henk A. M. J. ten Have, "Euthanasia in the Netherlands: the legal context and the cases," *HEC Forum* 1 (1989): 41, 44 (emphasizing that "euthanasia . . . requires that the patient be fully competent"). The requirements are "variously

stated." Battin, "Euthanasia," p. 299. This is probably because they de-
rive from a number of judicial opinions. However, as remarked in note 37
above, the very definition of "euthanasia" under Dutch law requires that
the patient request the intervention.

Legemaate states that the recent Dutch legislation on physician reporting when euthanasia has been performed "extends the notification
procedure to cases in which a doctor actively ends the life of a patient
without the latter's explicit request, . . . rais[ing] the question of when
such conduct is appropriate." Legemaate, "Legal aspects of euthanasia,"
p. 117. He states that this extension responds to data documenting cases
of active termination without patient request. Ibid.

41. See Battin, "Euthanasia," p. 302 ("The Dutch see Americans as
much further out on the slippery slope . . ., because Americans have
already become accustomed to second-party choices about other people. . . . [V]oluntariness is . . . central in the Dutch understanding of
choices about dying.").

42. See Marlise Simons, "Dutch doctors to tighten rules on mercy
killings: patient would administer drug," *New York Times,* September 11,
1995.

43. Though I focus in text on violation of the rules requiring the
patient's voluntary request, violations of other rules have been documented as well. See, e.g., Gerrit van der Wal et al., "Evaluation of the
notification procedure for physician-assisted death in the Netherlands,"
New England Journal of Medicine 335 (1996): 1706; M. T. Muller et al.,
"Voluntary active euthanasia and physician-assisted suicide in Dutch
nursing homes: are the requirements for prudent practice properly met?"
Journal of the American Geriatrics Society 42 (1994): 624; G. van der Wal
et al., "Euthanasia and assisted suicide. II. Do Dutch family doctors act
prudently?" *Family Practice* 9 (1992): 135.

44. There have been two primary teams of researchers. Publications by
the governmental team include Loes Pijnenborg et al., "Life-terminating
acts without explicit request of patient," *Lancet* 341 (1993): 1196; van der
Maas et al., "Euthanasia and other medical decisions," *Health Policy;*
Paul J. van der Maas et al., "Euthanasia and other medical decisions
concerning the end of life," *Lancet* 338 (1991): 669. The second team has
produced publications, including Gerrit van der Wal and Robert J. M.
Dillman, "Euthanasia in the Netherlands," *British Medical Journal* 308
(1994): 1346.

45. van der Maas et al., "Euthanasia and other medical decisions,"
Lancet, p. 670; Pijnenborg et al., "Life-terminating acts." These numbers
compare to the numbers for voluntary euthanasia (1.7 percent–2.6 per-

cent), assisted suicide (0.2 percent–0.4 percent), death from medication for pain and symptoms (18.8 percent–13.8 percent), and death from non-treatment decisions (17.9 percent–17.0 percent). van der Maas et al., "Euthanasia and other medical decisions," *Lancet,* p. 670.

46. See Paul J. van der Maas et al., "Euthanasia, physician-assisted suicide, and other medical practices involving the end of life in the Netherlands, 1990–1995," *New England Journal of Medicine* 335 (1996): 1699.

47. One thousand, the most frequently cited estimate, comes from van der Maas et al., "Euthanasia and other medical decisions," *Lancet,* p. 670. However, the same researchers in Pijnenborg et al., "Life-terminating acts," p. 1198, also venture a lower estimate of 270 per year.

48. Pijnenborg et al., "Life-terminating acts," p. 1197.

49. Ibid., p. 1198; van der Maas et al., "Euthanasia," *New England Journal of Medicine,* p. 1704

50. Pijnenborg et al., "Life-terminating acts,", p. 1199.

51. See Alan D. Ogilvie and S. G. Potts, "Assisted suicide for depression: the slippery slope in action?" *British Medical Journal* 309 (1994): 492; Tony Sheldon, "Reprimand for Dutch doctor who assisted suicide," *British Medical Journal* 310 (1995): 894 (disciplinary board reprimand).

52. Gomez, *Regulating Death,* p. 104.

53. For the 1990–91 analysis see van der Maas et al., "Euthanasia and other medical decisions," *Health Policy,* p. 144. For the subsequent analysis see van der Heide et al., "Medical end-of-life decisions," p. 253 (August–November, 1995, deaths excluding those by sudden infant death syndrome and other modalities precluding a medical decision concerning end-of-life care).

54. Orlowski et al., "Pediatric euthanasia."

55. Ibid., p. 1441.

56. Ibid.

57. Doyle, "Dutch doctors."

58. See Richard Fenigsen, "Euthanasia in the Netherlands," *Issues in Law & Medicine* 6 (1990): 229, 238; de Leeuw et al., "Foregoing intensive care treatment."

59. Gomez, *Regulating Death,* pp. 83–84.

60. See, e.g., Spreeuwenberg, "The story of Laurens"; Doyle, "Dutch doctors."

61. See Sheldon, "Dutch court convicts doctor of murder."

62. Orlowski et al., "Pediatric euthanasia," p. 1443.

63. Fenigsen, "Euthanasia in the Netherlands," p. 244 and n.65, citing "Arts geeft jongeren dodelijke pil mee" (Doctor supplies boys with deadly pills), *Brabants Dagblad,* October 10, 1987.

64. Fenigsen, "Euthanasia in the Netherlands," p. 244 and n.66, citing "Grote publieke steun voor Dokter Voute" (Broad public support for Doctor Voute), *Brabants Dagblad,* October 31, 1987.

65. See, e.g., Visser et al., "Medical decisions" (on Orlowski et al.); Letters, *Hastings Center Report,* November–December 1989, pp. 47, 47–50 (on Fenigsen).

66. Committee of the Section on Perinatology, "To do or not to do?" pp. 13–14. Other sources suggest more controversy. See Huibers, "Treating and non-treating," p. 241; Versluys and de Leeuw, "A Dutch report," p. 16.

67. See Committee of the Section on Perinatology, "To do or not to do?" p. 13: "Purposeful ending of life is only possible with the permission of the parents."

68. Royal Dutch Medical Association, *Vision on Euthanasia,* pp. 16–17. They had previously published a report entitled "Life ending treatment with incompetent patients: Part I: severely defective neonates." See E. van Leeuwen and G. K. Kimsma, "Acting or letting go: medical decision making in neonatology in the Netherlands," *Cambridge Quarterly of Healthcare Ethics* 2 (1993): 265, 265, citing Royal Dutch Medical Association Committee, "Acceptability of life ending treatment," *Medisch Contact* 43 (1988): 697. For additional Dutch institutional support of pediatric euthanasia, see note 10 above on the Dutch Health Council and a committee convened by the Ministers of Justice and Health.

69. According to Fenigsen, a March 1987 report of the Health Council agrees. See Fenigsen, "A case against Dutch euthanasia," S22, S23.

70. Royal Dutch Medical Association, *Vision on Euthanasia,* p. 17.

71. Orlowski et al., "Pediatric euthanasia," pp. 1444–1445.

72. Visser et al., "Medical decisions," p. 1430.

73. H. J. J. Leenen and Chris Ciesielski-Carlucci, "Force majeure' (legal necessity): justification for active termination of life in the case of severely handicapped newborns after forgoing treatment," *Cambridge Quarterly of Healthcare Ethics* 2 (1993): 271, 274.

74. See "Interview with Heleen M. Dupuis," p. 277.

75. Committee of the Section on Perinatology, "To do or not to do?" p. 11.

76. On the decisional standards applicable in pediatric cases see Angela Roddey Holder, *Legal Issues in Pediatrics and Adolescent Medicine* (2d ed. 1986); James M. Morrissey et al., *Consent and Confidentiality in the Health Care of Children and Adolescents: A Legal Guide* (1986). Note that although the best interests standard prevails for children, some authors argue for a special standard when the child is permanently unconscious. See, e.g., Hastings Center Project, "Imperiled newborns,"

p. 16 ("relational potential" standard). However, the work of such supplemental standards, which is to make life-sustaining treatment optional, seems accomplished by a best interests standard recognizing that a child correctly diagnosed as permanently unconscious will never experience any benefit from continued treatment. See generally President's Commission, *Deciding to Forego Life-Sustaining Treatment,* pp. 181–183.

77. See, e.g., Dellinger and Kuszler, "Infants," pp. 1216–1217; Hastings Center Project, "Imperiled newborns," pp. 17–18; President's Commission, *Deciding to Forego Life-Sustaining Treatment,* pp. 215–217. See generally Daryl Evans, "The psychological impact of disability and illness on medical treatment decisionmaking," *Issues in Law & Medicine* 5 (1989): 277.

78. Cf. Hastings Center Project, "Imperiled newborns," p. 24 ("Parents may advocate killing their infants to serve their own purposes rather than their infants' welfare."); President's Commission, *Deciding to Forego Life-Sustaining Treatment,* p. 216 ("[p]arents may be reeling"). For controversy over whether parents' interests have a proper role in termination of treatment decisions see, e.g., "Imperiled newborns," p. 16 ("Unlike the best interests standard, which is infant-centered, the relational potential standard allows the interests of others . . . to weigh in the decision. . . . "); Allen E. Buchanan and Dan W. Brock, *Deciding for Others: The Ethics of Surrogate Decision Making* (1989), 259–260.

79. See, e.g., Rebecca Dresser, "Missing persons: legal perceptions of incompetent patients," *Rutgers Law Review* 46 (1994): 609.

80. See, e.g., Charles S. Cleeland et al., "Pain and its treatment in outpatients with metastatic cancer," *New England Journal of Medicine* 330 (1994): 592; Mary D. Tesler et al., "Postoperative analgesics for children and adolescents: prescription and administration," *Journal of Pain and Symptom Management* 9 (1994): 85; Post, "History, infanticide, and imperiled newborns," p. 16 (recounting the history of physicians ignoring neonatal pain); Anne B. Fletcher, "Pain in the neonate," *New England Journal of Medicine* 317 (1987): 1347.

81. See, e.g., Philippe Ariès, *Centuries of Childhood: A Social History of Family Life,* trans. Robert Baldick (1962); John Boswell, *The Kindness of Strangers: The Abandonment of Children in Western Europe from Late Antiquity to the Renaissance* (1988), esp. 36–39 and n.83 (disputing Ariès).

82. See Post, "History, infanticide, and imperiled newborns," pp. 15–16; *Infanticide: Comparative and Evolutionary Perspectives,* pp. 427–520; Weir, *Selective Nontreatment,* pp. 5–19.

83. Laila Williamson, "Infanticide: an anthropological analysis," in *Infanticide and the Value of Life,* ed. Marvin Kohl (1978), 61, 64.

84. See Ruth Macklin, "Which way down the slippery slope? Nazi medical killing and euthanasia today," in *When Medicine Went Mad: Bioethics and the Holocaust,* ed. Arthur L. Caplan (1992), 173, 184–186; Robert J. Lifton, *The Nazi Doctors* (1986), 50–62.

85. See "Biomedical ethics and the shadow of Naziism: a conference on the proper use of the Nazi analogy in ethical debate," *Hastings Center Report,* August 1976, S1.

86. George J. Annas and Michael A. Grodin, The *Nazi Doctors and the Nuremberg Code: Human Rights in Human Experimentation* (1992), 25.

87. See Jerry Gray, "Through Senate alchemy, tobacco is turned into gold for children's health," *New York Times,* August 11, 1997; Merri Rosenberg, "Welfare reform spurs worry about effects," *New York Times,* March 16, 1997; Peter P. Budetti, "Health reform for the 21st century? It may have to wait until the 21st century," *JAMA* 277 (1997): 193; Robert Pear, "Overhauling welfare: a look at the year ahead," *New York Times,* August 7, 1996; "A sad day for poor children," *New York Times,* August 1, 1996 (editorial); Paul W. Newacheck et al., "The effect on children of curtailing Medicaid spending," *JAMA* 274 (1995): 1468; cf. Jack Lewin, "Protecting the health of children of immigrants: innocent victims of adult policy," *JAMA* 277 (1997): 672 (children bear the brunt of policy changes denying public services to immigrants).

88. See, e.g., Martha Minow, "What ever happened to children's rights?" *Minnesota Law Review* 80 (1995): 267.

89. Compare Orlowski et al., "Pediatric euthanasia," with Laurence Steinberg and Elizabeth Cauffman, "Maturity of judgment in adolescence: psychosocial factors in adolescent decision making," *Law and Human Behavior* 20 (1996): 249, and Elizabeth S. Scott et al., "Evaluating adolescent decision making in legal contexts," *Law and Human Behavior* 19 (1995): 221.

90. Holder, *Legal Issues in Pediatrics,* p. 120 (footnote with citations omitted).

91. Ibid., pp. 120–122, 127–128, 133–135.

92. See, e.g., American Academy of Pediatrics, "Guidelines," p. 535.

93. See, e.g., Lois A. Weithorn and David G. Scherer, "Children's involvement in research participation decisions: psychological considerations," in *Children as Research Subjects: Science, Ethics, and Law,* ed. Michael A. Grodin and Leonard H. Glantz (1994), 133, 152. Note that the division of my analysis by ages 14 and 7 echoes the old common law "rule of sevens" for determining the capacity of minors. See, e.g., Cardwell v. Bechtol, 724 S.W.2d 739 (Tenn. 1987).

94. See Weithorn and Scherer, "Children's involvement in research participation decisions," p. 144, citing the National Commission for the Protection of Human Subjects in Biomedical and Behavioral Research.

95. See "Model Aid-in-Dying Act," p. 167.

96. Orlowski et al., "Pediatric euthanasia," p. 1445.

97. For recent work, see, e.g., *Intending Death: The Ethics of Assisted Suicide and Euthanasia,* ed. Tom L. Beauchamp (1996); Susan M. Wolf, "Gender, feminism, and death: physician-assisted suicide and euthanasia," in *Feminism & Bioethics: Beyond Reproduction,* ed. Susan M. Wolf (1996), 282; Margaret P. Battin, *The Least Worst Death: Essays in Bioethics on the End of Life* (1994); Dan W. Brock, "Voluntary active euthanasia," in *Life and Death: Philosophical Essays in Biomedical Ethics* (1993), 202; Daniel Callahan, *The Troubled Dream of Life: Living with Mortality* (1993); Dworkin, *Life's Dominion;* and numerous journal articles.

98. See Alan Meisel, *The Right to Die,* vol. 2 (2d ed. 1995), §18.2.

99. See Leon R. Kass, "Neither for love nor money: why doctors must not kill," *Public Interest,* Winter 1989, p. 25.

100. See, e.g., ibid.; Wolf, "Gender, feminism, and death"; Susan M. Wolf, "Holding the line on euthanasia," *Hastings Center Report,* January–February 1989, S13, S15.

101. See Robert A. Burt, *Taking Care of Strangers* (1979); see also Wolf, "Holding the line on euthanasia."

102. See, e.g., Howard Brody, "Assisted death—a compassionate response to a medical failure," *New England Journal of Medicine* 327 (1992): 1384.

103. See Wolf, "Gender, feminism, and death," pp. 301–302.

104. See Cleeland et al., "Pain and its treatment."

105. See, e.g., The SUPPORT Principal Investigators, "A controlled trial to improve care for seriously ill hospitalized patients: the Study to Understand Prognoses and Preferences for Outcomes and Risks of Treatment (SUPPORT)," *JAMA* 274 (1995): 1591; Marion Danis et al., "A prospective study of advance directives for life-sustaining care," *New England Journal of Medicine* 324 (1991): 882.

106. See Washington v. Glucksberg, 117 S. Ct. 2258.

107. See Vacco v. Quill, 117 S. Ct. 2293.

108. See Wolf, "Gender, feminism, and death."

109. Cf. Leon R. Kass, "Is there a right to die?" *Hastings Center Report,* January-February 1993, p. 34 (answering no).

110. See Vacco v. Quill, 117 S. Ct. 2293; Washington v. Glucksberg, 117 S. Ct. 2258; Cruzan v. Director, Missouri Dep't of Health, 497 U.S. 261,

269, 278–279 (1990) and 287–289 (O'Connor, J., concurring), 302, 304–307, 309, 312 (Brennan, J., dissenting).

111. Some may respond that the claimed right to assisted suicide and euthanasia is not an affirmative right but a negative one, the right to be left alone with a willing physician. But this misconstrues what is required of the state. Medical practice is a product of the state's affirmative licensure and authorization of permitted practices. Thus the state must affirmatively empower physicians and insulate them from criminal prosecution if assisted suicide and euthanasia are to be legitimated.

112. For extensive development of this argument about social context see Wolf, "Gender, feminism, and death."

113. See Keith Bradsher, "Rise in uninsured becomes an issue in Medicaid fight," *New York Times,* August 27, 1995.

114. See Uwe E. Reinhardt, "Reforming the health care system: the universal dilemma," *American Journal of Law & Medicine* 19 (1993): 21, 30.

115. See van der Wal et al., "Evaluation of the notification procedure"; van der Maas et al., "Euthanasia and other medical decisions," *Health Policy,* pp. 46–48.

116. See the section in text on "The Dutch Embrace of Pediatric Euthanasia."

117. Weithorn and Scherer, "Children's involvement in research participation decisions," p. 148 (citations omitted).

118. Compare ibid., pp. 151–152, with Scott et al., "Evaluating adolescent decision making," and Elizabeth S. Scott, "Judgment and reasoning in adolescent decisionmaking," *Villanova Law Review* 37 (1992): 1607, and Steinberg and Cauffman, "Maturity of Judgment."

119. On the relationship between the gravity of the decision and the degree of competence required, see, e.g., Buchanan and Brock, *Deciding for Others,* pp. 51–57.

120. Weithorn and Scherer, "Children's involvement in research participation decisions," p. 160.

121. Ibid., p. 161.

122. Compassion in Dying, 79 F.3d at 820.

123. Ibid., pp. 832–833. The Supreme Court echoed this solicitude for the young in *Washington v. Glucksberg,* acknowledging their vulnerability to suicide and the state interest in preventing it. 117 S. Ct. at 2272.

124. Hoberman, "The impact of sanctioned assisted suicide on adolescents," pp. 202–204.

125. See American Academy of Pediatrics, Committee on Bioethics, "Informed consent, parental permission, and assent in pediatric practice," *Pediatrics* 95 (1995): 314.

126. Weithorn and Scherer, "Children's involvement in research participation decisions," p. 164 (citation omitted).
127. See Royal Dutch Medical Association, *Vision on Euthanasia,* p. 17.
128. Weithorn and Scherer, "Children's involvement in research participation decisions," p. 152.
129. Ibid., p. 144.
130. See Bill Wallace, "UC Hospital suspends 4 in mercy killing case," *San Francisco Chronicle,* March 28, 1995 (doctor allegedly gives a lethal injection to a 9-year-old California girl for whom life-sustaining treatment has been forgone, when she "continued to live"); "Doctor faces murder count in premature baby's death" (doctor allegedly removes 5 1/2-week-old Georgia infant from a ventilator then kills the child by holding her hand over his mouth and pressing the carotid artery "so that this will not drag on"). See generally van der Heide et al., "Medical end-of-life decisions," p. 253 ("Decisions to give drugs explicitly to end life were made for 48% . . . [of] infants among whom life-sustaining treatment had earlier been forgone.")
131. See on Baby Rianne, Sheldon, "Dutch court convicts doctor of murder" (3-day-old child "had at best a year to live as 'a sleeping plant'"); Dick Polman, "Euthanasia debated in Holland: doctor is charged in newborn's death," *Dallas Morning News,* January 22, 1995 (same case, quoting doctor as saying what bothered the parents was the child's pain, which could not be stopped). But see on the child's prognosis "Dutch bring a test case in euthanasia," *New York Times,* December 23, 1994 ("only weeks to live"). On Baby Maartje see "Trials signal Dutch headed for expanding euthanasia: severely deformed infants may be included in policy," *Rocky Mountain News,* December 26, 1994 (4-day-old child with spina bifida "and other deformities" and what the doctor described as "'unacceptable'" pain). The article implies that treatment was being foregone.
132. See, e.g., Brock, "Voluntary active euthanasia"; Quill v. Vacco, 80 F.3d 716.
133. See, e.g., Callahan, *The Troubled Dream of Life,* pp. 76–82; Meisel, *The Right to Die,* vol. 2, §§18.10–18.19; President's Commission, *Deciding to Forego Life-Sustaining Treatment,* pp. 60–89.
134. Just as "euthanasia" is sometimes used to cover forgoing life-sustaining treatment as well as active euthanasia, "infanticide" is sometimes used to cover both as applied to infants, as well as nonmedical forms of killing. See, e.g., Susan C. M. Scrimshaw, "Infanticide in human populations: societal and individual concerns," in *Infanticide: Compara-*

tive and Evolutionary Perspectives, ed. Glenn Hausfater and Sarah Blaffer Hrdy (1984), 439; Weir, *Selective Nontreatment,* pp. 3–28. Others use "infanticide" to denote only the direct and active killing of infants. See, e.g., Post, "History, infanticide, and imperiled newborns*";* Marvin Kohl, "Preface," in *Infanticide and the Value of Life,* ed. Marvin Kohl (1978), 5, 5. Earl Shelp comments on the definitional confusion that "all intentional deaths of infants tend to be classified as instances of infanticide. Killing by omission is not distinguished from killing by commission. . . . Thus it is difficult to be certain exactly what the literature means by the term 'infanticide.'" Shelp, *Born to Die?* p. 155. He also notes ambiguity about whether the term applies to older children up to 2 years old. Ibid., pp. 154–155.

135. Kuhse and Singer, *Should the Baby Live?* pp. 98–117. Others offering similar arguments include Shelp, *Born to Die?* pp. 154–166; Weir, *Selective Nontreatment,* pp. 3–28; Tooley, *Abortion and Infanticide,* pp. 309–322.

136. See Post, "History, infanticide, and imperiled newborns."

137. See Tooley, *Abortion and Infanticide.*

138. See Fletcher, "Abortion, euthanasia."

139. The Supreme Court's abortion jurisprudence has rejected the notion that a fetus is a person under the Constitution. As Justice Stevens remarked in *Webster v. Reproductive Health Services,* 492 U.S. 490, 568 n.13 (1988) (Stevens, J., concurring in part), "No member of this Court has ever questioned the holding in *Roe* . . . that a fetus is not a 'person' within the meaning of the Fourteenth Amendment." See also Planned Parenthood v. Casey, 505 U.S. 833, 912–913 (1992) (Stevens, J., concurring in part).

140. See Nancy Rhoden, "Trimesters and technology: revamping *Roe v. Wade,*" *Yale Law Journal* 95 (1986): 639, 643, 678–679.

141. See Planned Parenthood v. Casey, 505 U.S. 860; Roe v. Wade, 410 U.S. 113, 163–165 (1973).

142. Despite this technological constraint, commentators analyzing the law and morality of abortion have hypothesized future development of extracorporeal gestation. See, e.g., Frances M. Kamm, *Creation and Abortion: A Study in Moral and Legal Philosophy* (1992), 211–218; Rhoden, "Trimesters and Technology," pp. 665, 679. Rhoden discusses one current way to overcome the constraint: embryo transfer before implantation. See Rhoden, "Trimesters and Technology," pp. 670–671.

143. For a history of the law, policy, and clinical practice see, e.g., John Lantos, "Baby Doe five years later: implications for child health," *New England Journal of Medicine* 317 (1987): 444. See also note 77 above.

144. See note 77 above.

145. The requirement that treatment decisions be based on the child's best interests is clearest when the child is not permanently unconscious. See, e.g., Hastings Center Project, "Imperiled newborns," pp. 14–15, 17–18, 31; President's Commission, *Deciding to Forego Life-Sustaining Treatment*, pp. 216–217. Even then, exclusion of the interests of the family is not without controversy. See, e.g., Hilde Lindemann Nelson and James Lindemann Nelson, *The Patient in the Family: An Ethics of Medicine and Families* (1995), 88–90, 114–118. When the child is reliably diagnosed as permanently unconscious, some have argued that the interests of others become relevant and even decisive. See Hastings Center Project, "Imperiled newborns," p. 16; Buchanan and Brock, *Deciding for Others*, pp. 132–134, 236–237, 259–260.

146. Meisel, *The Right to Die*, vol. 2, §§15.6–15.9.

147. See, e.g., Buchanan and Brock, *Deciding for Others*, pp. 87–151; *Guidelines on the Termination of Life-Sustaining Treatment and the Care of the Dying* (1987), 3–4, 7, 9–10, 19; President's Commission for the Study of Ethical Problems in Medicine and Biomedical and Behavioral Research, *Making Health Care Decisions, The Ethical and Legal Implications of Informed Consent in the Patient–Practitioner Relationship, Volume One: Report* (1982), 41–51. As I have noted above, however, some make an exception for patients who are permanently unconscious. See, e.g., Buchanan and Brock, *Deciding for Others*, pp. 126–132.

148. See Buchanan and Brock, *Deciding for Others*, pp. 80–151; *Guidelines on the Termination of Life-Sustaining Treatment*, pp. 26–29; President's Commission, *Making Health Care Decisions*, pp. 177–181.

149. See Daniel Callahan, "Vital distinctions, mortal questions," *Commonweal* 115 (1988): 397.

150. On progress made toward recognizing children's pain and need for pain relief, see, e.g., Neil L. Schecter et al., "Pain in infants, children and adolescents: an overview," in *Pain in Infants, Children and Adolescents*, vol. 3, ed. Neil L. Schecter et al. (1993), 3; Patricia A. McGrath, *Pain in Children: Nature, Assessment, and Treatment* (1990), 355–356. There is a large literature on the history of children's legal and social status. On that history and progress see, e.g., Martha Minow, *Making All the Difference: Inclusion, Exclusion, and American Law* (1990), 283–311; Boswell, *The Kindness of Strangers; American Childhood: A Research Guide and Historical Handbook*, ed. Joseph M. Hawes and N. Ray Hiner (1985); Ariès, *Centuries of Childhood*. On recent setbacks, however, see Minow, "What ever happened to children's rights?"

151. See, e.g., Orlowski et al., "Pediatric euthanasia," p. 1445. I agree

with Orlowski et al. on children younger than 7. I go further than they on children 7 to 14.

152. See Wolf, "Gender, feminism, and death"; Wolf, "Holding the line on euthanasia."

153. See, e.g., Holl, "Profile of uninsured children"; Katherine L. Kahn et al., "Health care for black and poor hospitalized Medicare patients," *JAMA* 271 (1994): 1169; Council on Ethical and Judicial Affairs, American Medical Association, "Gender disparities in clinical decision making," *JAMA* 266 (1991): 559; Council on Ethical and Judicial Affairs, American Medical Association, "Black-white disparities in health care," *JAMA* 263 (1990): 2344.

154. See Judith C. Ahronheim et al., "Treatment of the dying in the acute care hospital: advanced dementia and metastatic cancer," *Archives of Internal Medicine* 156 (1996): 2094; Council on Scientific Affairs, American Medical Association, "Good care of the dying patient," *JAMA* 275 (1996): 474; Margo L. Rosenbach, "Access and satisfaction within the disabled Medicare population," *Health Care Financing Review* 17 (1995): 147.

6. Religious Viewpoints

1. The phrase "medical pacifism" comes from James F. Bresnahan, S.J., "Observations on the rejection of physician-assisted suicide: a Roman Catholic perspective," *Christian Bioethics* 1, no. 3 (December 1995): 256–284. The phrase "culture of death" is featured in Pope John Paul II, *Evangelium Vitae (The Gospel of Life)*, Origins 24 (April 6, 1995). Most subsequent references to the latter document will appear in the text with the section number in parentheses.

2. For an overview of Islamic thought, see Fazlur Rahman, *Health and Medicine in the Islamic Tradition: Change and Identity* (New York: Crossroad, 1989). For Buddhist and Hindu views, see Katherine K. Young, "Death: eastern thought," in *Encyclopedia of Bioethics,* vol. 1, pp. 490–491. The most comprehensive overviews of religious perspectives on suicide, assisted suicide, and active euthanasia include Campbell, "Religious ethics and active euthanasia in a pluralistic society," *Kennedy Institute of Ethics Journal* 2 (September 1992); The Park Ridge Center, *Active Euthanasia, Religion, and the Public Debate* (Chicago: The Park Ridge Center, 1991); and Gerald A. Larue, *Euthanasia and Religion: A Survey of the Attitudes of World Religions to the Right-To-Die* (Los Angeles, CA: Hemlock Society, 1985).

3. The Park Ridge Center, *Active Euthanasia, Religion, and the Public Debate,* p. 36.

4. In this essay, the term "euthanasia" without a qualifier will refer to voluntary euthanasia.

5. See Hessel Bouma III et al., *Christian Faith, Health, and Medical Practice* (Grand Rapids, MI: Eerdmans, 1989). For covenantal approaches within Jewish ethics, see Walter S. Wurzburger, *Ethics of Responsibility: Pluralistic Approaches to Covenantal Ethics* (Philadelphia: The Jewish Publication Society, 1994). See also David Novak, "Natural law, *Halakhah,* and the Covenant," and Elliot N. Dorff, "The Covenant: the transcendent thrust in Jewish law," both in *Contemporary Jewish Ethics and Morality: A Reader,* ed. Elliot N. Dorff and Louis E. Newman (New York: Oxford University Press, 1995). Paul Ramsey, *The Patient as Person* (New Haven, CT: Yale University Press, 1970). In various writings Ramsey interprets *agape* (love) as "covenant faithfulness."

6. On the imago Dei and relationality, see Courtney S. Campbell, "Religious ethics and active euthanasia in a pluralistic society," 269–271.

7. Robert N. Wennberg, *Terminal Choices: Euthanasia, Suicide, and the Right to Die* (Grand Rapids, MI: Eerdmans, 1989), pp. 225–226.

8. Ramsey, *The Patient as Person.*

9. Margaret Pabst Battin, *Ethical Issues in Suicide* (Englewood Cliffs, NJ: Prentice Hall, 1995), chap. 1.

10. U.S. Catholic Bishops, *Ethical and Religious Directives for Catholic Health Care Services, Origins* 24 (December 15, 1994): 458.

11. Henry S. Richardson's categories of application/deduction, specification, and balancing are useful for reflecting on the Roman Catholic and other positions. See "Specifying norms as a way to resolve concrete ethical problems," *Philosophy and Public Affairs* 19 (1990): 279–320.

12. *Catechism of the Catholic Church* (Mahwah, NJ: Paulist Press, 1994), #2281.

13. A similar summary of double effect appears in many places; see, for example, David Granfield, *The Abortion Decision* (Garden City, NY: Image Books, 1971).

14. *Ethical and Religious Directives for Catholic Health Care Services,* pp. 458–459. See also Richard A. McCormick, S.J., "Nutrition-hydration: the new euthanasia," *The Critical Calling: Reflections on Moral Dilemmas since Vatican II* (Washington, DC: Georgetown University Press, 1989), chap. 21.

15. *Catechism of the Catholic Church,* #2282.

16. Patricia Beattie Jung, "Dying well isn't easy: thoughts of a Roman Catholic theologian on death by choice," in *Must We Suffer Our Way to*

Death? Cultural and Theological Perspectives on Death by Choice, ed. Ronald P. Hamel and Edwin R. Dubose (Dallas, TX: Southern Methodist University Press, 1996), p. 177.

17. Richard McCormick, S.J., "Killing the patient," in *Considering Veritatis Splendor,* ed. John Wilkins (Cleveland: Pilgrim Press, 1994), p. 19. See the attacks on the proportionalists in *Veritatis Splendor* as well as, more indirectly, in *Evangelium Vitae.*

18. The Sacred Congregation for the Doctrine of the Faith, *Declaration on Euthanasia* (Rome: Vatican City, May 5, 1980). On suffering, see also B. Andrew Lustig, "Suffering, sovereignty, and the purposes of God: Christian convictions and medical killing," *Christian Bioethics* 1:3 (1995): 249–255, and Edmund D. Pellegrino, "Euthanasia and assisted suicide," in *Dignity and Dying: A Christian Appraisal,* ed. John F. Kilner, Arlene B. Miller, and Edmund D. Pellegrino (Grand Rapids, MI: Eerdmans, 1996), pp. 105–119. Pellegrino writes: "Christianity gives meaning to suffering because it is linked to the sufferings of God Incarnate, who willingly suffered and died for our redemption. In suffering, we humans follow in his ways, the way of the Cross. Through suffering, rightly confronted, we can grow spiritually" (p. 111).

19. See Paul Ramsey, *The Patient as Person,* and *Ethics at the Edges of Life: Medical and Legal Intersections* (New Haven, CT: Yale University Press, 1978).

20. Explicit theological convictions played only a modest role in Fletcher's later writings, as he moved more and more toward a humanistic orientation, and as he attempted to develop criteria of quality of life stated in terms of degrees of humanhood. See Fletcher, *Morals and Medicine* (Princeton, NJ: Princeton University Press, 1954); *Humanhood: Essays in Biomedical Ethics* (Buffalo, NY: Prometheus Press, 1979); and "In defense of suicide," in *Suicide and Euthanasia: The Rights of Personhood,* ed. S. E. Wallace and A. Eser (Knoxville, TN: University of Tennessee Press, 1981).

21. Arthur J. Dyck, *On Human Care* (New York: Abingdon Press, 1977).

22. See, for example, Stanley Hauerwas, "Rational suicide and reasons for living," in *Rights and Responsibilities in Modern Medicine: The Second Volume in a Series on Ethics, Humanism, and Medicine,* ed. Mark Basson (New York: Alan R. Liss, 1981). Stanley Hauerwas and Richard Bondi, "Memory, community and the reasons for living: reflections on suicide and euthanasia," in Hauerwas, *Truthfulness and Tragedy: Further Investigations in Christian Ethics* (Notre Dame, IN: University of Notre Dame Press, 1977), p. 111.

23. Allen Verhey, "Assisted suicide and euthanasia: a biblical and re-

formed perspective," in *Must We Suffer Our Way to Death?*, ed. Hamel and Dubose, p. 238. Hauerwas and Bondi, "Memory, community and the reasons for living," p. 114.

24. Gilbert Meilaender, "Euthanasia and Christian vision," *Thought* 57 (December 1982): 465–475. See also John F. Kilner, *Life on the Line: Ethics, Aging, Ending Patients' Lives, and Allocating Vital Resources* (Grand Rapids, MI: Eerdmans, 1992).

25. See Gilbert Meilaender, "On removing food and water: against the stream," *Hastings Center Report* 14 (December 1984): 11–13; contrast Ramsey, *Ethics at the Edges of Life.*

26. *Suicide: The Philosophical Issues*, ed. Margaret Pabst Battin and David J. Mayo (New York: St. Martin's Press, 1980). See James M. Gustafson, *Ethics from a Theocentric Perspective, vol. 2: Ethics and Theology* (Chicago: University of Chicago Press, 1984), chap. 6. See also Karl Barth, *Church Dogmatics* III/4., trans. A. T. McKay et al. (Edinburgh: T. and T. Clark, 1961), pp. 401–412. For a more critical view in different language, see Wennberg, *Terminal Choices.* These theologians also differ in their language of evaluation, whether suicide is tragic, etc.

27. Darrel W. Amundsen, "Suffering and the sovereignty of God: one evangelical's perspective on doctor-assisted suicide," *Christian Bioethics* 1 (1995): 285. Paul Badham, "Should Christians accept the validity of voluntary euthanasia?" *Studies in Christian Ethics* 8, no. 2 (1995): 8.

28. Lonnie D. Kliever, "Claiming a death of our own: perspectives from the Wesleyan tradition," in *Must We Suffer Our Way to Death?*, ed. Hamel and Dubose, p. 291. Daniel B. McGee, "Euthanasia and physician-assisted suicide: a believers' church perspective," in *Must We Suffer Our Way to Death?*, ed. Hamel and Dubose, p. 324.

29. See *Report of the Task Force on Assisted Suicide to the 122nd Convention of the Episcopal Diocese of Newark* (January 27, 1996). See also John S. Spong, Bishop of Newark, "In defense of assisted suicide," *The VOICE of the Diocese of Newark* (January/February 1996). One strong criticism is that, despite some qualifying comments, the Report defines euthanasia too broadly as "any intervention which lessens the suffering of illness; an intervention that at times carries with it the danger of terminating life prematurely." For this criticism and others see the balanced document prepared by the Committee on Medical Ethics, Episcopal Diocese of Washington, *Are Assisted Suicide and Euthanasia Morally Acceptable for Christians? Both Sides of the Question* (Draft Document, August 12, 1996).

30. Committee on Health, Human Values, and Ethics, Episcopal Diocese of Southern Ohio, *Response to the Resolution Concerning Assisted*

Suicide Adopted by the 122nd Convention of the Episcopal Diocese of Newark (February 23, 1996).

31. My discussion of Roman Catholicism and Protestantism does not exhaust the Christian tradition. Of particular importance is the Orthodox tradition, which is similar in many respects to Roman Catholic and Protestant approaches to bioethics but which differs in others. It too is generally opposed to suicide, assisted suicide, and euthanasia. For an overview see Stanley Samuel Harakas, "Eastern Orthodox Christianity," in *Encyclopedia of Bioethics,* rev. ed., ed. Warren T. Reich (New York: Simon & Schuster Macmillan, 1995), vol. 2, pp. 643–649. See also Vigen Guroian, *Life's Living toward Dying: A Theological and Medical-Ethical Study* (Grand Rapids, MI: Eerdmans, 1996).

32. Seymour Siegel, "Suicide in the Jewish view," *Conservative Judaism* 32 (winter 1979).

33. Ibid.

34. Ibid. See the discussion in Elliot N. Dorff, "Assisted death: a Jewish perspective," in *Must We Suffer Our Way to Death?,* ed. Hamel and Dubose, pp. 141–173.

35. *Sefer Hasidim* 723 [ed. Margaliot]; cited in Louis Newman, "Woodchoppers and respirators: the problem of interpretation in contemporary Jewish ethics," in *Contemporary Jewish Ethics and Morality,* ed. Dorff and Newman, p. 144. R. Moses Isserles *(Rema)* on *Shulchan Aruch, Yoreh Deah* 339:1; cited in Newman, "Woodchoppers and respirators," p. 145.

36. *American Reform Responsa,* ed. Walter Jacob (New York: Central Conference of American Rabbis, 1983), p. 254; quoted by David H. Ellenson, "How to draw guidance from a heritage: Jewish approaches to mortal choices," in *Contemporary Jewish Ethics and Morality,* ed. Dorff and Newman, p. 133.

37. Fred Rosner and Rabbi Moses D. Tendler, *Practical Medical Halacha,* 2nd ed. (New York: Feldheim Publishers, 1980), p. 56.

38. See Marc Kellner, "The structure of Jewish ethics," in *Contemporary Jewish Ethics and Morality,* ed. Dorff and Newman, pp. 12–24. See Elliot N. Dorff, "Assisted death: a Jewish perspective," in *Must We Suffer Our Way to Death?,* ed. Hamel and Dubose, p. 153.

39. Ellenson, "How to draw guidance from a heritage," p. 138. For a criticism of Ellenson's nonlegal approach from the standpoint of a legal approach, rooted in Conservative Judaism, see Elliot Dorf, "A methodology for Jewish medical ethics," in *Contemporary Jewish Ethics and Morality: A Reader,* ed. Dorff and Newman, pp. 161–176.

40. Newman, "Woodchoppers and respirators," p. 141.

41. Cited in ibid., p. 145.

42. Ibid., p. 146.

43. Fred Rosner, *Modern Medicine and Jewish Ethics* (Hoboken, NJ: KTAV, and New York: Yeshiva University Press, 1986), p. 200.

44. Newman, "Woodchoppers and respirators," p. 148. See Fred Rosner, "Euthanasia," in *Contemporary Jewish Ethics and Morality,* ed. Dorff and Newman, pp. 350–362.

45. See Byron Sherwin, "Euthanasia: a Jewish view," *Journal of Aging and Judaism* 2 (Fall 1987), rpt. in *Contemporary Jewish Ethics and Morality,* ed. Dorff and Newman, pp. 363–381. Baruch A. Brody, "A historical introduction to Jewish casuistry on suicide and euthanasia," in *Suicide and Euthanasia: Historical and Contemporary Themes,* ed. Baruch A. Brody (Dordrecht: Kluwer Academic Publishers, 1989), p. 74.

46. Immanuel Jakobovits, *Jewish Medical Ethics,* rev. ed. (New York: Bloch Publishing Co., 1975), p. 103.

47. On the role of experience in changes in moral doctrine in the Roman Catholic tradition, see John T. Noonan, Jr., "Development in moral doctrine," *Theological Studies* 53 (December 1993): 662–677.

48. See, for example, James Davison Hunter, *Culture Wars: The Struggle to Define America* (New York: Basic Books, 1991).

49. For a helpful typology of religious approaches to public policy regarding active euthanasia, see Campbell, "Religious ethics and active euthanasia in a pluralistic society."

50. Courtney S. Campbell, "Religious ethics and active euthanasia in a pluralistic society," *Kennedy Institute of Ethics Journal* 2 (September 1992): 253–277. Andrew Greeley, "Live and let die: changing attitudes," *Christian Century* 108 (1991): 1124–1125. See also Arthur J. Dyck, "North American law and public policy," in *Dignity and Dying,* ed. Kilner, Miller, and Pellegrino, pp. 154–164, which contends that "polls tend to exaggerate considerably the support that exists for legalizing physician-assisted suicide and euthanasia," but also concedes that "the change in attitudes toward these practices is real" (p. 156).

51. See *Evangelium Vitae,* passim.

52. Bouma et al., *Christian Faith, Health, and Medical Practice,* p. 300. McGee, "Euthanasia and physician-assisted suicide," p. 324. He also opposes physician-administered euthanasia. By contrast, Kliever argues for a regulatory approach along the lines of Dr. Timothy Quill's guidelines, and he contends that the opportunities for depriving the dying of proper medical care are as great with our unstructured practices of letting people die as "they might be with a properly administered system of helping people die." See Kliever, "Claiming a death of our own," pp. 297–298.

32. Allen Verhey, "Choosing death: the ethics of assisted suicide," *Christian Century* (July 17–24, 1996): 717. See also Verhey, "Assisted suicide and euthanasia," pp. 259, 261.

54. For example: "Although it is true that the envisioned dangers of the slippery-slope argument have been neither confirmed nor refuted, our knowledge of human nature and human history is sufficient to make us [resist] more permissive norms." Bouma et al., *Christian Faith, Health, and Medical Practice*, pp. 302–303.

7. Factual Findings

We would like to thank Drs. Ezekiel Emanuel, Agnes van der Heide, Hanny Groenewoud, Hillel Alpert, Johannes van Delden, Gerrit van der Wal, and Dick Willems for useful comments on previous drafts of this chapter, and Dr. Hans M. Lam for his valuable contributions to the section on culture.

1. P. J. van der Maas, J. J. M. van Delden, L. Pijnenborg, C. W. N. Looman, "Euthanasia and other medical decisions concerning the end of life," *Lancet* 338 (1991): 669–674. P. J. van der Maas, J. J. M. van Delden, L. Pijnenborg, "Euthanasia and other medical decisions concerning the end of life," *Health Policy* 22, nos. 1, 2 (1992): 1–26; also published as hardcover (Amsterdam: Elsevier Science Publishers, 1992). J. J. M. van Delden, L. Pijnenborg, P. J. van der Maas, "Dances with data: reports from the Netherlands," *Bioethics* 3 (1993): 323–329 (contains references).

2. K. L. Dorrepaal, N. K. Aaronson, F. S. A. M. Dam van, "Pain experience and pain management among hospitalized cancer patients: a clinical study," *Cancer* 63 (1989): 593–598. R. M. Kanner and R. K. Portenoy, "Are the people who need analgesics getting them?" *American Journal of Nursing* 86, no. 5 (1986): 589. R. M. A. Hirschfeld et al., "The National Depressive and Manic-Depressive Association consensus statement on the undertreatment of depression," *JAMA* 277 (1997): 330–340. Van der Maas, Delden, and Pijnenborg, "Euthanasia and other medical decisions concerning the end of life." D. S. Greer and V. Mor, "An overview of National Hospice Study findings," 39, no. 1 (1986): 5–7.

3. Van der Maas, van Delden, and Pijnenborg, "Euthanasia and other medical decisions concerning the end of life." G. van der Wal and P. J. van der Maas, *Euthanasie en andere medische beslissingen rond het levenseinde* (The Haag: Sdu Uitgevers, 1996). World Health Organization, *Cancer Pain Relief* (Geneva: WHO, 1986). E. J. Emanuel, D. L. Fairclough, E. R. Daniels, B. R. Clarridge, "Euthanasia and physician-assisted suicide: attitudes and experiences of oncology patients, oncologists, and the

public," *Lancet* 347 (1996): 1805–1810. S. E. Ward et al., "Patient-related barriers to management of cancer pain," *Pain* 52 (1993): 319–324.

4. Emanuel et al., "Euthanasia and physician-assisted suicide: attitudes." F. Y. Huang and L. L. Emanuel, "Physician aid in dying and the relief of patients' suffering: physicians' attitudes regarding patients suffering and end-of-life decisions," *Journal of Clinical Ethics* 6 (1995): 62–67. Emanuel et al., "Euthanasia and physician-assisted suicide: attitudes."

5. Van der Maas, van Delden, and Pijnenborg, "Euthanasia and other medical decisions concerning the end of life." A. L. Back, J. I. Wallace, H. E. Starks, R. A. Pearlman, "Physician-assisted suicide and euthanasia in Washington State: patient requests and physician responses," *JAMA* 275, no. 12 (1996): 919–923. Emanuel et al., "Euthanasia and physician-assisted suicide: attitudes." G. van der Wal, J. Th. M. Eijk, H. J. J. Leenen, C. Spreeuwenberg, "Euthanasia and assisted suicide, II: Do Dutch family doctors act prudently?" *Family Practice* 9 (1992): 135–140. W. Breitbart, B. D. Rosenfeld, S. D. Passik, "Interest in physician-assisted suicide among ambulatory HIV-infected patients," *American Journal of Psychiatry* 153 (1996): 238–242.

6. World Health Organization, *Cancer Pain Relief.*

7. L. Pijnenborg, "End-of-life decisions in Dutch medical practice," thesis, Erasmus University Rotterdam, 1995. P. J. van der Maas, G. van der Wal, I. Haverkate, C. L. M. de Graaf, J. G. C. Kester, B. D. Onwuteaka-Philipsen, A. van der Heide, J. M. Bosma, D. L. Willems, "Euthanasia, physician-assisted suicide, and other medical practices involving the end of life in the Netherlands, 1990–1995," *New England Journal of Medicine* 335, no. 22 (1996): 1699–1705. Van der Wal and van der Maas, *Euthanasie en andere medische beslissingen rond het levenseinde.*

8. Emanuel et al., "Euthanasia and physician-assisted suicide: attitudes." Back et al., "Physician-assisted suicide and euthanasia in Washington State."

9. Van der Maas, van Delden, and Pijnenborg, "Euthanasia and other medical decisions concerning the end of life." Van der Maas et al., "Euthanasia, physician-assisted suicide, and other medical practices involving the end of life in the Netherlands." G. van der Wal, P. J. van der Maas, J. M. Bosma, B. D. Onwuteaka-Philipsen, D. L. Willems, I. Haverkate, P. J. Kostense, "Evaluation of the notification procedure for physician-assisted death in the Netherlands," *New England Journal of Medicine* 335, no. 22 (1996): 1706–1711.

10. Van der Maas, van Delden, and Pijnenborg, "Euthanasia and other medical decisions concerning the end of life."

11. Ibid. Van der Wal and van der Maas, *Euthanasie en andere medische beslissingen rond het levenseinde*. P. J. van der Maas, L. Pijnenborg, J. J. M. van Delden, "Changes in Dutch opinions on active euthanasia, 1966 through 1991," *JAMA* 273 (1995): 1411–1414.

12. H. Kuhse, P. Singer, P. Baume, M. Clark, M. Rickard, "End-of-life decisions in Australian medical practice," *Medical Journal of Australia* 166 (1997): 191–196. R. K. Portenoy et al., "Determinants of the willingness to endorse assisted suicide: a survey of physicians, nurses and social workers," *Psychosomatics* (forthcoming April 1997). B. Koenig et al., "Attitudes of elderly patients and their families toward physician assisted suicide," *Archives of Internal Medicine* 156 (1996): 2240.

13. L. Pijnenborg, P. J. van der Maas, J. J. M. van Delden, C. W. N. Looman, "Life-terminating acts without explicit request of patient," *Lancet* 341 (1993): 1196–1199. N. L. Farberow, "Cultural history of suicide in N.L.," in *Suicide in Different Cultures,* ed. N. L. Farberow (Baltimore: University Park Press, 1975), pp. 1–15. E. M. Weyer, *The Eskimos: Their Environment and Folkways* (Hamden, CN: Archon Books, 1969; 1932). M. Pinguet, *La mort volontaire au Japon* (Voluntary death in Japan) (Paris: Edition Gallimard, 1984). G. Lienhardt, *Divinity and Experience* (Oxford: Clarendon Press, 1967).

14. S. Miles, "Physicians and their patients' suicides," *JAMA* 271 (1994): 1786.

15. President's Commission for the Study of Ethical Problems in Medicine and Biomedical and Behavioral Research, *Deciding to Forego Life-Sustaining Treatment* (Washington, DC: Government Printing Office, 1983). D. W. Brock, "Active voluntary euthanasia," *Hastings Center Report* 22 (1992): 10–27.

16. Van der Maas et al., "Euthanasia, physician-assisted suicide, and other medical practices involving the end of life in the Netherlands." B. J. Ward and P. A. Tate, "Attitudes among NHS doctors to requests for euthanasia," *British Medical Journal* 309 (1994): 1332–1334. C. A. Stevens and R. Hassan, "Management of death, dying and euthanasia: attitudes and practices of medical practitioners in South Australia," *Journal of Medical Ethics* 20 (1994): 41–46. P. V. Caralis and J. S. Hammond, "Attitudes of medical students, housestaff, and faculty physicians toward euthanasia and termination of life-sustaining treatment," *Critical Care Medicine,* 20, no. 5 (1992): 683–690.

17. L. Pijnenborg, P. J. van der Maas, J. W. P. F. Kardaun, J. J. Glerum, J. J. M. Delden, C. W. N. Looman, "Withdrawal or withholding of treatment at the end of life," *Archives of Internal Medicine* 155 (1995): 286–292. Dutch Pediatric Society, *Doen of laten? Grenzen van het medisch*

handelen in de neonatologie (To intervene or not? The limits of medical intervention in neonatology) (Utrecht, 1992). Van der Wal and van der Maas, *Euthanasie en andere medische beslissingen rond het levenseinde.* R. de Leeuw, A. J. de Beaufort, M. J. K. de Kleine, K. van Harrewihn, L. A. Kollée, "Forgoing intensive care treatment in newborn infants with extremely poor prognoses: a study in four neonatal intensive care units in the Netherlands," *Journal of Pediatrics* 129 (1996): 661-666. Agnes van der Heide, Paul J. van der Maas, Gerrit van der Wal, Carmen L. M. de Graaff, John G. C. Kester, Louis A. A. Kollée, Richard de Leeuw, and Robert A. Holl, "Medical end-of-life decisions made for neonates and infants in the Netherlands," *Lancet* 350 (1997): 251-255.

18. Van der Wal and van der Maas, *Euthanasie en andere medische beslissingen rond het levenseinde.*

19. Ibid. Emanuel et al., "Euthanasia and physician-assisted suicide: attitudes." B. D. Onwuteaka-Philipsen, M. T. Muller, G. van der Wal, J. T. M. van Eijk, M. W. Ribbe, "Attitudes of Dutch general practitioners and nursing home physicians to active voluntary euthanasia and physician-assisted suicide," *Archives of Family Medicine* 4 (1995): 951-955.

20. Miles, "Physicians and their patients' suicides." "Suicide patient discussed suing husband, sources say," *Boston Globe,* August 24, 1996. J. Rakowsky, "Welcome to the era of euthanasia chic," *Wall Street Journal,* May 1996.

21. P. J. E. Bindels, A. Krol, E. van Ameijden, D. K. J. Mulder-Folkerts, J. A. R. van den Hoek, G. P. J. van Griensven, R. A. Coutinho, "Euthanasia and physician-assisted suicide in homosexual men with AIDS," *Lancet* 347 (1996): 499-503. L. Sherr, F. van den Boom, "Aids and suicide," *Aids Care* 7, suppl. 2 (1995): 107-205. "Kevorkian chronology," Associated Press, September 7, 1996.

22. Royal Dutch Medical Association, *Position Paper on Euthanasia* (in Dutch) (Utrecht, RDMA, 1995). I. Haverkate and G. van der Wal, "Policies on medical decisions concerning the end of life in Dutch health care institutions" (Letter), *JAMA* 275, no. 6 (1996): 435-439

23. The table summarizes results from heterogeneous surveys, using different wordings for each question. Data sources and wordings of questions are summarized here.

Active Euthanasia Sometimes Acceptable

United States: Approve of euthanasia in situations with incurable cancer patients having unremitting physical pain. (In parentheses: Approve of physician-assisted suicide in situations with incurable cancer patients having unremitting physical pain.) *Netherlands:* Number reflects the percentage of physicians who have either performed euthanasia themselves (53%), or who could conceive of situations where they would be prepared to perform euthanasia (35%), or who would be prepared to refer patients with euthanasia requests to a colleague who would be prepared to perform euthanasia (9%). *Canada:* It is sometimes right to practice active euthanasia. *Australia:* Is it ever right to bring about death of a patient by taking active steps? *Denmark:* Ethically acceptable when a physician gives a lethal injection to a competent patient who repeatedly asks for it?

Law Should Permit Euthanasia

United States: Would vote to legalize euthanasia on a referendum. (In parentheses: Would vote to legalize physician-assisted suicide on a referendum.) *Netherlands:* In favor of some form of legalization. Number includes 20% who want to keep euthanasia punishable, but with specific exceptions. *Canada:* The law should be changed to permit patients to request active euthanasia. *Australia:* Do you think it should be legally permissible for medical practitioners to take active steps to bring about a patients' death under some circumstances? *United Kingdom:* Should the law on euthanasia in Britain be similar to that existing in The Netherlands? *Denmark:* A physician gives a lethal injection to a competent patient who repeatedly asks for it. Acceptable that this practice is legal/feel that this should be legal?

Performing Euthanasia Conceivable

Netherlands: Number reflects the percentage of physicians who have either performed euthanasia themselves (53%), or who could conceive of situations where they would be prepared to perform euthanasia or PAS (35%). *Canada:* I would practice active euthanasia if it were legalized. *United Kingdom:* If a terminally ill patient asked me to bring an end to his or her life, I would consider doing so if it were legal.

Ever Performed Euthanasia or Assisted in Suicide

United States: Ever performed euthanasia or PAS. *Netherlands:* Ever performed euthanasia or PAS. *Australia:* Have you ever taken active steps which have brought about the death of a patient? *United Kingdom:* Have you ever taken active steps to bring about the death of a patient who asked you to do so? *Denmark:* Ever given a lethal injection to a competent patient who repeatedly asked for it.

Ever Received a Request for Euthanasia or Physician-Assisted Suicide

United States: Have received requests for euthanasia or PAS. *Netherlands:* Have received requests for euthanasia or PAS. *Australia:* Have received a request from a patient to hasten death by taking active steps. *United Kingdom:* In the course of your medical practice, has a patient ever asked you to hasten his or her death? *Denmark:* Have you ever been requested by a competent patient to give a lethal injection?

United States Data

From Emanuel, Fairclough, Daniels, and Clarridge, "Euthanasia and physician-assisted suicide: attitudes and experiences of oncology patients, oncologists, and the public." Sample of 489 oncologists, 73% response rate. For other data from the United States, see (for Washington State) J. S. Cohen, S. D. Fihn, E. J. Boyko, A. R. Jonsen, and R. W. Wood, "Attitudes toward assisted suicide and euthanasia among physician in Washington State," *New England Journal of Medicine* 331, no. 2 (1994): 89–94; (for Michigan) J. G. Bachman, D. K. Alcser, D. J. Doukas, F. L. Lichtenstein, A. D. Corning, and H. Brody, "Attitudes of Michigan physicians and the public toward legalizing physician-assisted suicide and voluntary euthanasia," *New England Journal of Medicine* 334, no. 5 (1996): 303–309; (for Oregon) M. A. Lee, H. D. Nelson, V. P. Tilden, L. Ganzini, T. A. Schmidt, and S. E. Tolle, "Legalizing assisted suicide: views of physicians in Oregon," *New England Journal of Medicine* 334, no. 5 (1996): 310–315.

Netherlands Data

From: Van der Maas, Delden, and Pijnenborg, "Euthanasia and other medical decisions concerning the end of life"; Van der Wal and van der Maas, *Euthanasie en andere medische beslissingen rond het levenseinde;* Van der Maas et al., "Euthanasia, physician-assisted suicide, and other medical practices involving the end of life in the Netherlands." Face to face interview survey. Sample of 461 general practitioners, nursing home physicians, specialists in internal medicine, neurology, pulmonology, cardiology, and surgery. Response rate 88%.

Canada Data

From T. Douglas Kinsella and M. J. Verhoef, "Alberta euthanasia survey: 1. Physicians' opinions about the acceptance of active euthanasia as a medical act and the reporting of such practice; 2. Physicians' opinions about the acceptance of active euthanasia as a medical act and the reporting of such practice," *Canadan Medical Association Journal* 148 (1993): 1929–1933. Mail questionnaire survey. Sample of 2002 licensed physicians in Alberta, response rate 69%.

Australia Data

From Stevens and Hassan, "Management of death, dying and euthanasia: attitudes and practices of medical practitioners in South Australia." *Journal of Medical Ethics* 20 (1994): 41–46. Mail questionnaire survey. Sample of 494 medical practitioners in South Australia, response rate 60%.

United Kingdom Data

From Ward and Tate, "Attitudes among NHS doctors to requests for euthanasia," *British Medical Journal* 309 (1994): 1332–1334. Mail questionnaire survey of 424 general practitioners and hospital consultants in one area of England, response rate 74%.

Denmark Data

From A. P. Folker, N. Holtug, A. B. Jensen, K. Kappel, J. K. Nielsen, and M. Norup, "Experiences and attitudes towards end-of-life decisions amongst Danish physicians," *Bioethics* 10 (1996): 233–249. Mail questionnaire survey. Sample of 491 members of Danish Medical Association, response rate 64%.

24. Emanuel et al., "Euthanasia and physician-assisted suicide: attitudes." R. J. Blendon, U. S. Szalay, R. A. Knox, "Should physicians aid their patients in dying? The public perspective," *JAMA* 267, no. 19 (1992): 2658–2662. Van der Wal et al., "Euthanasia and assisted suicide, II." Van der Maas, Pijnenborg, and Delden, "Changes in Dutch opinions on active euthanasia."

25. Van der Wal et al., "Evaluation of the notification procedure for physician-assisted death in the Netherlands."

26. Van der Maas, van Delden, and Pijnenborg, "Euthanasia and other medical decisions concerning the end of life."

27. Van der Maas, Pijnenborg, and Delden, "Changes in Dutch opinions on active euthanasia."

28. Van der Maas, Delden, and Pijnenborg, "Euthanasia and other medical decisions concerning the end of life."

8. Why Now?

1. Anonymous, "It's over, Debbie," *JAMA* 259 (1988): 272.

2. *Compassion in Dying v. Washington,* 79 F.3d 790 (9th Cir. 1996).

3. J. Warden, "Euthanasia around the world," *British Medical Journal* 304 (1992): 7–10. W. Kondro, "Canada's euthanasia debate renewed," *The Lancet* 343 (1994): 534. C. J. Ryan and M. Kaye, "Euthanasia in Australia: the Northern Territory Rights of the Terminally Ill Act," *New England Journal Medicine* 334 (1996): 326–328. M. Spanjer, "Mental suffering as justification for euthanasia in Netherlands," *The Lancet* 343 (1994): 1630. D. Brahams, "Euthanasia: doctor convicted of attempted murder," *The Lancet* 340 (1992): 782–783. *Report of the House of Lords Select Committee on Medical Ethics* (London: HM Stationery Office, 1994).

4. D. W. Brock, "Voluntary active euthanasia," *Hastings Center Report* 22 (1992): 10–22.

5. L. Edelstein, "The Hippocratic Oath: text, translation, and interpretation," in *Ancient Medicine: Selected Papers of Ludwig Edelstein,* ed. O. Temkin and C. L. Temkin (Baltimore: Johns Hopkins University Press, 1967). D. W. Amundsen. "The physician's obligation to prolong life: a medical duty without classical roots," *Hastings Center Report* 8 (1978): 23–30. P. Carrick, *Medical Ethics in Antiquity* (Dordrecht: D. Reidel, 1985), chaps. 7 and 8. D. Gourevitch, "Suicide among the sick in classical antiquity," *Bulletin of the History of Medicine* 43 (1969): 501–518. R. Gillon, "Suicide and voluntary euthanasia: historical perspective," in *Euthanasia and the Right to Death,* ed. A. B. Downing (London: Peter Owen, 1969).

6. Pliny, *Letters and Panegyericus I,* trans. B. Radice (Cambridge: Loeb Classical Library, Harvard University Press, 1969), xxii.

7. T. More, *Utopia and Other Writings,* ed. J. J. Greene and J. P. Dolan (New York: New American Library, 1984).

8. D. Hume, *The Philosophical Works,* vol. 4 (Boston: Little, Brown, 1854), pp. 535–546.

9. W. B. Fye, "Active euthanasia: an historical survey of its conceptual origins and introduction into medical thought," *Bulletin of the History of Medicine* 52 (1978): 492–502.

10. C. F. H. Marx, "Medical euthanasia," in W. Cane, "Medical euthanasia," *Journal of the History of Medicine* 7 (1952): 401–416.

11. J. C. Warren, *Etherization: With Surgical Remarks* (Boston: Ticknor & Co., 1848), pp. 69–73.

12. J. Bullar, "Chloroform in dying," *British Medical Journal* 2 (1866): 10–12.

13. S. D. Williams, *Euthanasia* (London: Williams and Norgate, 1872). S. J. Reiser, "The dilemma of euthanasia in modern medical history: the English and American experience," in *The Dilemmas of Euthanasia*, ed. J. A. Behnke and S. Bok (Garden City, NY: Anchor Press, 1975).

14. Anonymous, "Essays of the Birmingham Speculative Club," *Saturday Review* 30 (1870): 632–634. Editorial, "Euthanasia," *Spectator* 44 (1871): 314–315. Editorial, "Our criminals," *Saturday Review* 34 (1872): 43–44. "Euthanasia," *Popular Science Monthly* 3 (1873): 90–96.

15. R. Hofstadter, *Social Darwinism in American Thought* (Boston: Beacon Press 1955). D. Ross, *The Origins of American Social Science* (New York: Cambridge University Press 1991). See also R. C. Bannister, *Social Darwinism: Science and Myth in Anglo-American Social Thought*, 2nd ed. (Philadelphia: Temple University Press, 1988).

16. "The euthanasia," *Medical and Surgical Reporter* 29 (1873): 122–123.

17. *Minutes on the Proceedings of the South Carolina Medical Association*, April 7, 1879, pp. 14–17. "The doctrine of euthanasia," *Medical and Surgical Reporter* 41 (1879): 479–480.

18. The Medical Jurisprudence Society of Philadelphia, *The Medico-Legal Journal* 2 (1885): 312–313. F. E. Hitchcock, "Annual oration: euthanasia," *Transactions of the Maine Medical Society* 10 (1989): 30–43. Editorial, "Permissive euthanasia," *Boston Medical and Surgical Journal* 110 (1884): 19–20. Editorial, "The moral side of euthanasia," *JAMA* 5 (1885): 382–383. Anonymous, "Euthanasia," *Medical Record* 28 (1885): 322.

19. Hitchcock, "Annual oration." Editorial, "The moral side of euthanasia."

20. P. Starr, *The Social Transformation of American Medicine* (New York: Basic Books, 1982), chap. 4.

21. C. B. Williams, "Euthanasia," *Medical Record* 70 (1894): 909–911. A. Bach, Medico-Legal Congress, *The Medico-Legal Journal* 14 (1896): 103–106.

22. S. E. Baldwin, "The natural right to a natural death," *St. Paul Medical Journal* 1 (1899): 875–889. Editorial, "May the physician ever end life?" *British Medical Journal* 1 (1897): 934. Editorial, "On the right of the physician to kill the incurable sick," *Interstate Medical Journal* 6 (1899): 488–490. R. Wilson, "A medico-literary causerie: euthanasia,"

Practitioner 56 (1896): 631–635. L. J. Rosenberg and N. E. Aronstam, "Euthanasia: a medicolegal study," *JAMA* 36 (1901): 10–110. Editorial, "Euthanasia," *JAMA* 41 (1903): 1094. Editorial, "Euthanasia for the defective and incurable," *JAMA* 43 (1904): 896–897.

23. Editorial, "Euthanasia," *Spectator* 88 (1902): 134–135. Editorial, "Euthanasia," *St. Louis Medical Review* 53 (1906): 66–69. "A silly bill in Ohio," *Medical Record* 69 (1906): 184–185. "To kill suffering persons," *New York Times*, January 24, 1906, p. 2. Editorial, "Euthanasia and civilization," *New York Times*, February 3, 1906, p. 8. A. Rupp, "Another view of euthanasia," *New York Times*, January 30, 1906, p. 8. G. Costigan, "Dr. Costigan on euthanasia," *New York Times*, February 6, 1906, p. 8. A. Tomlinson, "A case of euthanasia," *New York Times*, February 11, 1906, p. 8.

24. Editorial, "Euthanasia," *British Medical Journal* 1 (1906): 638–639. It was reported in the *British Medical Journal* in 1906 and by Reiser that an even more extreme bill to legalize euthanasia not just for incurable adults but also for "hideously deformed or idiotic children" was introduced into the Iowa state legislature at about this time by Dr. R. H. Gregory. I have tried to verify this report by searching through the *New York Times* and the *Times of London* indices as well as periodical indices of the time period. I could find no corroboration of the report. The law library at the Iowa State House confirms that a Dr. Ross H. Gregory was a representative in the Iowa legislature. However, the *Iowa House Journals*, which recorded the proceedings of the legislature, indicate that Dr. Gregory introduced bills on a lying-in hospital for pregnant women and licensing physicians from out-of-state but does not contain any record of a bill or an amendment to a bill proposing the legalization of euthanasia. These *Journals* are not verbatim records and are somewhat erratic in what they record, especially in regard to amendments to bills. In addition, the obituaries of Dr. Ross Gregory from November 1945 were searched for any mention of a euthanasia bill and none could be found. Proving a negative claim is difficult, if not impossible; nevertheless it seems unlikely—although cannot be absolutely refuted—that a bill was introduced into the Iowa legislature at the turn of the century to legalize euthanasia. Where the *British Medical Journal* and Reiser obtained their information I cannot explain.

25. "London Letter: Euthanasia," *JAMA* 72 (1919): 1557. S. R. Wells, "Is 'euthanasia' ever justifiable?" *Transactions of the Medico-Legal Society for the year 1906–7* 4 (1907): 1–14. A. Jacobi, "Euthanasia," *Medical Review of Reviews* 18 (1912): 362–363. V. Robinson, "A symposium on euthanasia," *Medical Review of Reviews* 19 (1913): 143–157. Editorial, "Euthanasia again," *JAMA* 87 (1926): 1491.

26. K. M. Ludmerer, *Learning to Heal: The Development of American Medical Education* (New York: Basic Books, 1985).

27. K. L. Garver and B. Garver, "Eugenics: past, present, and the future," *American Journal of Human Genetics* 49 (1991): 1109–1118. Rpt. and trans. of K. Binding and A. Hoche, "Permitting the destruction of unworthy life: its extent and form," in *Issues in Law and Medicine* 8 (1992): 231–265. Robert J. Lifton, *The Nazi Doctors: Medical Killing and the Psychology of Genocide* (New York: Basic Books, 1986).

28. This revival of interest seems to have occurred without any reference to the interest in euthanasia in Germany. For instance, I could find no review of or reference to either Jost's or Binding and Hoche's books in the *Lancet, British Medical Journal, JAMA,* or the *Boston Medical and Surgical Journal* in the five years after their publications.

29. C. K. Millard, "The legalization of voluntary euthanasia," *Public Health* 45 (1931): 39–47. Editorial, "The President, 1931–32," *Public Health* 45 (1931): 33–34.

30. Editorial, "Voluntary euthanasia: propaganda for legalisation," *British Medical Journal* 2 (1935): 856. Editorial, "Voluntary euthanasia: the new society states its case," *British Medical Journal* 2 (1935): 1168–1169.

31. Millard, "Legalization of voluntary euthanasia."

32. *British Medical Journal* 2 (1935): 1181. Medical Societies, Hunterian society, *Lancet* 21 (1936): 1215–1216. A. F. Tredgold, "Voluntary euthanasia," *British Medical Journal* 1 (1936): 33. C. E. Douglas, "Voluntary euthanasia," *British Medical Journal* 1 (1936): 3–34. R. A. Fleming, "Voluntary euthanasia," *British Medical Journal* 1 (1936): 86. J. S. Manson, "Voluntary euthanasia," *British Medical Journal* 1 (1936): 87. G. Griffiths, "Voluntary euthanasia," *British Medical Journal* 1 (1936): 134. P. J. McGarry, "Voluntary euthanasia," *British Medical Journal* 1 (1936): 134–135. W. G. Richards, "Euthanasia," *British Medical Journal* 1 (1936): 390. "The right to kill," *Time,* November 18, 1935, pp. 53–54. "The right to kill (cont'd)," *Time,* November 25, 1935, pp. 39–40. "The right to kill (cont'd)," *Time,* December 2, 1935, pp. 34–37. Anonymous, "Medicine: Britons would alter decalogue to end incurable pain," *Newsweek,* November 16, 1935, pp. 40–41.

33. "Parliamentary intelligence, voluntary euthanasia," *Lancet* 2 (1939): 1369. T. Helme, "The voluntary euthanasia (legislation) bill (1936) revisited," *Journal of Medical Ethics* 17 (1991): 25–29.

34. L. Alexander, "Medical science under dictatorship," *New England Journal of Medicine* 241 (1949): 39–47. G. Williams, *The Sanctity of Life and the Criminal Law* (New York: 1957). Y. Kamisar, "Some non-religious

views against proposed 'mercy killing' legislation," *Minnesota Law Review* 42 (1958): 969–1042. G. Williams, "'Mercy-killing' legislation: a rejoinder," *Minnesota Law Review* 43 (1958): 1–12. J. Rachels, "Active and passive euthanasia," *New England Journal of Medicine* 292 (1975): 78–80. M. A. M. de Wachter, "Active euthanasia in the Netherlands," *JAMA* 262 (1989): 3316–3319.

35. K. M. Ludmerer, *Genetics and American Society* (Baltimore: Johns Hopkins University Press, 1972). D. J. Kevles, *In the Name of Eugenics* (New York: Knopf, 1985). "The purpose of eugenics," *British Medical Journal* 1 (1924): 397–398.

36. "Euthanasia," *The Lancet* 1 (1899): 489. W. G. Burnie, "Euthanasia," *The Lancet* 1 (1899): 561.

37. A. E., "Voluntary euthanasia," *British Medical Journal* 1 (1936): 186.

38. E. J. Emanuel, *The Ends of Human Life* (Cambridge: Harvard University Press, 1991), chap. 1.

39. C. E. Rosenberg, *The Care of Strangers* (New York: Basic Books, 1987), pt. 2.

40. P. Drinker and C. F. McKhann, "The use of a new apparatus for the prolonged administration of artificial respiration, *JAMA* 92 (1929): 1658–1660.

41. J. G. Williamson and P. H. Lindert, *American Inequality: A Macroeconomic History* (New York: Academic Press 1980), chaps. 3–5.

42. D. Gourevitch, "Suicide among the sick in classical antiquity," *Bulletin of the History of Medicine* 43 (1969): 501–518. "Permissive euthanasia," *Boston Medical and Surgical Journal* 110 (1884): 19–20. Costigan, "Dr. Costigan on euthanasia." Bullar, "Chloroform in dying."

43. A. Bach, Medico-Legal Congress, *The Medico-Legal Journal* 14 (1896): 103–106. Editorial, "Euthanasia," *American Medicine* 10 (1905): 1093–1095.

44. E. Foner, "Introduction," in Hofstadter, *Social Darwinism*. C. N. Degler, *In Search of Human Nature: The Fall and Revival of Darwinism in American Social Thought* (New York: Oxford University Press, 1991). C. K. Cassel and D. E. Meier, "Morals and moralism in the debate over euthanasia and assisted suicide," *New England Journal of Medicine* 323 (1990): 750–752. P. A. Singer and M. Siegler, "Euthanasia: a critique," *New England Journal of Medicine* 322 (1990): 1881–1883. R. A. Knox, "Poll: Americans favor mercy killing," *Boston Globe* November 3, 1991, pp. 1, 22.

45. Kevles, *In the Name of Eugenics.* Ludmerer, *Genetics and American Society.*

46. "The doctrine of euthanasia," *Medical and Surgical Reporter* 41 (1879): 479–480. Kevles, *In the Name of Eugenics.* Editorial, "Permissive euthanasia," *Boston Medical and Surgical Journal* 110 (1884): 19–20. Editorial, "Euthanasia," *American Medicine* 10 (1905): 1093–1095. Rupp, "Another view of euthanasia."

47. *Bouvia v. Superior Court,* 225 Cal. Rptr. 297 (1986).

48. D. W. Brock, "Voluntary active euthanasia," *Hastings Center Report* 22 (1992): 10–22. Rosenberg, *The Care of Strangers.*

9. The Bell Tolls for a Right to Suicide

1. Major portions of this chapter are adapted from G. J. Annas, "The promised end: constitutional aspects of physician-assisted suicide," *New England Journal of Medicine* 335 (1996): 683–687, and G. J. Annas, "The bell tolls for a constitutional right to physician-assisted suicide," *New England Journal of Medicine* 337 (1997): 1098–1103. I also filed an amicus brief on behalf of a group of Bioethics Professors when these cases went before the U.S. Supreme Court. The brief, which was co-authored with Leonard Glantz and Wendy Mariner, argued that neither the right to refuse treatment nor abortion provided a constitutional precedent supporting a right to physician assistance in suicide. The full text of the brief is available at http://www-busph.bu.edu/Depts/HealthLaw.

2. *Compassion in Dying v. Washington,* 79 F.3d 790 (9th Cir. 1996). *Quill v. Vacco,* 80 F.3d 716 (2d Cir. 1996). See for example Derek Humphry, *Final Exit* (Eugene, OR: Hemlock Society, 1991).

3. T. Quill, "Death and dignity: a case of individualized decision making," *New England Journal of Medicine* 324 (1991): 691–694.

4. *Planned Parenthood v. Casey,* 505 U.S. 833 (1992).

5. *Cruzan v. Director,* Missouri Dept. of Health, 497 U.S. 261 (1990).

6. *Matter of Eichner,* 52 N.Y. 2d 363 (1981).

7. *Compassion in Dying v. Washington,* 49 F.3d 586 (9th Cir. 1995).

8. See S. Kreimer, "Does pro-choice mean pro-Kevorkian? An essay on Roe, Casey and the right to die," *American University Law Review* 803 (1995): 44; and Susan Wolf, "Physician-assisted suicide, abortion, and treatment refusal: using gender to analyze the difference," in *Physician-Assisted Suicide,* ed. Robert Weir (Bloomington, IN: Indiana University Press, 1997).

9. S. Sontag, *AIDS and Its Metaphors* (New York: Doubleday, 1988). T. Preston and R. Mero, "Observations concerning terminally ill patients who choose suicide," *Journal of Pharmacology Care and Pain and Symptom Control* 4 (1996): 183–192. G. J. Annas, "Death by prescription: the

Oregon initiative," *New England Journal of Medicine* 331 (1994): 1240–1243.

10. Y. Kamisar, "Against assisted suicide, even a very limited form," *University of Detroit Mercy Law Review* 72 (1995): 735–769.

11. *Lee v. Oregon,* 891 F. Supp. 1429 (D. Or. 1995), and see Annas, "Death by prescription." S. M. Wolf, "Holding the line on euthanasia," *Hastings Center Report* 19, no. 1 suppl. (1989): 13–15.

12. *U.S. v. Rutherford,* 442 U.S. 544 (1979).

13. *Washington v. Glucksberg,* 117 S.Ct. 2302 (1997).

14. *Vacco v. Quill,* 117 S.Ct. 2293 (1997).

15. *Roe v. Wade,* 410 U.S. 113 (1973)

16. In *Glucksberg* the Court summarizes the position of the American Medical Association and its conclusion that "physician assisted suicide is fundamentally incompatible with the physician's role as healer" (Code of Ethics, sec. 2.211), saying "the State . . . has an interest in protecting the integrity and ethics of the medical profession." The AMA deserves credit for this strong statement; nonetheless had the Court looked more carefully at sec. 2.211 it would have seen that the definition the AMA had adopted of physician-assisted suicide is much broader than any legal definition any court or legislature has adopted ["Physician-assisted suicide occurs when a physician facilitates a patient's death by providing the necessary means/or information to enable the patient to perform the life-ending act (e.g. the physician provides sleeping pills and information about the lethal dose, while aware that the patient may commit suicide)"]. As explained in more detail in note 17 below, the conduct so described cannot by itself ever constitute "assisted suicide" because: (1) assistance in suicide *requires* that the patient actually commit suicide; and (2) provision of drugs and information about lethal doses has nothing to do with suicide, unless provided to a suicidal patient with the intent that the patient commit suicide (as the Court makes clear in its opinion). It is probably this gross misunderstanding of the law (and ethics) that led the AMA to mistakenly lump Kevorkian's suicide machine and carbon monoxide poisoning with Quill's prescription to Diane. See AMA Council on Ethical and Judicial Affairs, "Decisions near the end of life," JAMA 267 (1992): 2229–2232. These are readily distinguishable acts, and the AMA should take the occasion of the Supreme Court victory to reassess both its definition of physician-assisted suicide and its application to Timothy Quill-type drug prescriptions. G. J. Annas, "Physician-assisted suicide: Michigan's temporary solution," *New England Journal of Medicine* 328 (1993): 1573–1576.

17. My colleagues and I made this point in some detail in a footnote to

the brief of the Bioethics Professors: It should be noted that no case has ever held that a physician who prescribes drugs a patient later uses to commit suicide is guilty of assisting suicide. No physician has ever been charged with such an offense. It is surprising that the Ninth Circuit Court of Appeals could simultaneously find that the doctors in Washington run a "severe risk of prosecution" (79 F.3d at 795) and that there is "no reported American case of criminal punishment being meted out to a doctor for helping a patient hasten his own death" (79 F.3d at 811). In its footnote 54, it describes two cases where physicians were charged with directly administering lethal injections to patients. While the court refers to these as assisted-suicide cases, they were in fact homicide cases. Both physicians were acquitted. It is unlikely that the mere prescription of drugs for a patient constitutes assisted suicide. The named plaintiff in the Second Circuit Court of Appeals case, Dr. Timothy Quill, admitted in an article published in a prestigious medical journal that he had prescribed a lethal dose of sleeping pills for a patient so she could decide at some future time whether or not to commit suicide with these pills. Based on this admission, a Grand Jury investigated the case and refused to indict. Furthermore, the New York Board for Professional Medical Conduct conducted an investigation to determine if Dr. Quill should be disciplined for his actions. The panel found Dr. Quill acted lawfully and appropriately. It noted that he could not determine with certainty what use the patient might make of the drugs he prescribed. Even if Dr. Quill prescribed the drugs believing they might be used by the patient to commit suicide, he did not participate in the taking of her life. The panel did not wish to interfere with the good medical practice of physicians who prescribe drugs to relieve a terminal patient's anxiety, insomnia, or pain because the physician suspects the patient may later use the medication to terminate his or her life. See John Alesandro, "Comment: physician assisted suicide and New York law," *Albany Law Review* 57 (1994): 820, 823 nn. 19 and 21. Thus, in the only case ever investigated that resembles the activities the plaintiffs claim are illegal in New York, the authorities ruled that the actions were lawful.

It must be kept in mind that the activity in question is the prescription of drugs by physicians. Once the prescription is written, the patient must decide whether to fill it, and then must decide whether to use the drugs for the lawful purpose for which a prescription is written, such as relief of insomnia, or to take these drugs to commit suicide. These decisions all occur over a lengthy period of time. Thus, there is a long and tenuous chain of events between the writing of the prescription and its use for suicidal purposes.

This is quite different from prosecuted assisted-suicide cases, where there is a close link between the assistance and the act of suicide. In one case a defendant helped her sister to commit suicide by attaching a vacuum cleaner hose to the end of an exhaust pipe of a car, gave her sister the other end of the hose, said good-bye, and closed the garage door as she left. In another case a husband helped his cancer-ridden wife commit suicide by preparing an overdose of sedatives, sitting with her while she ate it, and helping her put a plastic bag over her head. Catherine Shaffer, "Note: criminal liability for assisting suicide," *Columbia Law Review* 86 (1986): 348, 366, n. 77. In these cases, and others cited in the article, the "assistance" that was found to be unlawful was much more direct than writing prescriptions, much closer in time to the commission of the suicide, and led directly to the suicide. At least three of the six patient-petitioners in these two appeals were not suicidal at the time they signed their declarations but rather wanted exemptions from the drug laws so that they could have their physicians write them prescriptions for lethal drugs that they might use at some time in the future to commit suicide if their suffering became intolerable (79 F.3d 794–5; 80 F.3d 720–21).

It is notable, given the relief sought in this case by the plaintiffs, that no court has actually concluded that writing a prescription constitutes assisting suicide. Perhaps the federal courts should have remanded the issue to the state courts for a definitive interpretation of the statutes in question. Both statutes are written in general terms and neither explicitly forbids physicians from writing prescriptions for their patients. Furthermore, it may have been possible for the federal courts to have interpreted the statutes in a way that would have made it unnecessary for them to decide the constitutional question. *Communications Workers of America v. Beck,* 487 U.S. 735, 762 (1988).

Interestingly, the Ninth Circuit opinion states, "We are doubtful that deaths resulting from terminally ill patients taking medication prescribed by their doctors should be classified as 'suicide.'" This is likely to be correct, and if it is correct then there is no need to resolve whether there is a constitutional right to assistance. If writing a prescription for drugs a patient may or may not use at some unspecified future time to commit suicide does not constitute assisted suicide under state law, then physicians may prescribe such drugs for their terminally ill patients without any constitutional determination by a federal court.

18. T. Quill, "The ambiguity of clinical intentions," *New England Journal of Medicine* 329 (1993): 1039–1040.

19. *When Death Is Sought: Assisted Suicide and Euthanasia in the*

Medical Context (New York: State Task Force on Life and the Law, 1994); and Supplement to the Report (April 1997).

20. See above note 17.

21. The SUPPORT Investigators, "A controlled trial to improve care for seriously ill hospitalized patients: the Study to Understand Prognoses and Preferences for Outcomes and Treatments (SUPPORT)" *JAMA* 274 (1995): 1591–1598.

22. G. J. Annas, "How we lie," *Hastings Center Report,* November 1995, S12–14.

ACKNOWLEDGMENTS

I thank Pamela Barron, Shannon Smith, Katherine Rouse, Kathryn Blatt, Cheryl Brooks, Susan Wallace Boehmer, and Michael Fisher for essential assistance in the logistical and editorial demands of this volume. I also thank the Culpepper Foundation for support of an important portion of my work on this book.

Index

Fourteenth Amendment *(continued)*
244–245; Due Process Clause, 205,
207, 211, 217–218, 220, 223, 225,
245–246; Equal Protection Clause,
207, 215, 220–221, 223

Genocide, 189
Germany: Nazi euthanasia programs,
53–54, 63–64, 95, 102, 146, 189, 246,
247; advocacy of mercy killing,
187–188; policies on euthanasia, 200
Glucksberg, Harold/*Washington v.
Glucksberg,* 108, 111, 204, 217–218,
221, 229
Good death concept, 145
Green, Ronald, 140
Guilt, 81, 82; of patient, 84; of physician, 89–90
Gustafson, James, 141

Harm, 55–56, 57, 58; future, 34; to physician, 38; benefit *vs.* harm debate, 54,
71, 90–91, 133; refusal to help as, 56;
noncompliance with patient's wishes,
78
Hauerwas, Stanley, 133–134
Health care, 118, 133, 146, 200, 244, 247,
248, 254, 255; facilities, 40, 46, 250;
costs, 87, 94; for children, 102; coverage, 108, 246; and patient's rights,
232–233
Hemlock Society, 175, 204, 205
Home care, 232, 250
Hospice care, 76, 153, 213, 229, 232, 246,
250
Hospitalization, involuntary, 27
Hospitals: patient's rights and, 232
Hospitals, teaching, 230–231

Ideal minimal rate for assisted suicide
and euthanasia, 157–158, 161–162
Individualism as social value, 198, 199
Informed consent, 4, 8, 97, 218, 223, 233,
242
Intent issue, 213–214, 216, 221, 222, 225,
226, 228, 230, 239, 245, 257–258

Justification for killing, 30; religious
perspectives on, 122, 135, 136–137,

142; by euthanasia, 193–194. *See also*
Capital punishment; Self-defense;
War

Kevorkian, Jack, 13, 14, 72, 74, 85, 86,
94, 175, 205, 212, 222, 255
Killing: different from letting die, 71,
72, 144; benefit/beneficence concept,
72; desensitization to, 89–90; intrinsic
wrongness of, 144

Lane v. Candura, 7–8, 10, 11, 12
Law(s): against euthanasia and assisted
suicide, 14, 15, 66, 146, 175, 204, 218,
220; pediatric euthanasia, 117; liberal, 144–146; regulation, 145–146;
drug, 215, 228; on right to refuse
treatment, 215–216; against suicide,
218, 225; against assisted suicide, 223,
225; state, 227, 228
Legalization of assisted suicide or
euthanasia, 15–16, 18, 46, 48, 59,
65–66, 78, 102, 186, 229, 248, 255,
259; obligation of physicians and,
39–40; slippery slope argument and,
71–72, 78, 147; overtreatment issues,
76–77; increased power of physician
and, 80, 82; issues concerning children, 92–94; debate issues, 117–119;
referendums and initiatives,
144–145; moral issues, 145–146; suicide rates and, 152; trust in physician/patient relationship and, 152;
empirical data and, 168; historic
campaigns, 196
Letting die, 62, 125, 130, 140, 194; different from killing, 71, 72, 144
Living wills, 5, 10, 76–77, 78, 80, 214, 226

Managed care facilities, 231
Medical ethics, 7, 23, 62–63, 76, 80, 228,
233; assisted suicide and, 85–86;
euthanasia and, 85–86
Medical holocaust, 29, 34
Medical technology advances, 140,
141–142, 143, 174, 179; effect on withholding treatment, 134–135; linked to
euthanasia and assisted suicide,
196–198